MW00607734

Writing a Romance Novel

2nd Edition

by Victorine Lieske and Leslie Wainger

FOREWORD BY Linda Howard

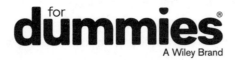

for **dummies**®

A Wiley Brand

Writing a Romance Novel For Dummies®, 2nd Edition

Published by: **John Wiley & Sons, Inc.,** 111 River Street, Hoboken, NJ 07030-5774, www.wiley.com

Copyright © 2023 by John Wiley & Sons, Inc., Hoboken, New Jersey

Media and software compilation copyright © 2023 by John Wiley & Sons, Inc. All rights reserved.

Published simultaneously in Canada

For general information on our other products and services, please contact our Customer Care Department within the U.S. at 877-762-2974, outside the U.S. at 317-572-3993, or fax 317-572-4002. For technical support, please visit https://hub.wiley.com/community/support/dummies.

Wiley publishes in a variety of print and electronic formats and by print-on-demand. Some material included with standard print versions of this book may not be included in e-books or in print-on-demand. If this book refers to media such as a CD or DVD that is not included in the version you purchased, you may download this material at http://booksupport.wiley.com. For more information about Wiley products, visit www.wiley.com.

Library of Congress Control Number: 2022951779

ISBN 978-1-119-98903-5 (pbk); ISBN 978-1-119-98904-2 (ebk); ISBN 978-1-119-98905-9 (ebk)

SKY10040980_010923

Table of Contents

PART 3: PUTTING PEN TO PAPER

CHAPTER 8: Finding Your Own Voice

CHAPTER 9: Letting Your Characters Speak

CHAPTER 10: Pacing: The Secrets of Writing a Page-Turning Romance

Foreword

I admit it: When I wrote my first romance book, I didn't know what I was doing. Of course, I was only nine years old and didn't know what I was doing most of the time. What I did know was that I loved writing, and I took great joy in creating these rambling, clichéd stories that swooped in and out of different characters' points of view as the plot galloped from one country to another — all without a single chapter break. I *knew* what chapters were; I just didn't care. All that mattered was telling the story.

My love of writing never faded. I eventually learned to break the tale into chapters (just as I learned the rules of grammar), although I still hate all that wasted white space on a page. Margins are for sissies. Do you know how many words you can get on one sheet of paper when you make your handwriting really, really tiny so you can actually get two lines of prose inside one ruled line of notebook paper, and write from one side of the paper to the other? A lot. And I wrote on both sides of the paper. I think one sheet held close to 1,500 words. Ah, the good old days. Now stories have to be typed and double-spaced on only one side of the paper; not only is a lot of white space wasted, but the challenge of seeing how small I can write and having the words still legible is gone.

But fast-forward a couple of decades, roughly. I was still writing. I had never stopped, and writing was the great private joy of my life. I wrote westerns; I wrote science fiction; I wrote fantasy; and I wrote thrillers — but they all had one thread in common: They all had romances in them. I *connected* to romances, but I wrote everything by the seat of my pants. I hadn't researched or studied anything and had no idea of any do's or don'ts — I just had the stories. Finally, one morning I woke up and decided to see whether I was good enough to be published. Then I did some research. I found out how to prepare a manuscript (margins were required) and how to submit it. Everything else, I did the usual way: by the seat of my pants.

I wrote a book and sent it to Leslie Wainger, my dear friend and editor of over 20 years now, who bought it. That's how she became my dear friend and editor. I was a newbie in the business; she was fairly new herself. What I knew about writing would have rattled around in a peanut shell, but I loved what I did know. Leslie loves books, and she taught me the publishing lingo, how a manuscript gets into book form, and all the other details that become part of a writer's life. Her editing — good heavens, how I needed editing — taught me more about the *structure* of writing than anything else I'd learned since learning the English language.

Little did I know that my chosen genre, romance, was the toughest one to write. It can't be, you say; so many romance books are out there — it can't be difficult. Oh, yeah? Try it. Romance readers are probably the most prolific readers on the face of the earth, and they don't read just romance. They read everything. As a group, they're frighteningly knowledgeable. They know their genre, they know what they expect, and they like being surprised. How do you give them what they expect and surprise them at the same time? Sheer dumb luck, and a lot of hard work.

Romance is the best discipline for writers. It forces you to learn how to make your characterization so strong that the characters not only live on in the readers' minds, but the readers also have a personal connection to the books. A romance writer has to learn pacing, how to tell a coherent, cohesive, and engrossing story in 80,000 words or less, depending on the category line. It's a tough challenge. Any tips are appreciated.

There weren't any tips when I started writing, back in the dark ages B.C. (Before Computers). No one had analyzed the hearts and parts of numerous romance books and broken them down for me to study so I could polish my craft, tighten my plot, and otherwise get a head start.

I feel cheated. Why wasn't this book written 25 years ago????

But it's written now, by an expert in the romance publishing field, for you to enjoy and learn from. Have fun!

I still feel cheated.

— Linda Howard

Introduction

Romance is far and away the best-selling genre in all of fiction. The specific numbers are constantly changing, but on average, romance book sales exceed one billion dollars every year. Just take a look at the best-seller lists: They're filled with romance novels!

Romance is a something-for-everyone genre. Looking for a quick read to pull up on your phone whenever you have a few minutes free? A 55,000-word category romance may give you just what you want. Want a complex story that can keep you turning pages for days as you relax on the beach or the porch of a mountain cabin? Try a 150,000-word mainstream romance. Whether you like history, the here-and-now, or even the future, whether you're looking for comedy, suspense, something spooky, or an inspirational read, the romance genre has something for you.

Because romance is so popular with readers, it's also popular with would-be writers — many of whom started out as readers and then suddenly decided that they had a story to tell, too. If you're one of these aspiring writers, this book is for you, because there's always room for one more.

A lot of outsiders have a very clear — and clearly wrong! — image of the typical romance writer. They picture her as someone dressed all in pink (boa included) who taps computer keys with the long, red nails of one hand while devouring bon-bons with the other — unless she's writing in the tub, artfully camouflaged by bubbles and probably shorting out a laptop per day.

The real truth, as insiders know, is that romance writing is hard work done by both men and women. It's also extremely rewarding work, allowing successful authors to express their creativity and earn money for it, all the while making millions of readers happy. Not a bad job if you can get it, and if you've read this far, I'm betting it's a job you want. So welcome to the *inside* of the romance business. It's time to start your new career!

About This Book

The romance industry has changed a lot over the years. Subgenres come in and out of popularity, and we see some shifting over time. Some things, though, never change. Readers are always looking for *a good story.* I've heard that phrase more times than I can count, and when I probe a little deeper, it always comes down to the same things. Readers are looking for strong, compelling characters; a story that makes them feel things right along with those characters; and a happy ending that lets them experience the thrill of falling in love all over again with each book.

As a writer, your job is simple: Give your readers what they're looking for. I tell this to writers all the time. The secret to selling a lot of books is knowing what readers want, and giving it to them. It may seem simple, but the practicalities of that are complex. You not only need to know the basics of writing any novel, but you also need to know — and master — the specifics of writing a romance. You need to put emotion on the page, and that can be a bit like catching lightning in a bottle.

In this book, I distill everything that I've learned about writing romance into a step-by-step, topic-based guide to help aspiring romance authors take an idea and grow it into a published novel. I'm not big on rules and regulations when it comes to writing a romance novel, because I think too many do's and don'ts make a writer self-conscious and stifle their creativity. And writing a romance novel is all about finding creative ways to make the reader happy. Instead of dictating to you or using the dreaded F-word, *formula,* I'm going to do for you what I've done for writers throughout my career: I'm going to give you the tools you need to write well, and to understand what a reader wants and how to give it to them. Then I'm going to turn you loose to tell the story of *your* heart so you can touch *your reader's heart.*

Foolish Assumptions

Every author — whether they're writing a romance novel or *Writing a Romance Novel For Dummies* — has to make assumptions about their audience. And I've made a few, at least one of which I suspect is true of you:

>> You're interested in making a serious effort at writing a romance novel and either publishing it yourself or getting it traditionally published.

>> You're sitting down to write your first book, and you're looking for advice on everything from writing the manuscript to finding the perfect agent or publisher to how to be successful in self-publishing.

>> You have a stack of unpublished manuscripts under your bed.

>> You've published a few romance novels, but they're not selling as well as you'd like.

>> You've had some success in the romance-publishing world, but, like most authors, you're always looking for tips, tricks, or advice to help you improve your craft.

If any of these descriptions sound familiar, you've come to the right place! You can find something here to help you improve your writing skills and guide you to success in your career.

Icons Used in This Book

I've scattered some icons throughout the book for easy reference. Here's a sneak preview along with their descriptions, so that you know what to keep your eyes peeled for in the rest of the book.

TIP

This icon clues you in to bits of romance-writing wisdom, some advice that's definitely worth checking out — and putting to use.

WARNING

This icon gives you advice on things to avoid to keep your romance writing on the right track.

REMEMBER

This icon flags important bits of information that can really help you in your quest to write the perfect romance — and create the perfect romance-writing career. Even if you skim through the text of a chapter, stop and check out these points.

TECHNICAL STUFF

This icon points out text that, while interesting, is a bit more technical in nature. If you want to skip over this info, know that your romance-writing potential won't suffer!

Beyond the Book

Check out this book's free online Cheat Sheet for quick tips and information on addressing reader's expectations, setting up a space for writing, choosing the publishing path that works for you, and more. To access it, go to dummies.com and type **Writing a Romance Novel For Dummies Cheat Sheet** in the Search box.

Where to Go from Here

You can read this book from cover to cover as an overview to help you get started, or you can pick and choose just those chapters that are relevant to or of interest to you. If you've been a romance reader all your life, for example, you may opt to skip Chapter 2, but you may find the chapters on plotting (Chapter 5) and pacing (Chapter 10) key. If you don't know how you're going to publish, you might want to look at the pros and cons of indie and traditional publishing in Chapter 15. If you already have a manuscript and it's time to start submitting it, you'll want to check out Chapter 17. Scanning the Table of Contents and the Index can help you pinpoint a specific area of interest.

Bottom line? The only right way to read this book is the way that works best for you. But in the end, wherever you start in *this* book, I hope your ultimate destination is the shelves of your local bookstore — as the published author of your *own* book.

1

Welcome to the World of Romance Writing

Get an overview of the world of romance writing and your place in it.

Identify your options in the multifaceted romance market.

Organize your life and surroundings to optimize your writing.

Chapter **1**

Romance Writing at a Glance

The world of romance writing and publishing is rewarding. There's nothing better than hearing back from a reader that they laughed and cried while reading one of my books. Pulling out those emotions in readers is always my goal, and I get excited and happy when I know I've hit my mark. But romance publishing can also be complex — even daunting — especially when you're approaching it for the first time. So, I've taken up the challenge of demystifying this world for you. Whether this book marks your first foray into writing romance novels or you've been hard at work honing your skills for years, I'm glad you're here. As you read, you'll find lots to interest you and, most of all, help you write a winning romance novel.

In this chapter, I provide you with a snapshot of the romance-writing process and the romance industry as a whole: from the different types of romance novels, to the elements that all good romance novels possess, to the pros and cons of indie versus traditional publishing. So let's dive in!

Tuning in to the Market

Many aspiring writers set out to tell a story without a clear idea about what kind of story they're writing, whether (and where) a market exists for it, or what they'll do with the manuscript when they're done writing. Now, I won't tell you that an unplanned approach to writing never works, because a lot of books get published every year, and some of them undoubtedly follow that path.

TIP

But if you want to write popular fiction in general and romance novels in particular, you can cut down on the time you spend on writing, as well as increase your odds of success, by researching the marketplace and paying attention to what readers and editors are looking for.

Defining a romance

A large portion of the fiction books on store shelves — from mysteries, to science fiction, to horror, and pretty much everything else — have romantic elements in them. But they're not considered romances. If you want to define your book as a romance novel, you need to keep certain things in mind.

At its heart — pun intended — a *romance* distinguishes itself from other forms of fiction because the romantic relationship is the focus of everything that happens — it's the driving force behind the story, the one thread that makes the entire tapestry fall apart if it's removed.

REMEMBER

Romance readers are knowledgeable. They're very aware of the elements in a book that make them happy and the elements that make them *un*happy. Romance readers have specific expectations for every book that they pick up. They want to identify with the heroine and love the hero. They want to root for the relationship to overcome the seemingly insurmountable obstacles in its path, and at the end of the day, they want an interesting plot that delivers a happy ending. When you meet these expectations and focus on the central romantic relationship, your book becomes a romance novel. (See Chapter 2 for more details on meeting readers' expectations.)

Contrary to popular belief (a belief you've probably run up against, if you've been a romance reader for a while), romance novels do *not* follow a prescribed formula. Instead, writers of this genre have a lot of freedom in how these expectations are satisfied.

Subdividing romances into genres

Approximately one-third of all fiction novels sold in the mass market are romance novels, making romance one of the top genres of all time. But not all romances are the same. Within romance publishing in general, all kinds of distinctions exist. Each type of romance comes with its own set of reader expectations that must be met. In Chapter 2, I go into detail about the different types of romances. But every writer needs to know the major distinctions:

>> **Contemporary versus historical romances.** The first big decision you need to make — one that affects every page of your novel from first to last — is whether to set your book in the past or the present.

- **Historical romance:** Your readers expect your research — into clothes, everyday life, occupations, social structure, language, and everything else — to be accurate and your characters to behave in ways that are appropriate to their world and its society. (I devote Chapter 13 to research specifics.) Certain story lines and plot twists work perfectly in historical contexts, while others are completely out of place — and it's your responsibility to know which is which.

- **Contemporary romance:** These novels are set in your reader's own time, so they're often subject to even closer and more knowledgeable scrutiny. Slang that's even slightly out of date or characters that feel like they're from the 1950s (when women were expected to cook, clean, and do just what the man said), for example, will turn a reader off faster than you can type "Chapter 1."

>> **Category versus mainstream romances.** This concept is based on the ways that books are packaged and marketed to the reader.

- **Category romance:** Also known as *series romances,* these novels are published on a monthly schedule in groups, which usually consist of four or six novels. The groups are referred to as *lines* or *series,* and all the books in a given series are similar in certain basic ways such as length, editorial focus, and cover design. Series books appear together on store shelves and are marketed to readers as part of a series rather than as individual titles. Most series are contemporary romances, but that's always subject to change.

- **Mainstream romance:** These novels are also known as *single titles,* which is an accurate description of how they're perceived and sold. Each book stands alone and fits its own individual vision, though that vision often identifies the book as belonging to a subgenre like romantic suspense, western, or Regency. A single title has unique packaging and is placed on the book racks separately, usually in alphabetical order by the author's last name. Single titles almost always have larger page counts — sometimes substantially so — than series books, which allow them to have more complex plotting and a bigger cast of characters.

>> **Sweet romance versus steamy romance.** There are different "steam levels" in romance:

- **Sweet romance:** In these clean and wholesome romances, the steam level focuses on emotion rather than the sexual aspect of the relationship. There can be sexual tension in a sweet romance, but it's kept mostly off the page and implied. If there is sex, it's behind closed doors. Think Hallmark romance movies. Inspirational or Christian romances fall in this category.

- **Steamy romance:** If a romance doesn't mention it's sweet, then it probably falls somewhere within the steamy spectrum. Different publishers have different ways to show the steam levels, ranging from one hot pepper to five hot peppers, to naming the levels different things. Just be aware of your steam level and take note what a publisher wants for a particular romance line.

Beyond these basic distinctions, the romance genre is also divided into all kinds of more specific *subgenres.* Subgenres can include romantic suspense, inspirational romance, western romance, romantic comedy, and others I detail in Chapter 2, where I also help you figure out where you — and your novel — fit into this spectrum.

Practicing Your Craft

After you know the marketplace and what kind of romance you want to write, you have to take care of a few everyday matters before you start hitting the keyboard. Writing is a creative profession, and after you and your muse get in "the zone," the last thing you want is to be yanked back to reality because your kids are fighting over the remote, or you have a question about grammar or British history and have no idea where to go for the answer. Here are a few suggestions to help limit the number of distractions you may encounter (I include many more in Chapter 3):

>> Set up a workspace for yourself, even if it's only a corner of your bedroom or family room.

>> Get your family invested in your writing so that they're happy to pitch in so you can succeed.

>> Dedicate a specific time each day or week when your writing is given first priority.

Only after you have the mundane under control can you sit down, face that blank screen and blinking cursor, and *start* telling your story. After that it takes dedication and commitment to *finish* telling your story.

REMEMBER

No one can make you a storyteller or magically inject you with talent, but if you have the drive and creativity to be a writer, you *can* hone your craft so you make every book as strong as it can possibly be. Writing has many practical aspects, and the bulk of this book focuses on helping you master them. Here's a quick look at just a few of the topics I tackle.

Everything starts with characterization

Let me note here that while there are other types of romances, this book focuses on heterosexual romance, with one man and one woman. This is an important distinction as we move into talking about characterization in later chapters.

REMEMBER

Without compelling characters to win over the reader, a romance novel simply won't succeed. The heroine, in particular, is key, because she becomes the reader's alter ego. Your heroine needs to be strong, smart, and attractive, but also vulnerable and emotionally accessible. She needs to be an interesting and admirable woman who your reader enjoys spending time with. Your hero needs to be just that: heroic. But that doesn't mean he has no flaws. He definitely needs to be vulnerable, otherwise he won't have a place for the heroine in his life or his heart. Your hero has to be a man that your heroine — and your reader — can fall in love with. (Chapter 4 covers creating characters, making it one of the most important chapters in this book.)

Both your hero and heroine should be fully realized human beings, with complete and complex inner lives. They need to have more going on than just sexual attraction — although, as I discuss in Chapter 11, sexual attraction and emotionally involving love scenes are important, too. Every character also needs an individual voice. Chapter 9 sets you on the right path to creating unique ways of speaking — ways that are also distinct from your *own* voice — for all your characters, especially the star couple.

It's all about emotional tension

REMEMBER

Emotional tension is the driving force of every romance. Your hero and heroine are more than just attractive faces. Make their relationship the driving force of your novel, because your reader's main reason for picking up a romance novel is to experience the roller-coaster thrills of falling in love.

To keep that roller coaster going, you need to create emotional tension between your hero and heroine, something that comes from who they are that can believably keep them apart for the course of the book. Maybe your wealthy hero has a hard time believing that the heroine's not just like all the other gold diggers. Maybe the heroine thinks no man can be trusted to stay for the long haul because her father left her mother, and her own relationships have never lasted longer than six months. In every book, the emotional tension is unique to that heroine and hero, grows out of who they are, and is enhanced by their situation.

I explain how to use emotional tension to propel your plot and create momentum in the hero and heroine's relationship in Chapter 5. Compelling emotional tension gets your reader involved even more deeply in your characters, and the more deeply involved your reader feels, the more quickly she'll turn the pages to see what happens next. (Bestselling novels aren't referred to as page-turners for nothing!)

Plotting, pacing, and point of view

Once you have your characters and their conflict down, your job is to plot out, and then tell, their story. Think of your novel as the context in which the hero and heroine can work out their issues. But plotting is more than just figuring out what happens in the story. You need to structure events in a way that keeps your reader's interest. You need an *external conflict* — something that gives your hero and heroine something to argue about and deal with when they can't talk about the emotional conflict that's *really* bugging them.

In Chapter 5, I give you tips on how to use conflict to build the reader's involvement as the action escalates. In Chapter 10, I focus on pacing, especially achieving the all-important balance between showing and telling: knowing when to let your characters show the readers what they're doing and thinking, and when using narrative is the most effective tool for getting the reader from point A to point B.

WARNING

When you're telling your story, guard against letting *your* voice call too much attention to itself, which can overshadow the characters, their voices, and their points of view. I provide strategies for finding your own voice and using it for greatest effect in Chapter 8.

Finding the right spot to begin your book and knowing how to start and stop every chapter and every scene for maximum effect are crucial aspects of structuring your plot. As you work on these mechanics, creating cliffhangers and knowing how to resolve them is likely to become one of your most effective strategies. For more information on beginnings and endings, not to mention on how to leave your reader dangling (but in a good way), check out Chapter 12.

Choosing Indie Publishing or Traditional Publishing

In today's world, many romance authors are finding success with indie publishing, also called self-publishing. Some are even making six-figure incomes and beyond. This is due largely to the invention of the Kindle (a wireless electronic reading device, aka "e-reader") and ebooks (short for "electronic books"). Other authors find success in the traditional way, by submitting their work to agents and editors. I also know hybrid authors who are doing both. But, how do you know which path is right for you, and where to start?

Exploring the pros and cons of each

REMEMBER

There is no one right way to publish. Indie publishing is generally a much faster process than traditional publishing. Yes, there are things you must do in order to publish, like hire an editor, but I know successful indie authors who write and publish a book in just a few months. This allows indie authors to follow trends and keep up with the market at a breakneck speed. But the downside is you must do everything yourself, or assemble your own team to help you do everything yourself. Traditional publishing can take up to two years, or longer in some cases, but you have a whole ready-made team of professionals to help you along the way.

In the end, though, you can decide to do both for different books. Some projects are simply better suited for indie publishing, while others will do much better traditionally. It all depends on what you want to achieve. It's wonderful that we live in a world where authors can choose hybrid alternatives. Chapter 15 gives you an in-depth look at each avenue to help you decide where to start.

Choosing your path

If you are the type of person who loves control and wants to be involved in every step of publishing, you might be more suited to indie publish. This option gives you more freedom. You are your own boss, you create your own deadlines, and you get a larger percentages of royalties. But keep in mind you also pull all the weight, supply all the upfront costs, and have to make all the decisions.

If your goal is to see your book on the shelf of every bookstore, you might want to try for a traditional contract. Yes, it can be difficult to sell a manuscript to an editor, but you will most likely get an advance, and they pay for all the costs involved. It's possible your publisher will provide some marketing, and they may set up things like book signings for you. Yet, your royalties are apt to be small, and unless you are quite lucky, you may need a full-time job to support yourself. If you're unsure about your path, we touch on both options here to help you decide. Part 5 explores indie publishing and traditional publishing in detail.

Best Practices of Indie Publishing

If you decide you're best suited for the indie-publishing route, Chapter 16 helps you learn what to do to put your book ahead of the game. No one can promise you massive sales. But there are things you can do to better position your book in the market — the most important is creating a well-written book that pulls the reader in. Nothing can kill your career faster than putting out a book that wasn't ready. Editing, formatting and design, and marketing are some of the areas where indie authors may encounter some pitfalls and where it might make sense to hire professionals.

REMEMBER

When you publish, you are putting forth an introduction to you, as a writer. First impressions are of paramount importance. You will never again get the chance to introduce yourself to that reader. Make sure your first impression is a good one.

Packaging your romance in a professional way is also very important. Everyone knows the saying, "You can't judge a book by its cover." Yet, everyone does. Your cover will be the very first thing people will see, and if it looks homemade, you will lose many potential sales. If you decide now that you're going to spend the necessary money to hire a graphic designer in order to publish a professional product, you'll be ahead of many writers who try to do everything themselves. There are many ebooks languishing in the bottom of the sales pool. Don't let your book be one of them.

Working with editors and graphic designers

Working with industry professionals can be rewarding, and can help your book reach that next level. It's not difficult, and you'll get many tips in this book to set you on the right path. Just be aware that even though you are hiring these jobs out, it's also important for you to know the market. You must be well-read in your genre to know when a developmental editor is steering you in the right direction. You also need to be aware of what kinds of covers sell better than others. Don't stress, you probably already read books in your genre, and you probably subconsciously pay attention to covers without even realizing it. The next step is to study them and look for clues of good design.

Marketing and selling your book

Marketing is often the thing that authors are most afraid of. No one likes to shout, "Buy my book!" The good news is, this is not necessary to have a successful launch. In fact, market research is probably more important to sales than anyone realizes. You won't have to spend as much time trying to convince others to buy your book if you've written the book to sell from the beginning. That doesn't mean you won't ever have to advertise. You will. But your ad dollars will go much further if you've prepped your book for success before you've published. I walk you through how to market your book in Chapter 16.

Submitting Your Manuscript

If you decide to publish traditionally, you will need to send query letters and eventually submit your manuscript. This is generally considered a lot more nerve-wracking than the writing process. Although you can't control the process after your manuscript leaves your hands, you *can* take steps beforehand to weight the odds in your favor.

Choosing the right publisher

REMEMBER

You can give your book its best shot at being published by targeting the most appropriate publisher for your genre, and, when possible, a specific editor whose taste runs to books like yours. You can't ensure a sale, but finding an appropriate publisher helps you on two fronts:

» It increases your chances of success.

» It saves a lot of time.

Once again, you need to research the market. Look past what's out there and focus on who's publishing it and which agents are involved. I provide tips on how to compare what you're writing to what each house is publishing, how to know if you need an agent, how to figure out what a particular editor likes to see, and other helpful strategies in Chapter 17.

Putting together a selling submission

Every publisher has its own rules about submissions, what they look at, and what they buy. Those rules often vary based on whether an author has an agent and whether an author's brand-new or has been published elsewhere, even if in a different genre. Whatever you submit, you want it to be as perfect as possible to increase your chances of making a sale.

You can submit your manuscript in three types of formats: complete manuscript, partial manuscript, and query letter. A complete manuscript is self-explanatory, but the latter two require some explanation. Query letters and partial manuscripts both involve a synopsis of your manuscript (I discuss them in greater detail in Chapter 17). In a query letter, your synopsis has to be brief, and it's all an editor sees of your novel. The good news is you don't need to convince the editor to buy your book based on your query; you only need to convince them that they want to see more of it. And in the scheme of things, it's easier to get an editor to invest their own time rather than the company's money. A partial manuscript consists of a longer synopsis and chapters — usually the first three chapters. This manuscript gives an editor a fuller look at what you're capable of.

In most cases, an editor likes to see a complete manuscript before going to contract with a brand-new author. Getting a request for a complete manuscript, based on your query letter or partial manuscript, is no guarantee that you're going to make a sale, but you're that much closer.

REMEMBER

Submitting a complete manuscript also means that you have to make sure every possible detail of your manuscript is perfect. For tips on formatting and advice on grammar and spelling — two aspects of writing and manuscript preparation that every author thinks they have under control but which many authors are wrong about — check out Chapter 14. My biggest suggestion on that score? Use or ignore spell-check — whatever makes you happy — but *always* proofread your work. It's also helpful to have a fresh set of eyes on your manuscript, so if you can, ask another author to read your work, too.

Somewhere along the way, you're almost certainly going to deal with rejection, either when submitting your manuscript for traditional publishing or in the form of low sales or bad reviews when indie publishing. Every writer has faced rejection, and dealing with it can be the hardest time in their career. The good news is that rejection won't kill your career. If you take every rejection as a learning experience, you will go far. Above all, never give up writing. There's always hope that the next book you write will sell well and make you into a bestselling author.

Chapter **2**

Romancing the Marketplace: Identifying Your Options

The single most important decision you can make, after you've decided to be a romance writer in the first place, is what kind of romance to write. Despite what skeptics, non-romance readers, and plain old killjoys believe, romances are *not* all the same.

Not only do their settings range from the past to the present and even into the future, but the books themselves also range in length from around 50,000 words to 150,000 words or more. They can be highly sexy or sweet and tender; suspenseful, humorous, or glitzy; highly realistic, populated by vampires, ghosts, and werewolves, or filled with barely dreamed-of technology.

But all romance novels share one thing in common — they're all built around the romance between two people who find their way past all obstacles in order to live happily ever after together.

In order to choose what to write, you need to know what kinds of romances publishers are releasing, who's reading them and why, and where your own interests and strengths lie. In this chapter, I introduce you to the average romance reader and the vast array of choices you both have, and I give you tips for figuring out where you can best fit in.

Knowing Your Reader

REMEMBER

Romances are popular fiction, with the emphasis on *popular.* That means the entire romance industry is driven not by *literary* concerns, but by a desire to make as many readers as possible as happy as possible. It's a market-driven genre.

I'm not saying that creativity and talent aren't important, because they definitely are — very important. With literally thousands of romance novels being published every year, it's incredibly difficult to stand out — to give the readers what they want while still maintaining a unique voice and approach.

Your creativity and talent come from within. You're born with the talent and desire to tell stories. But you can acquire craft and the ability to write what readers want to read. That part of the equation starts with knowing your market, which boils down to knowing your readers and what they want.

Meeting the romance reader

Writing is a solitary profession, especially when you're unpublished and don't have an editor to talk things over with. Published authors have an editor, but even they don't really have a boss. Instead, you, like all writers, have thousands of bosses — all the readers you're hoping will one day be your readers. No two romance readers are exactly alike, but as a group, they have a lot in common.

Not surprisingly, a recent survey conducted by Romance Writers of America (RWA) states that 82 percent of romance readers are women. The youngest readers are somewhere in their teens, and the oldest are in their 80s and 90s. But the bulk of readers range in age from their 30s into their 50s. A few more characteristics:

>> Most romance readers have at least some college education (and plenty of them are doctors, lawyers, and other highly educated professionals).

>> Most readers work outside the home part or full time, and their median income is slightly above the national average.

>> Most readers are or have been married, and many of them have children.

Most romance readers are strong, smart women who know what they want and, in terms of fiction, expect you to give it to them.

Meeting the romance reader's expectations

In my opinion, way too many people think of romances as formula books. As far as I'm concerned, a formula is something scientific. Toothpaste, laundry detergent, and nail polish all have formulas, but romance novels come in too many styles and sizes to be based on something as limiting as a formula.

Romance novels are built around reader expectations. Every romance reader picks up a book — contemporary or historical, mainstream or category, Regency, romantic suspense, or inspirational — with certain expectations firmly in place, and the author has to satisfy those expectations with *every* book. The five basic expectations that every romance reader shares — and that you, as an author, implicitly promise to fulfill — are simple and leave you a lot of room for creativity:

>> **A sympathetic heroine:** The heroine is the key to every romance. The reader's sense of identification with the heroine draws the reader into the book and keeps her reading. Your heroine needs to be sympathetic — strong without being hard, vulnerable without being weak, intelligent, ethical, interesting, capable (but not perfect), beautiful (but not unreal) — in short, a surrogate for your reader as she wants to see herself. (See Chapter 4 for more information on both heroines and heroes.)

>> **A strong, irresistible hero:** Both your heroine and your reader need to fall in love with the hero. He has to be strong without being overbearing (or borderline abusive), yet vulnerable enough to need the heroine; as intelligent, ethical, and capable as she is; fascinating; and, of course, good-looking.

>> **Emotional tension:** The heart of every romance is the emotional conflict that keeps the hero and heroine from being together, even though they both want to be. You need to create a source of tension that's complex, interesting, and believable, and that grows intrinsically from the characters you create; then allow the characters to deal with their issues as the book unfolds (check out Chapter 5 to find out more about plotting, including creating conflict and tension).

>> **Sexual tension:** Whether you're writing on the sweet side of the steam scale or an all-out erotic romance, your story needs sexual tension. Physical intimacy is part of every romance, and romance readers expect it even if it stops with a kiss. The sexual tension in your book comes from the emotional intimacy you create mixed with the conflict that is keeping your lovers apart.

>> **A believable plot:** Though your plot is the context for the characters' all-important emotional journeys, not the point of the story itself, it still needs to be believable, logical, and interesting, so that your reader stays immersed in the world you've created.

>> **A happily-ever-after ending:** Every romance novel ends with the hero and heroine together. They commit to a future as a couple, with marriage generally somewhere in the offing (if they're not already married or engaged). In a romance novel, happiness is part of the promise.

Fulfill these five expectations, and you're well on your way to writing a successful, and publishable, romance novel. Of course, your reader may have secondary expectations stemming from the type of romance you're writing — expectations for an inspirational and a Gothic romance, for example, will be quite different — and you have to keep them in mind, too. (For more on the different types of romance, see the "Getting to Know Your Genre" section and the "Secondary expectations" sidebar, both later in this chapter.)

Starting from Square One: Reading

If you want to be a successful writer, there's no substitute for reading. That fact holds true no matter what you want to write. Whether you look at reading as a way to learn the so-called rules, figure out where the publishing industry has set the bar, or scope out the competition, you need to know something about your chosen genre and the elite company of published authors you're hoping to join. Reading is the best way to do that.

TIP

Many authors don't like to read in their genre while working on a book, afraid of being subconsciously influenced in their own writing. That decision is understandable, and you may feel the same way while you're writing. But you should read extensively before you start writing and when you're in between manuscripts. You're not writing in a vacuum, and romance is *popular* fiction, which means you need to use every tool you can to figure out what can make you popular, too. The more you read, the more you know what works.

Drawing up a reading list

REMEMBER

When you start reading within the romance genre as an aspiring writer (rather than as a normal reader simply looking for enjoyment), read broadly, across a number of different time periods and subgenres, quite possibly also moving between mainstream and series romances. Take this broad approach, even if you've been reading romances for years, because you need to become objective about the market and your best chance for fitting into it.

After you've read broadly and decided what you may want to write, narrow your focus and concentrate your reading on the type of book you're thinking of writing — contemporary or historical, series or mainstream, or a particular subgenre.

TIP

You can also keep an eye on the bestseller lists to see what's selling and then focus on reading the books that draw in the most readers. You may find this approach especially helpful if you have a limited amount of time for reading. The following publications have some of the most well-respected bestseller lists:

>> *The New York Times*

>> *USA TODAY*

>> *Publishers Weekly*

Or go to the Romance Writers of America (RWA) website (rwa.org) to see a number of bestseller results all gathered in one place.

Reading like a writer

REMEMBER

As an aspiring author, don't just read for pleasure. Instead, read like a critic, like an analyst. As you read, look at every aspect of the novel considering all the things that I talk about in this book: characterization, plotting, writing style, pacing . . . everything you can think of counts. Constantly ask questions:

>> Where does the author get it right, and where do they go wrong?

>> What can you do better? What do you already know how to do well?

>> What does the author do better than you can? How can you improve in that area?

When you read a book you like, think about what made it work for you. When you read a book you don't like, think about what didn't work. Recognizing and avoiding pitfalls before you make them can save you a lot of time and disappointment. Also, think about why a book you didn't like may have sold a lot of copies. Something in it spoke to the readers, so try to spot that element. You can often learn more from the books that you consider creative failures, or at best only semi-successful, than from the ones that are letter perfect. Even after you've published a book — or 20 — you'll find that you can still learn from reading other authors, just as someday aspiring writers will be able to learn from you.

You can easily look at a traditionally published book you don't like and think, "If *that* got published, I can throw together *anything* and still find a publisher." Don't count on it. No editor sets out to publish a weak book, but sometimes a book just never pulls together the way the editor hoped, or perhaps practical needs — time constraints, the need to publish a certain number of books, and so on — mean putting out a book that isn't as strong as the publishing house had hoped. Or you may dislike a book that other people like a lot simply because everyone's tastes are unique.

In any case, you owe it to yourself to write the best book you can every time you sit down and type "Chapter 1." Aiming to do your best work improves your chances of finding success and gives you your best avenue to winning the readers' hearts — and getting them to spend their money on you.

Getting to Know Your Genre

You need to know the different types of romance novels so that you can define what you're writing and discuss your work like a professional when you talk to other writers and, eventually, when you publish or submit your book to an editor or an agent. Plus, readers have differing expectations for every general romance type and specific subgenre.

In many cases, there's nothing mutually exclusive about the distinctions within the genre and between the subgenres I discuss in this section. A book can be a mainstream historical romantic suspense, for example, or a mainstream contemporary paranormal romantic comedy. You can mix and match to your heart's content. Just make sure to choose elements that work together, target a house that can publish your book, and keep things simple (not trying to do too many things at once). And never forget that, whatever the trappings, you're writing a romance, so your focus needs to stay on your hero and heroine and their developing relationship.

Historical versus contemporary

You need to make several important big-picture distinctions and a lot of smaller ones that will help you place your romance in the correct category. First, you have to decide whether to write a historical or a contemporary romance. To make this decision, you need to know what each consists of. The basic distinction is obvious, and I feel a little silly pointing it out: Historical romances are set in the past, and contemporary romances are set in the present. But the differences don't end there.

Contemporary romances account for the bulk of sales, in large part because most series romance lines are contemporary, but historical romances (including the Regency subgenre) are also extremely popular.

Paging through history

Technically, any book set between the Stone Age and today is a *historical* book because it's set in the past. But readers and publishers define a historical romance more narrowly than that.

REMEMBER

There are exceptions, but the earliest era that shows up regularly in historical romances is the medieval period (knights and chivalry are quite popular). At the other end, publishers used to set the late 1800s as the cutoff point for historical romances, but you could still find books set as late as the San Francisco earthquake of 1906 or the days of Pancho Villa (who was active from around 1910 to 1920). Now that we're in the 21st century, the cutoff date may continue to shift, with individual editors deciding, based on individual books, what they feel comfortable with.

That definition leaves a big chunk of the recent past in limbo, including both World Wars, the '50s, and the '60s. These time periods are too recent to be considered historical but too far in the past to be considered contemporary. (Check out the "Mainstream versus category" section later in this chapter for more about this limbo period.)

Also, most historical romances are set in one of two places: the United States, especially the West (due to the cowboy mystique, though Native Americans are quite popular, too), or Europe, especially England. Plenty of exceptions exist (just off the top of my head, I can recall books set in ancient Rome, Asia, Egypt, and South America), but offbeat settings can make for a harder sell. I'm not saying that you should choose a different setting if you have a great story you're dying to tell. You just need to know that you may have a tougher time when you're ready to publish or submit your manuscript.

Living in the present

Contemporary romances are pretty much what they sound like: books that feel as if they're taking place at the same time that the reader is reading the book. I like to say they're happening in the *eternal present.*

In the "Mainstream versus category" section that follows, I talk about the distinction between mainstream and series romance and explain that the definition of *contemporary* varies a bit between the two. In contemporary series romance, the books *must* take place in the eternal present. You can't do a prologue set in 2021 and then headline Chapter 1 "Three Years Later." (If you need to make the time-line clear, headline the prologue "Three Years Ago" and Chapter 1 "Today.")

In mainstream romance, you have a bit more flexibility. You can go back a few years or indicate a specific year and still consider the book contemporary. As with the cutoff date in historical romances, nothing's hard and fast in contemporary romances. One editor may let you go back to the '90s, another only to the 2010s.

If you choose the eternal present, you need to keep certain things in mind as you write so that you don't date your book:

>> **Never mention the year in which the book is taking place.** This tip sounds like common sense, but you can easily forget and mention the hero's brand-new 2023 Porsche.

>> **Don't talk about current events.** Don't talk about the current presidential election or refer to specific big events you read about in the papers or see on the news. If you need that kind of dramatic background, make something up. Invent a president and his challenger, make up a global conflict, name your own hurricane . . . whatever you have to do to avoid tying your story to a time that'll be long gone when your book comes out.

>> **Be careful about pop-culture references.** Today's hit is tomorrow's trivia question. So when it comes to pop culture references — music, movies, television, bestselling books, and even computer games — you're better off having your characters stream a classic like *Casablanca* or *M*A*S*H,* or listening to a standard artist like Billie Holiday, rather than something that's current (and will probably be forgotten by the time the book comes out). Or, just as good, mention that they rent/stream a *just-released hit* or tune the radio to *a station playing all the latest hits,* which lets you avoid mentioning any specifics.

>> **Don't try too hard to sound too cool.** Slang changes overnight. Avoid using slang as much as possible, and when you do use it, try not to be too cutting edge. Use expressions that have been around for a while and are still in use, like "cool" or "awesome." Slang is also highly generational, so you'll want to be careful your teenager doesn't sound like she's 50.

>> **Set trends instead of following them.** This tip holds especially true when you're talking about fashions. Luckily, the fashion magazines or the latest teen-angst nighttime soaps probably don't dictate to your heroine, but those influences may be important for secondary characters, especially younger ones. So don't get too specific about what people are wearing if you want their clothes to be cutting edge. The same holds true for whatever else your characters share with the in-crowd. Talk in general terms, or create a fashion statement or a trend of your own. That way, you can never be behind the times.

Mainstream versus category

The second big distinction publishers, readers and, of course, writers make is between mainstream (single title) romances and category (series) romances. The main differences involve length and the way the books themselves are marketed to the reader. While these distinctions are highly important for traditionally published authors, even if you're planning to self-publish I would suggest learning about the differences and striving to write within these guidelines, because this is what readers are used to.

Making the most of mainstream

REMEMBER

Mainstream romances are the genre's "anything goes" books. You still need to satisfy the basic tenets of any romance and give readers what they want, but you have a lot of freedom in how you do that. Mainstream romances can be contemporary or historical, and they can belong to any subgenre: western, futuristic, inspirational, romantic suspense, or anything else. Most mainstream novels are 100,000 words or longer, but they don't really have a limit, upper or lower — other than what an editor and a publishing house think that they can market.

Publishers also refer to mainstream romances as *single titles* because of the way they market them — singly. In contrast to *category romances* (see the next section, "Keeping track of category"), which publishers market in related groups, called *series,* single titles stand on their own. Publishers sell each one into stores individually, and then, in most cases, stores put them on shelves alphabetically by the author's last name, so readers generally need to know who they're looking for in order to find your book.

REMEMBER

You have a lot of freedom when you write a single title. Your creative instincts have plenty of room to play, and every born storyteller finds that freedom exciting. You don't have any restrictions (other than those restrictions based on subgenre, if you're working in one) on:

>> The kind of story you can tell (tone, genre, etc.)

>> The language you and your characters can use

>> Your characters' behavior in the bedroom (or anywhere else that appeals to them)

And you can incorporate gritty realism, way-out fantasy, or anything in between that you want. You have the freedom, and the room, to create more fully realized subplots and a larger cast of characters, and to use additional points of view to tell your story. (See Chapter 9 for details on using different points of view in your novel.)

A mainstream editor can feel free to publish books set in that limbo period between where historical romances leave off and contemporary romances pick up, and books from that period definitely get published. It *is* a tough sell, though, in part because you don't have an easy way to define the book in terms of a larger grouping, so it's harder for editors, marketers, PR people, and sales reps to talk about the novel. You shouldn't look at this limbo period as impossible for you to work with, but it *is* more difficult. It's also harder for indie authors to sell books set in a limbo period.

The bestseller lists almost exclusively contain mainstream books, and most of the well-known names in the business got so well known by writing single titles (though most of them didn't become stars with their first books). Very few romance novels get made into big Hollywood films or even made-for-TV movies, but most of the ones that do are mainstream romances. Those six- and seven-figure advances you read about? They go to mainstream writers, too. However, most six-figure indie authors are making those incomes through series writing.

WARNING

The rewards of writing single titles in traditional publishing can be huge, but it's a tough market to crack and very competitive. Far more authors aspire to sell a mainstream than there's room for in the market, and actually getting published is no guarantee of the kind of success and fame most authors dream of. For every giant advance and matching print run, a dozen or more mainstream authors get advances that don't pay the mortgage for more than a few months. Most books don't get the advertising and PR push to support the big print runs that turn a novel into a bestseller. Luck, as much as talent, is often what makes a star.

Don't let the challenges turn you away. I firmly believe that a good book can always find a home. Know going in, though, that you need to have a clear idea of what you're up against, because the road to your first sale is likely to be long and paved with rejection letters. If you're aware of the challenges, you're less likely to get deterred if things are hard, and you'll be pleasantly — even ecstatically — surprised if things go unexpectedly easily.

Keeping track of category

In traditional publishing, *category romances,* often called *series romances,* sit at the other end of the spectrum from single-title romances. Series romances are published, as their name implies, in a series. Each series, or *line* (and there are many), puts out the same number of titles (usually four or six) every month.

All the books in any given series have the same number of pages and the same approximate word count (as of this writing, different series range from 50,000 to 100,000 words), which is necessary so they'll fit the prescribed page count. Each series has a consistent look — with a particular art style, graphic design, and the series name featured almost as a brand — so that readers look not (or not only) for particular authors but for particular series, because they know that each series can be counted on to provide a particular reading experience.

REMEMBER

Each line has a *strongly defined* editorial personality, shared by all the books in the series. Some series are so sexy that they're just short of erotica, and others feature a low level of sensuality but with sexual tension so thick you can cut it with a knife. Some series feature a wide range of plot types, while others are defined by subgenre (see the "Subgenres and niche markets" section later in this chapter).

Most category romance series are contemporary romances, but historical romances are represented, too, and more could enter the category marketplace at any time.

Publishers have so well defined the different series' personalities that they have *tip sheets* to describe the specifics of each series, including its editorial focus, level of sensuality, and length requirements. Tip sheets frequently also include specific editors' names and information on how to prepare and submit a manuscript. When a publisher offers tip sheets, they're available from the publisher, online, and at conferences.

The category approach, with its use of tip sheets to guide aspiring authors, is completely different from mainstream, where you're left to your own devices to decide what you write and where to submit it. Category romance requires creativity of a different sort than mainstream does, because you have definite and clearly defined requirements and expectations, and you need to be creative and establish your unique style and abilities within those boundaries.

Writing for series has both upsides and downsides, just as writing mainstream does. Category-only writers can never earn the huge advances that some mainstream writers receive, and they rarely star on the national bestseller lists or become household names. On the other hand, most mainstream authors can publish only one book per year, either because of the time it takes to write a long novel or because most single-title publishers find that a one-book-a-year schedule works for them. But publishers encourage series authors to write multiple titles per year. Plus, series authors can often contribute to several different series. So the advances may be smaller, but several per year, plus royalties, can add up.

REMEMBER

Another huge plus to writing for series romance is that it provides a great point of entry into the business, for two reasons:

>> **Large need for books:** Most romance readers don't just read, they read voraciously! Every month, the large publishing houses put out many original titles in series romance.

>> **Migration from series to mainstream:** Many mainstream authors, including some of the biggest and most successful, got their starts in series. As authors move on to mainstream romances, they either stop writing series books altogether or cut down on the number of series titles they produce, making room for new stars in the category world. This migration is constant, so publishers constantly need new authors.

Writing in a series as an indie author

Many indie authors today are creating full-time incomes for themselves by writing in their own series. I've seen authors tie books together with location, theme, or cross-over characters. Just be aware, the fundamental aspects of the romance novel isn't going to change when doing this. If your couple doesn't have a happy ending at the end of book one, you aren't writing a romance novel. The mistake I see many first-time authors making is trying to continue the story of the couple spanning several books. While this may work when your romance is a side-plot, it doesn't work when trying to write a romance novel. Instead, introduce a new couple in book two who can have their own set of obstacles that keep them apart and come together for a happy ending, following the same pattern for the rest of the series.

Subgenres and niche markets

REMEMBER

The biggest distinctions in the romance genre are the ones I describe earlier: historical versus contemporary romances, mainstream versus series, and sweet versus steamy romances. But romance also has all sorts of subgenres. *Subgenre* refers to books that are intended to appeal to a specific niche within romance as a whole. Some subgenres can be historical or contemporary, while others (those tied to a specific era) can only be historical. Some are subject-based, while others are defined by their approach to storytelling, and most can be mainstream or category romances. You can even combine several subgenres if that's what makes your story work. Some subgenres are widely popular, and others appeal to a smaller but devoted group of readers. Not every book fits into one of these subgenres; plenty of romances are just contemporaries or historicals, and the writer gets to decide the specifics. But every editor and experienced author knows the subgenres, so you need to know them, too.

You may be tempted to aim for the themes with the broadest possible appeal, but niche markets can be profitable, too. What a niche market lacks in numbers of readers may be made up for by the devotion of those readers it does have, who buy virtually everything in their area of interest. You can make a name for yourself more easily in a niche market, too. It's the old big-fish-small-pond situation.

TIP

Keep an eye on what subgenres are currently popular, but remember that things change. Just like in Hollywood, you only need one big success to change the face of the industry. An unexpected bestseller puts every publisher on alert to the marketing possibilities, and suddenly every editor is looking for good books to appeal to the same readers who drove "That Book" onto the bestseller lists.

Ultimately, you should make your decision about what type of romance to write based on a combination of factors, with one of them being your knowledge of the market's possibilities and its relative popularity.

Futuristic: Looking ahead

Futuristic romances aren't true science fiction, because you emphasize the characters and their relationship, just as you would in every other romance and not the science. No strange, monstrous aliens need apply, and futuristic romances are usually set here on Earth — just Earth in the future. You set the book in the future for a reason, though, whether because technology plays a part (maybe someone is developing computer technology to bring world governments to their knees), or because it's set in a post-apocalyptic world. You may even set it in space or on another planet, but both of those settings can make for a tougher sell.

REMEMBER

Whatever futuristic trappings you put on your story, though, those trappings are not the point of the book. You still need to structure your story like any romance. The setting should help drive the plot and create an atmosphere, but it's never the story.

Check out the work of Ilona Andrews, a pseudonym for a popular husband-and-wife team, who writes in this subgenre.

Gothic: Simply sinister

Gothic romances used to be widely popular. Every one of these books had a similar cover: a woman, at night, running away (often along a cliff-edge path, with one scraggly tree leaning ominously into the abyss) from a menacing castle or a huge, turreted Victorian house. And a light was always shining from a single window. Rumor — never substantiated, as far as I know, but intriguingly believable — says that one publisher left out the light in the window on one cover, and sales tanked.

In the Gothics' heyday, from the '60s to the '70s, the basic plotline involved an innocent heroine who found herself living in the sinister hero's equally sinister house, falling in love with him — sometimes even already married to him — while wondering whether he was actually out to kill her, because clearly someone was, judging by the "accidents" and outright attempts on her life that kept on happening.

The popularity of Gothic romances has waned, but they've never quite died. These days, the covers don't give away the subgenre as they once did, and the heroines are less innocent and have more backbone, but the heroes are still dark and sinister, even scary. The defining characteristics remain the spooky (but rarely paranormal) setting and the sense of encroaching menace, which is tied to the hero, though ultimately someone else turns out to be the real threat. The romance world has room for a good Gothic every now and then, though they're often disguised as so-called psychological thrillers, which may contain romance but aren't necessarily romances themselves.

Prolific author Phyllis A. Whitney is often referred to as the "Queen of the American Gothics."

Inspirational: Relying on faith

Inspirational romances are non-denominational Christian romances, and they feature faith and faith-based issues as an important element of every plot, in addition to the developing relationship. Whether the characters' lives are simply shaped by their religious beliefs, which feature in all their actions and decisions, or one character has lost faith and finds it again, or anything in between, this faith-based thread is what runs through every inspirational romance.

The books aren't sermons, however. Like every romance, they feature strong, sympathetic characters who must overcome their own emotional issues on the way to happily ever after. They don't feature sex or even a level of sensuality that would be out of place in a '50s TV show. You don't just close the bedroom door and keep the reader from peering inside. Your characters — especially unmarried couples — don't go into the bedroom at all.

Inspirational romance is a growing niche market with a devoted (no pun intended) readership. For many years, inspirational romances were almost all historical romances, but in recent years, contemporary romances have entered the mix in increasing numbers. You can find both inspirational single titles and series, and romantic suspense is popular. This subgenre is expanding all the time, both in terms of the kinds of books it includes, and in the number of readers.

Julie Klassen is one of the top authors in the inspirational romance category.

Paranormal: Hauntingly good

Paranormal romances, with their mystical, even mythical, elements, have become quite popular. While a haunted house, a heroine with ESP, or maybe even a reincarnation story — along with the hero and heroine fated to complete a romance set into motion a century ago — can be found in the paranormal section, the biggest draw to the paranormal are shapeshifters, vampires, witches, and angels.

Paranormal novels combine elements of fantasy, science fiction, and horror, leaving you with a suspenseful story filled with romance. You will often see a human falling in love with a paranormal being, and fated love is a strong theme in many of these books. The settings for the paranormal romance tend to lean toward an alternate form of our own world.

J. R. Ward is a top author in the paranormal romance subgenre.

Regency: Crowning success

Regency romances are a subgenre of historical romance that is set in a specific time period. A traditional Regency romance is different enough from most historical romances that it's given its own category and discussed separately. The actual Regency period was quite short (1811–20) and got its name from the fact that George, Prince of Wales (later to be King George IV), was appointed Regent due to his father's increasing insanity. Prinny, as he was called, lived a lavish lifestyle that the titled class aspired to share. He ascended to the throne in 1820, marking the literal end of the period.

ROMANCE BY INVITATION ONLY

What about traditionally published anthologies and continuities? *Anthologies* usually consist of three novellas (occasionally more) on a similar theme, frequently holiday-based. *Novellas* are shorter than full-length novels, often 30,000 to 40,000 words. Sometimes the novellas are editorially connected, but most of the time a common theme ties them together. *Continuities* are series of linked books, usually 12, with an umbrella story that runs from the first to the last alongside each individual romance. Continuities are Bible-driven, with all the authors working from an editorial blueprint.

Story-wise, anthologies and continuities are quite different, but they share one key element in common: They're contracted by invitation only. If you are aspiring to be traditionally published, don't waste your time attempting to write for either of these formats. Concentrate on becoming a successful multi-published romance novelist, which provides your best chance of being invited to participate in one of these exciting projects.

Indie authors have also seen the benefit of creating anthologies. Coming together to produce one book with similar stories can introduce new readers to your work, help advertise your other work, and create something fun for readers. This, too, is by invitation only, but as an indie author you have the opportunity to be the one inviting other authors to join you. Don't be afraid to approach other indie authors who are selling well to see if they would be interested in a collaboration. This is where spending time in author groups can pay off. They are much more likely to say yes if they know you from an author group than if they have no idea who you are and what you write.

In romances, English novelist Georgette Heyer (1902–74) popularized the period, and her name is still synonymous with the Regency romance. Her books, more than any histories, continue to inform the subgenre.

Two things distinguish a traditional Regency romance:

>> **Length:** Most historical romances are at least 100,000 words long (Harlequin Historicals, with a minimum length of 90,000 words, are an exception), but the traditional Regency is shorter, around 65,000 words.

>> **Tone:** The traditional Regency is also generally lighter in tone, often almost a comedy of manners, and both the author and the characters pay a great deal of attention to the ins and outs of society and the social whirl. Though Regencies were once very low-key in terms of sensuality, a lot more variety exists these days, and some can be quite sensuous.

In more recent years, Regencies have expanded, so publishers have put out full-length (in historical-romance terms) Regencies, many of them darker stories that explore the underside of the society of the time and allow their characters to face heavier issues.

Indie publishing has also changed the landscape, with many authors, such as Sally Britton, publishing shorter Regencies with more frequency. While the average indie published Regency spans 50,000 to 65,000 words, I've seen many novella-length books (30,000 to 40,000 words) on the top of the charts as well. It is always best to research the market for yourself to see the current landscape.

Romantic comedy: Looking for laughs

Romantic comedy isn't only a box-office draw, it's also a growing presence in romance fiction. Real-life romance makes people happy — lovers have fun in each other's company. *Romantic comedies* capture that sense of fun while simultaneously throwing up emotional roadblocks between the lovers.

Although humor can have a place in pretty much any book, a romantic comedy is humorous throughout and at every level: characters, plot, and writing style. In my experience, romantic comedies are always contemporary; with a hip, flip tone; and usually feature characters on the younger end of the spectrum — 20s and 30s rather than 40s — who are frequently unattached and child-free. The books are upbeat, with a sense of fun throughout, and while some characters may deal with emotional trauma, the tone of the book is lighter and does not dive deeply into those matters.

WARNING

If you write romantic comedy, avoid slapstick and physical comedy, or joke telling. Let the humor come from the characters themselves, from their reactions to situations, rather than from bizarre setups that would throw anyone for a loop.

Carole Matthews and Emma St. Clair are two successful authors of romantic comedy.

Romantic suspense: Thrills and chills

This subgenre is one of the most popular, as of this writing. It's also one of the fastest growing. As its name implies, *romantic suspense* is a mix of romance with suspense and mystery, so you propel the reader through the story not only by her desire to see the romance reach a happy conclusion but also by her need to make sure everyone lives, and the danger, whatever form it takes, is averted.

WARNING

One of the challenges of writing successful romantic suspense is that you need to write a strong, complete, and compelling romance *and* a strong, complex, and believably threatening suspense plot. Too often, writers feel that they can slack off on one or the other, so either the emotional conflict gets settled too soon, leaving the hero and heroine as romantic allies for the rest of the book as they work together to solve the mystery; or the suspense angle is too simplistic and the solution transparent. One failing I see constantly is that either the hero or heroine is a suspect in whatever's going on, and there's only one other possible villain. Because the reader knows (despite her willing suspension of disbelief) that the hero or heroine will turn out to be innocent, there ends up being no mystery at all, and any feeling of suspense is severely compromised, if not totally lost.

True romantic suspense novels shouldn't be confused with suspense novels that include an element of romance, which don't need to satisfy a romance reader's expectations (see the "Meeting the romance reader's expectations" section earlier in this chapter) in dealing with the relationship. Both of these kinds of novel have one thing in common, though — both men and women like to read them. Romantic suspense is the genre most likely to attract a crossover readership, and that's partly why many of the romances you see on national bestseller lists are romantic suspense.

Nora Roberts is one of the queens of romantic suspense, as well as one of the top romance authors of all time.

Western: Riding the range

Western romances have been popular forever and continue to sell well. Westerns are set in the American (and sometimes Canadian) West. They can be either contemporary or historical romances. The key is that they're decidedly non-urban in tone and usually in setting. Dallas, Denver, and Santa Fe are all western cities, but books set in these cities often have just as much, if not more, in common with books set in New York, Chicago, and Los Angeles. In this subgenre a rough-and-tumble landscape of sorts, such as a ranch setting or during a cattle drive, is of intrigue to the reader.

The real draw of the western lies in the hero — usually a cowboy, a rancher, or a Native American. He's a quintessential American type: rugged, strong, usually solitary, and very definitely not a touchy-feely sensitive, new-age guy. He lives in a rugged land that tests men's courage, and he passes the test every time. He can tame a wild horse, rope a runaway steer, and sleep as comfortably on a mountain-side as in his own bed. In Chapter 4, I talk about alpha heroes, and this guy is alpha to the max. You may sometimes find the western hero in a boardroom, but it's usually not by choice, and he's probably still wearing his broken-in boots, hoping to get out of the office and back on horseback long before the end of the business day.

WARNING

Westerns are less appealing to overseas publishers, where readers see the fantasy these books depict as quintessentially American and not as appealing as some of the other subgenres. But because North America is the single biggest romance-buying market in the world, you can still make plenty of money if you write a successful western, even if your overseas rights never sell.

SECONDARY EXPECTATIONS

Depending on what kind of romance you're writing, your reader may have secondary expectations you need to keep in mind (in addition to the big five I outline in the "Meeting the romance reader's expectations" section earlier in this chapter). This list is far from comprehensive, but here are some things you may want to think about:

- **Historical accuracy:** Every historical romance needs to stay true to its period while still satisfying a modern reader's desire for characters she can identify with and writing that doesn't sound stiff to her ear.

- **An appropriate level of sensuality:** Mainstream romances don't dictate a sensuality level, but many category romance series do, and so do inspirationals. So it's up to you to live up to what's expected.

- **A convincing mystery/level of suspense:** Romantic suspense readers aren't easily fooled. They're good at picking up on clues and spotting red herrings. It's your responsibility to plot out the suspense side of your book believably, to put your characters in real jeopardy, and to make any mystery sufficiently mysterious to keep the reader guessing.

Australian outback romances have picked up in popularity, and these romances fall under the western umbrella, with many similarities. They embody the same feeling of taming the wild, and often carry the same tropes and plotlines.

Liz Isaacson has built a massive career writing inspirational westerns.

Related women's fiction markets

A number of non-romance genres, often grouped together as women's fiction, are closely related to romance and sometimes referred to in the press and by readers as romances. All these genres contain elements of romance, even though they're different in terms of structure and focus. Because you're likely to run into them as you navigate the publishing maze, I want to quickly cover these related genres.

Chick lit

Chick lit focuses on young (mostly 20-something) heroines navigating the perils of single life. These books are very heroine-focused, and the author often tells the story in first-person point of view, which differs from the usual third-person approach of romance novels (see Chapter 8 for more on voice). Key themes include men and how to deal with them, but the heroine's entire life and its travails (often humorous) form the backbone of the plot, and a happily-ever-after ending isn't required and is often pointedly avoided. Most chick-lit novels are published in trade paperback.

Mom lit has emerged as a spinoff genre of chick lit. It deals with slightly older characters who are at a different place in life — married (or divorced) with children. Again, the book focuses on the heroine's whole life, with romantic relationships playing only one small part in the whole.

Sophie Kinsella is a popular and bestselling author of chick-lit books.

Erotica

Many romances are sexy, even extremely sexy, but they're still romances, with a focus on the characters' emotions and their ultimate union in every sense. *Erotica* focuses on sexual relationships rather than emotional ones, and the plot makes no pretense that the relationship will be a lasting one. Erotic novels are about sexual thrills, not emotional highs. And although they do have actual characters and plots (something pure — a very strange term, under the circumstances — that pornography lacks), the real point of these books is to explore the characters' sexuality in great detail, at great length, and often in ways (kinks and multiple partners, separately and simultaneously) that even highly sensuous romances don't.

Sylvia Day is a successful international author who writes in the erotica genre.

Family sagas and multigenerational novels

Family sagas and *multigenerational novels* are the miniseries of the publishing world, painted on a broad canvas and covering the lives and loves of several generations of the same family, though in slightly different ways.

>> **Family sagas:** These novels cover many years, so the first generation that the reader meets will get old, maybe even be long dead, by the time the most recent generation takes center page.

>> **Multigenerational:** The story in these novels covers far less time, but members of several generations feature prominently.

In both types of novels, you usually find strong, and strongly drawn, romances of the same sort that any romance novel features, but those romances are only pieces of a much bigger story. Family relationships, births and deaths, the economic ups and downs of a family, the way a marriage evolves over time . . . these life moments are all of equal importance and help define the broad canvas against which the romances also play out.

Elana Johnson is a bestselling author who writes in several genres, including family sagas.

Young adult

Young adult, or YA, novels come in all forms, and some of them are romances. Because the characters are in their teens — the same age as the readers, maybe even slightly older — they're almost always dealing with the challenges of first love, along with all the issues that go along with adolescence. This very different focus, a simple function of age, makes YA romances too different from romances aimed at the adult market for me to discuss them in tandem. In addition, even if a book ends with the young couple still together and planning to stay that way, it's unlikely, given their ages, that they really will live happily ever after the way an adult couple can.

Nicola Yoon and Colleen Hoover are two popular authors of young adult novels.

LGBT Romance

The romance world is rapidly changing. While this book's main focus is heterosexual romance, I would be remiss to not mention the rise in *LGBT romance*. Many LGBT romances are quite steamy; however, you can find lower steam levels in this genre as well. Just as the varying subgenres in male-female romance are highly specific in their tropes and expectations, so are the books in the LGBT category. Reading widely in this space will give you the best information about what readers are expecting when they pick up an LGBT romance.

Check out Casey McQuiston's work in the LGBT genre.

Choosing Your Subgenre

After you know everything the romance genre offers a writer and a reader, you need to focus and choose what kind of romances you want to write. Making that choice is important, because your success depends on striking the right match between your interests, your talents, and the market's needs.

TIP

Too often, I hear an aspiring author say that they have several ideas: a historical romance, a sexy series title, and a romantic suspense. It's clear that their creative energies and attention are divided among the three, that they have no idea what to write first or how to move forward. I always tell them to focus, to look at all the ideas objectively, and start with the strongest one — whether it's the premise they like the best or the one they think is the most salable.

REMEMBER

Making a choice now also affects future choices. If you sell your manuscript, you'll have a good reason to continue writing more of the same, to develop a readership who's willing to follow you into another subgenre. Even if you don't sell this one, any success (like getting feedback from an editor) may merit sticking with that subgenre so you can follow up on the contacts you've made.

You may have a particular idea that just won't let you go, in which case you need to write it and give it a chance. But often aspiring authors are torn, knowing they want to write romances but not sure exactly what kind. If that sounds like you, you need to ask yourself questions like those I pose in the following sections, and then let the answers combine with practicality to illuminate your path to publication and success.

By comparing what you like, what you're good at, and what the market's up to, you can probably arrive at the answer to "What should I be writing?" without even having to stress. Then let your mind start wandering, see what idea captures your imagination, sit down at the computer, and get started. Your romance-writing career has begun!

What do you like to read?

Sometimes the answer to this question is simple. You're strongly drawn to something specific — inspirational romantic suspense, for example. But a lot of writers like many kinds of books. Historical *and* contemporary romances. Series *and* mainstream romances. The first step to choosing what you should be writing is to narrow down your options. Use this list of questions to help you figure out what direction you may want to go:

>> Do you read more of one type of book than another?

>> Who are your favorite authors, and what do they write?

>> Do you like to do research?

>> Does the past fascinate you?

>> Do you enjoy solving puzzles?

>> Do you ever read outside the romance genre for fun? What kinds of books do you read? Mysteries? Science fiction? Nonfiction?

>> What kinds of movies and TV shows are your favorites?

REMEMBER

Follow your heart — at least, as much as possible — in choosing what kind of romance to write. Romances are all about the heart, so if yours isn't engaged, your reader's won't be, either. Loving what you write helps you write the best book you're capable of, and only your best has a chance to sell.

WARNING

If you don't like romance novels, can't love your hero and heroine, or only want to write a romance because you know they're popular and you think you can sell a few to make some money before moving on to "real" books, do us both a favor and put this book down now. Don't waste your time on the impossible, because love can't be faked — and that includes the kind of love found between the covers of a romance novel. Choose a genre that *does* appeal to you and start exploring *those* possibilities.

By asking yourself the preceding questions, you may be able to pinpoint a single type of romance that you're meant to be writing, in which case you've taken your first important step on the path to publication. If your interests are very specific, you need to be aware of what the market looks like, but don't let that be the only factor in choosing what to write. But maybe you've just narrowed things down to a few possibilities that appeal to you, in which case, it's time to bring practicality to bear on creativity, and that's what I discuss next.

How do you fit into the market?

After you have a sense of what you want to write, you need to get practical: Look at your own strengths, compare them to the state of the market, and see where the two come together to give you your best shot at publication if you're going for traditional publishing, or your best chance at selling well if you're going to indie publish. It all comes down to asking questions and analyzing the answers.

Knowing your own strengths

Knowing what you're good at is more than just knowing what you like — though knowing what you're interested in is certainly a big part of it. I love to watch equestrian show jumping, but if you put me on a horse and aim me at a 5-foot fence? Just watch me faint dead away.

You may love to read long, complicated romantic suspense novels, but writing something similar that's complex and tightly plotted enough to fill 150,000 words may be more than you feel up to right away. On the other hand, a 75,000-word Harlequin Intrigue romance may feel much more within your reach. Or maybe plotting suspense isn't your strong suit, in which case, you can always enjoy reading romantic suspense, but need to look for something more romance-centric to write.

REMEMBER

Based on your answers to the questions in the preceding section about what you like, ask yourself whether what you like and what you can do are the same thing. Take a practical look at the realities of your life, too. Are you working full time and also taking care of children and a spouse? How much time can you realistically expect to steal for yourself so that you can write? If the answer is "not very much," you may want to think about series romance, even one of the shorter series, rather than a lengthy mainstream romance that takes much longer to complete.

The following list of questions can help you narrow down your choices, helping you figure out what kind of romance is the best choice for you because you not only enjoy it, but it also plays to your existing strengths:

>> Have you always been fascinated by history, maybe even one period in particular? Do you sometimes think you were born a hundred years too late and that you'd fit in so much better if the world moved a little slower? Historical romances probably fit you just right.

>> Do you feel uncomfortable writing love scenes — the more explicit they are, the more uncomfortable you feel? Inspirational or sweet romance might be for you. Or do you love to write them, looking on each one as a reward for your hard work writing the rest of the book? Let your own comfort level with sensuality guide you, because writing compelling love scenes is an important

part of writing a steamy romance, but some subgenres, like inspirational, don't focus on the physical relationship.

>> Do your friends think you're the funniest thing on two feet? Romantic comedy might be a natural match for you. Or can you screw up a simple knock-knock joke? Romantic comedy as an option? Not so much.

>> Is religion a key component of your life, or have you forgotten the last time you went to church? You're going to have a hard time going against your natural inclinations, so why not make things easy for yourself and follow them?

Matching yourself with the market

REMEMBER

After you have a sense of what you'd be good at, figure out that particular market's strengths and weaknesses. This step can be challenging, because the romance market shifts constantly. No matter how much info you gather, you can never be sure where things will stand even a month or two in the future, much less by the time you get your finished book in front of an editor, which can be a year or more away. You can try to track and predict trends and collect as much helpful information as possible. I have a number of rock-solid avenues for you to take when the time comes for your market research.

>> **Writing resources:** In Chapter 3, I talk about writing resources, and many of those resources — writers' organizations, writers' conferences, magazines, and websites — are great sources for market information, giving you a timely idea of what's hot and what's not.

>> **Bestseller lists:** Keep an eye on the bestseller lists and watch top indie authors to see what kinds of books are represented.

>> **Media:** Read the papers and the pop culture magazines to see what's selling and getting critical acclaim, and who's getting paid the big bucks.

>> **Retailers:** Talk to your local booksellers and get their take on things. They not only know what's selling, but also what kinds of books publishers are pushing for the future.

>> **Online writers' communities:** Indie authors often have their eyes on the market. You can get a lot of great information about what's going on in the world of publishing just by keeping an eye on some of the larger writing communities, especially those social media groups where successful authors hang out. These groups tend to come and go, so Google is your best friend when it comes to finding the top indie author groups currently in operation.

When you're gathering information, don't just look at what's selling in the stores. Look beyond the sales to learn what the publishers are up to. Find out who's buying manuscripts and what kind of stories they're looking for. The category market is always hungry for new writers, and you may find a perfect fit in one of the many different series. Mainstream houses and editors often have more specific needs, and it never hurts to know whether one editor or a dozen are looking for what you want to write.

TIP

Never make your decision about what to write based solely on what's selling the best or the hot new trend. Just as you shouldn't be writing a romance novel at all if you don't love the genre, you shouldn't choose a plot type or a subgenre that you don't enjoy just because you think that's where the money is. You need to write the best book possible if you want to sell, and that requires an emotional and creative commitment on your part.

Chapter **3**

Setting Up for Writing Success

On TV and in the movies, romance writers always seem to wear frou-frou negligees, spend about five minutes a day writing, and forego a desk and a computer for the sake of a bubble bath and a notebook. Unfortunately, the reality is a bit different. In real life, you have practicalities to consider, like carving out space and time for writing, as well as figuring out what kinds of supplies you need to keep on hand. Taking care of those practical considerations before you start writing is important, because when you get into your creative zone, you won't want to break your concentration to run out for thumbtacks or sticky notes.

Another important part of getting yourself ready to write is knowing what writing-related resources are available. Organizations, publications, websites, and more offer information and instruction for writers. Some resources are more general, while others are romance-specific.

The exact realities of your situation are going to differ from everybody else's, but your basic needs are similar, and that's where this chapter can help. Here I talk about all these real-world concerns, so you can get set, forget . . . and just write!

Finding the Perfect Time to Write

Some successful writers (or writers who start out with money to burn) rent out-of-the-home offices that let them get away from all the interruptions of day-to-day life so they can write full-time. Most writers, however — especially just-getting-started writers — aren't so lucky. Most romance readers are women, and that is probably why most romance writers are women as well — women who are busy holding down a job and/or taking care of a family. Pursuing your writing may not always be easy, but you're starting out with two big advantages:

>> **You're creative.** That means you can find clever, unique solutions to challenges, including finding time.

>> **You're good with people.** Romances are all about people and their emotions, and if you can deal with the emotions of fictional people, you can also deal with the real emotions of your family.

Making time to pursue your dream

These days, everyone seems to be on the go from the moment they get up to the moment they go to bed. Every minute is crammed full of something. Mothers of toddlers know all too well that sometimes privacy only comes in the bathroom. In order to get that manuscript done, you need to make time for your writing.

Reconciling your family to the new you

Nowadays most women work outside the home, and when they are home they juggle tending to the needs of the children and making sure the house doesn't look like it's been ransacked. Standing up for yourself and insisting on some time for what you want — and for something that may not have any immediately obvious benefit, financially or otherwise — is difficult. But if you want to be a writer, you're most likely going to have to stand up and insist. And, because your boss probably won't pop the cork on a celebratory bottle of champagne if you tell them that you can work only five hours a day from now on, your writing time is going to have to come from the rest of your schedule.

If you're married with kids, your decision to write will affect your husband and children — sometimes in ways that don't make them very happy. Fancy dinners may give way to plainer fare, and your husband and children, depending on their ages, may have to start doing more to help out around the house (cooking, cleaning, and the older kids helping to take care of the younger ones). If you're single, you may have to cut back on your social activities, or carve out time that you'd normally spend doing something else. No matter what, expect to change a few things in order to make time for your writing.

TIP

If you get serious about your writing, you may not have as much time for helping with homework or driving your children everywhere, and at first that may make you feel bad — like you're letting your family down. At the risk of sounding hard-hearted, get over it. I'm not advocating ignoring your family, because they are — and should be — the most important people in your life. But, like most women, you've probably structured your life so that every spare minute is spent taking care of them and your house. Let them take some responsibility for themselves. Their reward? A happy wife and mother who's doing something that makes her feel fulfilled and makes her even better than ever to have around.

Factoring in your new priorities

TIP

So how can you find time to write and keep your family happy at the same time? Here are some tips for balancing your time:

>> **Schedule everything you can.** Most of us move through the day without a hard and fast plan, playing a lot of our tasks by ear or as they arise. Instead, make yourself a to-do list and set aside specific amounts of time for specific chores. Keep track of your time and keep to your schedule. Streamline your housework and plan your errands so you don't have to zigzag all over town.

>> **Simplify mealtime.** Make quick and easy meals, or prepare meals ahead of time; plenty of cookbooks are available that can give you mealtime hints and hacks. Slow-cookers are a great invention and free up time for other things. Not all takeout is bad or bad for you, and there's nothing wrong with scheduling and budgeting a weekly dinner out somewhere inexpensive and fun.

>> **Bring in some help.** If you can afford it, hire someone to help around the house, even if it's just once a month or every couple of weeks. You can hire a teenager to help with childcare for an hour or two once or twice a week. Think of it as an investment in your future — financed perhaps by giving up small luxuries that you could live without or find for free, like an online subscription, buying books (support your local library!), or even curtailing a habit such as cigarettes or your daily coffee shop purchase.

>> **Trim your TV-watching.** Most folks (like me) have favorite TV shows, and I'm not advocating that you give them up. But you may find you can add several hours to your week by cutting back on how much television you watch. Cutting out the nonessential TV, watching one or two fewer movies a week, or taking a break from watching the nightly news can buy you valuable writing time.

» **Stay up late or get up early.** I've lost track of how many authors have told me that they wrote their first books by getting up an hour or two early and writing when everyone else was still asleep. You can also stay up later than everyone else to get in some writing time. This strategy is especially helpful if you have young children who can't be on their own as much as older ones.

» **Say no.** You don't always have to be the one to drive to and from lessons, sports, the mall, or the movies. Your kids' friends have parents, too. Work out a fair division of labor — which may demand compromise from your kids as well as other parents — and stick to it. If you're a full-time mom, you're probably used to doing all the driving because the working moms figure that you have nothing better to do. Well, that was never true, but you're writing now, so this assumption is even more off base. Writing is your job, and you're going to have to tell people you need time to do it.

» **Make your time with family count.** Quality instead of quantity really does count. When you're with your family, be present in the moment; don't cook dinner and help with homework at the same time. When you take a break to play a game or go prom-dress shopping, get into it wholeheartedly.

» **Share the responsibilities.** Your family can probably help out more than they have been. I don't want to sound like a broken record, but the point bears repeating. Older kids can learn to cook and can certainly help clean up, no matter who did the cooking. Your husband can pitch in, too. You may discover that your husband actually likes having more one-on-one time with the kids. Let him do a driving shift, too. The more involved he is in his kids' lives, the better for all of them.

» **Make finishing your book a family goal.** Plan to have a special family outing or take a real family vacation after you complete your writing. If you get your family invested in your dream, you can bet they'll be more willing to give you time to accomplish it. You can even break things down incrementally, promising a favorite meal, a special dessert, or a family trip to the movies at the end of every chapter.

Creating your writing routine

No matter what time of day you've found works best for you, I've found creating a writing routine helps get me into the right mindset so I can be the most productive with the time I have. Setting a routine, no matter what it is, helps train your brain that now is the time to write, and you will spend less time staring at a blank screen.

TIP

How can you create a routine that works for you? Here are some tips:

>> **Find your writing space.** Whether you have a home office you can claim as your own or a simple desk in the corner, find a quiet space that works for you. For me, it's a favorite recliner. Other authors leave home and write at the coffee shop or the library. No matter where it is, find that place where you can concentrate and get into the zone, even if it's in your living room with earbuds in place.

>> **Create a playlist.** Songs inspire me, and certain songs bring out certain emotions for me. I love to create writing playlists for the books I'm writing that help me get into the headspace of the characters I'm writing.

>> **Set the mood.** No matter what it is, if you always make a cup of coffee, light a candle, or let the dog out to give you quiet time, setting your writing mood can help you get your creative juices flowing. Sometimes the small things can make a big difference. Allow yourself a few prep moments before diving in so you can be in the right zone.

>> **Eliminate distractions.** Turn off your phone or put it out of reach so you're not tempted to check the latest status of a friend on social media or scroll aimlessly through the Internet looking for funny videos. The fewer distractions you have, the more words you'll be able to get down on the page.

>> **Set goals.** Set small writing goals and give yourself rewards when you hit them. I like to put a sticker on my calendar when I hit 500 words. When I'm feeling even less motivated to write, I'll reward myself with a sticker every 100 words. Giving yourself incremental, bite-sized goals and being able to achieve them helps you hit those larger goals.

>> **Try writing sprints.** Set the timer for 20 minutes, and write as much as you can. You'll be surprised at how many words you can write when you're trying to beat the clock. Sprinting with friends is even more fun, if you can find a writing buddy. After the timer goes off, tell each other how many words you got down. A little friendly competition can be a great motivator.

>> **Set your office hours.** Decide what time of the day you'll be writing, and set aside those hours for working on your manuscript. Let your family know you'll be working during these hours so they can get on board with you treating this like a business, not a hobby. It's okay to hang a "Do not disturb" sign during your office hours.

>> **Utilize technology.** Bear Focus Timer, Freedom, and 4thewords are just a few of the apps that can help you manage your time, structure tasks, calendar events, take notes, track submissions, help with writer's block, and get rid of distractions. If you use Scrivener, try using Composition Mode, which cuts out everything but what you're working on, helping you to focus.

>> **Don't stress about perfection.** Writing your first draft can be daunting. Don't spend a lot of time revising what you have, or worrying about each sentence. Get the story down first, and then go back and edit it later.

Building a Writer's Tool Kit

After you've created a writing routine and found a writing space that works for you, you need to furnish it so you can take advantage of the time you carve out for your writing. You don't need me to tell you the basics of getting a desk, chair, printer, and bookshelf. Just get what fits in your space (with emphasis on a comfortable chair, because you'll spend plenty of time in it). The following sections discuss some other items to consider.

Finding the best software for you

There are plenty of software options out there for writers to take advantage of. While I won't go over all the options, here are the ones I see most used by authors today. With the exception of Google Docs, which is free to use, all of these programs offer a free trial period before purchasing the software or paying a monthly fee.

>> **Scrivener:** This word processing software is the one I see used and talked about most, with good reason. Scrivener is versatile, with many options that are helpful for writers, like a virtual corkboard, outliner, a place to keep your research notes, photos, and more.

>> **Atticus:** Created by Dave Chesson, Atticus gives you a writing platform and a formatting tool in one. Packed with powerful features, this cloud-based software can help you collaborate with other authors, build your own templates, and format your manuscript when it comes time to publish.

>> **Google Docs:** Many authors find it useful to write in Google Docs. It's free, you can access it from any computer if you log into your account, and it has some free tools that can help you organize your document.

>> **Dabble:** If you're looking to simplify the writing process, Dabble might be a great fit for you. It's a cloud-based writing software that cuts out all the complications leaving you free to just write.

>> **Plottr:** Plotting a novel can be difficult. Plottr can help you organize your thoughts, outline your story, and build your characters. My favorite feature is the timeline where I can keep track of my story beats, or pieces of plot, which subplot they belong to, and even move them around if needed.

Sharpening up your office supplies: More than just pencils

You're probably not going to need a lot of supplies, and most of the ones you do need are pretty basic. (You don't want to be scrambling around looking for a pencil when an editor calls.) Here's a list of basic office supplies to get you started:

>> **Bulletin board and thumbtacks:** If you're old school, I recommend getting a bulletin board and a good set of thumbtacks. Bulletin boards can be helpful in all kinds of ways: keeping track of timelines, listing character traits, listing key research facts, and so on.

>> **Paper and pads:** Keep plenty of paper on hand for your printer; you also want to keep pads handy for taking notes. Always keep a pad near the phone. You may also want some quality stationery for making letterhead. (Preprinted letterhead is an unnecessary expense now that quality printers are widely available.)

>> **Pens, pencils, and erasers:** Computers are great, but sometimes you need to write things down the old-fashioned way. Keep a few red pencils and pens around, too, so you can write notes on the hard copy of your manuscript.

>> **Sticky notes and index cards:** These are handy because you can put them on your bulletin board, computer monitor, your husband's forehead, or anywhere else.

>> **Other stuff:** You also need such basics as tape, a stapler, binder clips, paper clips, folders, and so on.

TIP

Keep your supplies organized (and don't let your children raid your desk drawers), so they're always at hand when you need them.

Stocking the shelves: Your home library

Whether you prefer print or ebook, or using online resources, having certain books around is useful. As a romance writer, you'll want some or all of the following:

>> Grammar reference

>> Dictionary

>> Thesaurus

>> How-to books and guides on writing romance, writing in general, and marketing book-length fiction

>> Research books for topics covered in your romance (see Chapter 13 for more information about research)

Don't overload yourself with writing references. Find a few that work for you and stick with them. (*The Elements of Style* by Strunk and White is a good one to start with.)

Booking it: Accurate financial records

Most creative writers don't like thinking about money and numbers because those are so, well, *uncreative*. But you have to think about finances, because they're part of having a home office and earning money (which you're planning to do with your writing). You need to think about how writing and its attendant costs affect your tax status, and you probably also want to keep an eye on your expenses. In this section, I give you a few basics so you can start thinking in the right direction, but what you really need is expert advice, which you can get from books, a financial planner, an accountant, a tax advisor, or any combination of these options. Tax laws vary from state to state, and your specific situation needs to be examined individually, because getting it wrong can have legal and financial repercussions.

Treating your writing like a business and looking at how the money flows in and out will help you make better decisions. Keeping good financial records can also help you meet the tax filing deadline with less stress. Here's the minimum you should plan to do to keep your finances straight:

>> **Find a way to track revenues and expenses that works for you.** A basic accounting software, Excel workbook, or written ledger will help you keep track of the numbers you'll need when it's time to file your taxes.

>> **Find a way to capture receipts.** Whether you save paper receipts or scan them, keeping proof of your expenses, and keeping them well organized, will help you support your numbers in the event of an audit (heaven forbid!).

Err on the side of caution. If you think that something may be relevant to your writing finances, save it or write it down. You can decide later whether or not to write it off on your taxes.

What kinds of expenses may be tax-deductible? This list is far from comprehensive, and different types of expenses are covered for one person and not for another. (See why I told you to get expert advice?) As a start, though, you might keep track of:

>> **Capital expenses:** These expenses are the big goods, like furniture or a computer.

>> **Home office expenses:** In some cases, you can write off a portion of your mortgage or rent, utilities, and repairs.

>> **Phone:** You may be able to deduct a portion of your cell phone bill based on the amount you use it for business.

>> **Office supplies:** Paper, printer cartridges, sticky notes, and so on fall into this category.

>> **Books:** Other romance novels, books on writing (like this one), or research books may also be written off on your taxes.

>> **Software/Internet:** Any software you purchase or subscriptions you have along with a portion of your Internet bill may be deductible.

>> **Entertainment and news:** Depending on what you're writing, you may be able to deduct the cost of some streaming services, or subscriptions that give you an idea about contemporary society and concerns.

>> **Travel:** You may travel for research or attend conferences that are related to your writing. Travel-related expenses can include gas mileage, car rental or transportation, airfare, hotel, and meals.

Accessing Resources for the Would-Be Writer

Many writing–related resources are available that give you a chance to interact with other writers, both aspiring and published, or to find guidance and instruction for your craft. I can't give you a complete list, but I can offer you some places to start and tips for finding more resources.

Joining writers' organizations — romance-related and otherwise

Here are a few organizations that you can check out:

>> **Romance Writers of America (RWA),** rwa.org. A professional organization for romance writers, RWA publishes a monthly magazine and has an annual conference.

>> **Alliance of Independent Authors (ALLi),** allianceindependentauthors. org. This organization is a nonprofit professional association for indie authors.

>> **Novelists, Inc.,** ninc.com. This organization is for published authors, although you don't necessarily need to be published in romance fiction. Novelists, Inc. puts out a newsletter and holds an annual conference.

>> **National League of American Pen Women (NLAPW),** nlapw.org. This organization fosters women's participation in the arts; specifically letters, art, and music. The organization has several hundred local branches in the U.S. and sponsors writers' workshops and conferences.

Going where the writers are: Conferences and more

Writers' conferences are located all over the U.S. and Canada throughout the year. Some conferences are specifically for romance writers, while others cover multiple genres. RWA and other writers' organizations sponsor many of these conferences; check the organization's website for more up-to-date information.

TIP

If your goal is to traditionally publish, be sure to make the most of an appointment with an author or editor. If you can arrange a conference-sponsored one-on-one appointment with an editor, make sure you request your appointment with an editor who handles the type of book you're writing. Go prepared with a project to pitch or specific questions to ask. Don't take up an editor's time just to say "hi" (even if your agent, your mom, or anyone else told you to) or to pitch a project that's already on a fellow editor's desk.

Informal local writers groups are another option for meeting and interacting with other writers. To see whether there's a group in your area, check local college or library bulletin boards or ask around in likely places, such as colleges, bookstores, coffee shops, and libraries. You can also put up your own notice in the same places, asking for information on existing groups or even volunteering to start your own if enough like-minded people are interested.

Taking advantage of courses and critique groups

Many community colleges and adult-education programs offer writing courses. You may have a tough time finding a class specifically for writing romance novels, but you should have much less trouble finding a class for fiction writers. You may luck out and find one specifically for popular fiction.

Because editors are not writing teachers and because they can respond only to specific manuscripts, many aspiring writers find it helpful to take a course in learning and practicing the basics of story structure, character development, and so on in a very feedback-heavy environment. Many writers also find having a critique partner or being part of a larger critique group to be invaluable, again because of the hands-on feedback. There are some wonderful websites for meeting potential critique partners and setting up what is, essentially, your own self-directed writing course. Here are two I recommend:

>> Critique Circle (critiquecircle.com)

>> Scribophile (scribophile.com)

CRITIQUE GROUPS: PROS AND CONS

Many authors find working with critique partners both helpful and enjoyable. In a critique group, members present their works-in-progress to each other for constructive feedback and provide moral support at every stage of the writing process. The decision to join a critique group is an individual one. Writing is a very personal process, and for some, it's a private one; others love to share their work. Either approach can be successful; go with the one that makes you most comfortable and frees your creativity. But make an informed decision. Talk to people who are already in critique groups to get a firsthand opinion about how they work. Here are some additional points to consider:

- **Are you comfortable sharing your work while it's still in progress?** Each writer works on her own manuscript, but being a member of a critique group means being part of a collaborative process. Do you feel comfortable letting others see what you're working on, and are you open to making changes based on others' opinions?

- **How well do you handle criticism?** In a critique group, your work is subjected to a variety of close readings and comments. You'll hear some compliments, but you're also likely to hear a lot of criticism. If negative comments, even when phrased constructively, cause you to become defensive or hurt, a critique group may be difficult for you. Another part of handling criticism is determining which critique-based changes will help your book and which won't.

- **Do you work and play well with others?** It's a two-way process. You can benefit from others' attention to your work, but you need to cede the spotlight so that every member's work gets equal attention and be able to comment on other manuscripts with a combination of diplomacy and honesty.

(continued)

(continued)

- **Do you have the time?** Groups meet on a regular basis, though the frequency varies, and meetings can be long. Plus, some groups require members to read manuscripts ahead of time, rather than reading and critiquing passages on-site.

- **Will you be bothered if other members sell their manuscripts before you do?** Everyone in the group is working toward publication, and everyone makes that journey at her own pace. You need to be able to handle others' successes without letting it get you down.

One last thing: Critique partners can help strengthen a manuscript, but they can also weaken it by watering down a book's strengths or creating problems. I've seen examples of both. As a writer, you may have difficultly discerning if a suggestion helps or hurts. You must decide whether this is a risk you feel comfortable accepting.

Online resources

Nothing seems to shift faster than the online environment. Sites that were old faithfuls suddenly disappear without a trace, while new sites spring up, just waiting to be discovered. It's always important to know how to find websites that meet your individual needs:

>> **Use well-defined, narrow searches.** When searching for writing-related sites, try narrowing your search to get the best results. For example, don't just search for "romance writers"; instead, search for "Silhouette Intimate Moments authors" or "historical romance writers medieval." The more keywords you put into your search phrase, the more specific your results will be. And if one word doesn't work, try substituting another. For example, change "writers" to "authors" and see what you get.

>> **Follow the links.** If your favorite author has a website, look around it for suggested sites — you can often find useful links. Many authors also provide a "Contact Me" page so you can write to them. I've found that romance writers are incredibly generous, so a politely worded (and brief — don't ask for the moon) request for direction is very likely to receive a response. Some authors even offer writing advice on their sites.

Checking in with publishers

Major publishers have official websites, and most sites provide information on submission procedures and, in some cases, editorial guidelines or tip sheets. A direct link for submission guidelines may be supplied, but in many cases the "About Us" or "Contact Us" link can get you to that information. You can find out a lot about companies' needs just by looking around their websites and noticing what they're currently publishing.

Helpful websites

Since websites come and go, it's best to search for what is currently the most helpful out there. It can be difficult to search when you don't know what to look for. Here are my favorite current resources to help you along your journey:

» **AgentQuery:** agentquery.com. This website not only gives you a searchable database for agents to query, but it also helps with things like how to write a great query letter, how to beware of scammers, and when to submit.

» **QueryTracker:** querytracker.net. This is a great website for searching agents and keeping track of your submissions.

» **Writer's Digest:** writersdigest.com. Writer's Digest has many resources for writers, including linking to the best websites for writers, writers' workshops, and more.

» **Kindlepreneur:** kindlepreneur.com. This website for indie authors offers fantastic articles on book marketing, giving you valuable information to help you succeed.

» **K-lytics:** k-lytics.com. K-lytics reports are in-depth genre reports that show you which books are the best performing in your genre, which tropes are underserved, and how the market is doing in general. Most helpful for indie authors, these reports can help you know what to write, how to package it, and who to target when you buy ads.

2
Laying the Foundation: The Building Blocks of a Great Romance

Chapter **4**

Creating Compelling Main Characters: Alpha Males and Fiery Females

E veryone dreams of falling in love, and it's the reason romance novels exist: so readers can experience the vicarious thrill of falling in love as if for the first time with every new book. More than anything — more than a clever plot, an exotic setting, or beautiful prose — what makes that possible are the characters.

In this chapter, I talk about why characterization is so important, and I also offer tips on creating sympathetic heroines and irresistible heroes, so your readers find themselves caught up in your book and eagerly turning pages. Of course, your hero and heroine don't exist in a vacuum, so I provide some tips for handling secondary characters, too, because they make your book's world seem real, and add color and complexity to your novel. Finally, I give you some general tips on characterization to help you create rounded, interesting characters, no matter how large or small their roles.

Depending on Your Characters

Romances are all about emotion, and emotion comes from people. In real life, our family and friends bring emotion into our lives. In a romance novel, your characters, especially your heroine and hero, are responsible for fueling the emotional fire.

REMEMBER

Romance, by definition, involves two people. And in a romance novel, those two people are the entire reason for the book's existence. In other genres, a romance can exist in the background or as a secondary element in relation to a mystery, a family drama, a battle against evil aliens from outer space, or any other scenario that the author dreams up. But in a romance novel, the hero and heroine's relationship takes center stage. Their romance isn't just part of the action — it *is* the action. And your readers view every other plot development through this lens. (For that reason, I devote most of this chapter to stand-alone heroine and hero sections.)

REMEMBER

The heroine is the reader's alter ego. She's key, the gateway for the reader to get involved in the novel on a personal level. The reader's identification with the heroine keeps the reader involved in your story because everything that happens to the heroine also happens to the reader. And the hero? Not only does the reader vicariously fall in love with him as the book progresses, but she also feels the excitement as he falls in love with the heroine.

Your hero and heroine must be interesting enough to capture the reader's imagination, strong enough to move the plot forward, and admirable enough to deserve a happy ending. They don't have to be 100 percent perfect; in fact, as I discuss later in this chapter, perfection is a problem. But your hero and heroine must deserve being called a hero and a heroine. You can define your supporting cast by moral ambiguity, but your hero and heroine need to be genuinely good people, even if they've made mistakes or are on a journey of redemption from something in their past.

A romance requires more than an interesting and appealing couple. For one thing, the characters have to find each other interesting, too. Their interest in each other has to strike several kinds of sparks. They must have romantic sparks — that wonderful, almost indefinable electricity that two people feel for each other — that tell them they have a shot at something wonderful. I talk more about this type of spark in Chapter 11, when I discuss love scenes. A second kind of spark is also crucial — and that spark comes from conflict. I talk in detail about conflict in Chapter 5. Because you need to keep conflict-based sparks in mind when creating your characters, and because all good conflict is character-driven, I also touch on it in this chapter.

The Key to Every Romance Is the Heroine

Most romance readers are women, and naturally, they want to see themselves reflected in their choice of reading. That desire for reflection doesn't mean that every heroine has to be straight from everyday life (even everyday life in, say, the 1800s); however, the heroine does have to feel real and be interesting and emotionally complex enough to keep the reader interested in your story.

REMEMBER

Your heroine needs to be at the center of the plot. Your story is really *her* story. Sometimes her point of view is the only one, but even in duel point of view novels, she's the character your reader will identify with the most. Every romance novel is still the story of the *heroine's* romance — she's the focus, the pivot on which all action turns. In the end, the happy ending comes because she literally gets her man.

Drawing the reader into your story

TIP

Because she's the reader's alter ego — the reader's avenue into the story — your heroine directly controls everything the reader feels, and dictates whether or not she keeps reading. To get your reader involved in the novel, convince her that your heroine's not only someone she would like to know, but also someone she would like to *be*.

When the reader identifies — whether consciously or subconsciously — with the heroine, she takes on the heroine's thoughts and feelings as her own. As she reads the story, the reader feels everything's happening to *her*, not just to a fictional character.

REMEMBER

The reader's identification is your secret weapon to make the reader fall in love with the hero. He has to be appealing on his own merits. But suppose you make him a cowboy, and your reader generally goes for suit-and-tie guys? Your heroine's thoughts and feelings — as she falls for the hero — become the reader's thoughts and feelings, too, until suddenly the reader has fallen in love with her first cowboy.

Making your heroine feel real

REMEMBER

To foster the reader's identification with the heroine, you need to make your heroine feel real. Making her feel real doesn't necessarily mean depicting her as someone your reader could be or might know. Instead, it means giving her character reference points that readers recognize, which let your readers easily slip into the heroine's role and internalize her thoughts and feelings. In the following sections, I line up five rules for creating believable heroines.

Responding realistically

Make your heroine's emotional responses realistic. She's certainly going to experience things in the course of the book that most women never experience in real life, so your reader can't say, "I remember how I felt when that happened to me." So how do you get the reader to go along for the ride when your heroine's in the protective custody of a handsome detective, or marrying a handsome billionaire she just met because he needs a fake wife? Simple. Just make her respond as the reader would. If a woman would be scared or shocked (and also attracted to the hero, of course) in real life, let your heroine feel that way, too. Her realistic response to a seemingly unrealistic situation will make sense to the reader and keep her caught up in your story.

Sowing the seeds of conflict

The sparks of all conflict come from your characters, and the best conflict is emotional. Your heroine's the key character, so root the novel's conflict in your heroine's emotions. When the heroine's emotions feel real, her emotional conflict also feels real.

The circumstances may be unrealistic — like my previous example of the woman marrying a billionaire — but her conflict can still be one the reader identifies with. What if your heroine has always been unsure of her ability to attract — and hold — the attention of a man, so she's afraid that when the hero finds out who she really is, he'll lose interest in her? This conflict is emotionally based and is one your reader can empathize with.

Exhibiting identifiable traits

Give your heroine character traits that feel real. She often has a job or lifestyle that your reader will never have. Maybe your heroine is a spy, a federal judge, a minister, or the daughter of a millionaire and her first car was a Mercedes. On the surface, she may seem too far outside the reader's realm of experience for that crucial sense of identification to occur, but a few well-chosen character traits can change that. Maybe she likes to drive too fast or is always playing with her hair. Maybe she has a soft spot for stray dogs or coos at babies in the supermarket.

TIP

Something small and human that you briefly mention just once or twice can resonate with the reader and make them realize that, for all their differences, they aren't so dissimilar after all. For example, many heroines are often quite stubborn. While this can be a trait we identify with, it also presents us with opportunities for conflict between the heroine and the hero (who is often equally stubborn). Just don't mention these traits over and over again, because then they seem forced, which will distance your reader instead of drawing them in.

Keeping complexity in mind

Make your heroine a complex and interesting human being. You may think that having a complex and interesting heroine goes without saying, but not all writers realize this necessity. I've seen many heroines who were just plain boring. They had whatever character traits the author decided were necessary for the plot — curious, lonely, and intelligent, for example — but that was it. I didn't feel I was reading about a real person who had quirks, contradictions, and layers worth uncovering.

I think I'm a pretty interesting and complicated woman, and for me to identify with a heroine, she needs to be pretty interesting and complicated, too. And believe me, your readers feel the same way I do. Of course, don't go to such extremes that your heroine feels like a mass of tics, insecurities, and disconnected enthusiasms. She needs to be strong, admirable, and intelligent, and she should definitely feel like herself and no one else.

Overlooking her own great looks

Don't let your heroine realize she's beautiful. This tip may seem like a small point, but especially in our visually driven society, it's actually an important one. Most women are very critical of their own appearances. I look in the mirror and see flaw after flaw, not my good points — even though I know I have them!

TIP

Most romance heroines are quite attractive, but if all your heroine does is admire her own beauty, readers aren't able to identify with her. So, instead of working your heroine's description into the story through her point of view, let the reader see her through the hero's eyes. After all, no one can object if *he* finds her beautiful. Giving her a flaw or two doesn't hurt, either. Maybe her hair is a beautiful shade of red but has a tendency to frizz in the humidity, or maybe she needs glasses to read. Little touches like these make her more human and easier for the reader to empathize with.

Introducing imperfection

True heroines are strong but flawed. An imperfect heroine makes a perfect heroine. At first glance, I know that doesn't seem to make any sense, but trust me, it does, and for several reasons:

>> **Readers can't identify with a perfect heroine.** No one is perfect. So if you make your heroine perfect, without flaws, fears, or vulnerabilities, your reader won't feel the bond that keeps them inside the heroine's head and turning the pages. By introducing weaknesses and vulnerabilities, you let the reader create that all-important bond with the heroine.

>> **Static characters are boring.** Your heroine (and yes, your hero, too) can't remain static over the course of the book. As the plot progresses, you need to make your heroine develop, change, grow, and discover things about herself and her abilities — especially how to love and live with her hero. If your heroine starts out perfect, she has nowhere to go. But if she has insecurities, past failures to put to rest, doubts about herself and her abilities, or an out-and-out bad habit — maybe a quick temper, or impatience that leads to rash, unwise decisions — she has room for progress, and readers will want to see how she masters the challenges of the plot and the romantic relationship.

>> **Imperfections call for complementary strengths.** Part of what makes a couple right for each other is that they complement each other; they need each other, and bring out the best in each other. The same must be true of your hero and heroine, so the reader believes they belong together.

Your heroine's insecurities and flaws allow room for the hero in her life and in her heart. As an example, perhaps your heroine comes from a broken family, which left her doubting her ability to succeed in a relationship, much less be a successful mother. Pets are the most she can manage, she's decided. So who moves in next door? A single father whose 5-year-old daughter just can't stay away from the heroine's golden retriever. Suddenly she finds herself playing mom at unexpected moments — not to mention having dinner at the hero's house so he can thank her for her help, where she discovers that maybe she does have what it takes to win the love of a good man after all. Without her insecurities, you wouldn't have a story — *or* a romance.

Naming your heroine

I've never heard of an editor turning down a manuscript because they didn't like a character's name, but the names you choose for your characters can subliminally express whether you have an ear for language or a knack for doing thorough research. Although a rose by any other name might smell as sweet, the idea of buying a dozen skunk cabbages doesn't appeal to most people. Names carry both connotations and information, so as a writer, you want to make your characters' names work for you, not against you. And because your heroine is your key character, her name is also key.

REMEMBER

Ultimately, select the name that simply *is* your heroine's name, the name that belongs to her as an individual. Listen to your instincts as an author. At the same time, know the consequences of your decision, so you can make them work for you as you write your romance.

Choosing an accurate name

REMEMBER

Taking accuracy into account when naming a character may sound odd, but the idea is important. You want your heroine's name to fit seamlessly into her world. Her name is part of the illusion that makes her feel real.

For example, if you're writing a medieval romance, don't name your heroine Tawanna or Tiffany. In any historical romance, choose a name that's appropriate to the period. When you don't choose a historically accurate name, the reader may question the accuracy of *all* your research. Research — especially in a historical novel, where most readers have to be told how people dressed, what they ate, and any other details of their lives — is crucial, so your readers know they can rely on you to get it right.

The accurate-naming rule applies to ethnicity and region, too. If your heroine's Scandinavian, the names Ellie and Rose aren't appropriate first names, and Smith and Weinstein aren't suitable surnames. If your heroine's from New England, she's unlikely to go by Sarah Kate, because that double-name construction is more indicative of the American South.

WARNING

Watch out for place-based stereotypes, such as Sarah Kate from down South. If your heroine's name sounds like a cliché, your reader may think the heroine herself is a cliché, too. You also want your heroine's name to sound unique so she'll stand out from the other characters in your book, who may need to be defined by their names more than your heroine does.

Connotations count: Pretty is as pretty does

Some names just sound nicer than others, like *rose* versus *skunk cabbage.* Every generation has its own standards of beauty — in clothes, cars, and names. With no offense meant to anyone who has a mother, aunt, or sister named Blanche, it's a tough name to pull off for a heroine these days. Younger generations are conditioned to think of Blanche as an old-fashioned name, so if you choose it, you're fighting an uphill battle to convince the reader that the name isn't an accurate indication of the heroine's personality. That's not to say you can't choose a name that creates challenges for you, just know what those challenges are so you can overcome them and even incorporate them.

TIP

Be aware of any connotations the name you choose carries so you can work with them or against them to create your heroine. Choose a name that has no real connotations, so you can create your heroine from scratch, or pick one that communicates *what you want to convey* about your heroine. Is she brash and iconoclastic? Bree (with its echo of "breezy") may work. Quiet and feminine? Perhaps Emma or another name that hints at the past and has a soft sound. A tomboy? Try Meg or Becky — something that has a playful lilt. Or, if you choose a name that has connotations that clearly don't fit your heroine — Emma for a tomboy or Mabel for an adventurous astronaut, for example — be aware of the mismatch so you can work to counter it. You may even have another character comment on her name, so you can bring it out into the open and get it out of the way.

Covering gender

WARNING

Unisex names are awesome, just be aware they can mislead the reader if they scan your blurb and can't tell if you're writing a heterosexual or homosexual romance. You can correct this by wording your blurb in such a way that makes it clear, just be aware this could be an issue for you. Unisex names are less of a problem in the books themselves, but know that you're creating a challenge on the marketing end.

Is exotic erotic?

The short and oh-so-definitive answer is . . . sometimes. Exotic (meaning different, not necessarily from an exotic locale) names can be beautiful, musical, romantic, and enticing. Romina. Michelline. Shoshanna. But exotic names can also be so strange, attention-getting, and unpronounceable that they stop the reader in her tracks, pulling her out of the story to sound out a name. Shivareena. Caledonia. Briganta. Don't try so hard to choose something different that you work against your own best interests.

TIP

Figure out what age you want your heroine to be, and Google the top baby names for her birth year. This can help you choose a name that fits the age of your character. You'll have a lot of choices, or you can use that as a springboard to come up with your own name that still sounds on point for your character.

Creating Your Hero

Your hero's almost as important as your heroine, because a one-person romance is . . .well, not a romance. Every heroine needs a hero. Your reader needs to empathize with your heroine, but she needs to fall in love with your hero. Don't worry. This prerequisite doesn't mean that you have to create some too-true-to-life (boring!) man your reader may run into in the course of everyday life. This guy isn't called a hero for nothing. Like the heroine, he doesn't have to be perfect; he just has to be perfect for *her,* and that's something altogether different.

Heroes are for loving

The heading sums up what you need to know about your hero. In the rest of this section, I talk about how to make him worthy of your heroine's — and your reader's — love. Think of your hero as a prize, the prize the heroine wins after all the conflict is resolved. (And of course, vice versa.) From the moment he appears, something about him has to affect the heroine in a way no other man ever has — even if she (thinks she) hates him.

REMEMBER

Because conflict is the driving force of a romance novel, you can't let your heroine love your hero (or vice versa) right away. But you *do* need to demonstrate immediately that your characters have a connection and an excitement between them that marks him as the hero and tells the reader that these two characters are going to be madly in love by the end of the book.

So how can you show that special something that tells the heroine this guy is different — and special? The possibilities are as limitless as your imagination, but in the following sections, I present a number of sure-fire ways to show that your hero's special.

Selling the sizzle

Make him gorgeous. Sure, this approach has been used literally a million times, but it works. A big part of what makes a fictional romance appealing is something that works in real life: chemistry. And a big part of chemistry is finding your partner physically irresistible.

Maybe he's a millionaire who's just stormed into your heroine's flower shop to accuse her of buying the neighboring property to mess up his business deal. She's furious because she had no idea he was even looking at the property, and she needs it to expand her flower shop. And yet, as angry as she is, she can't help noticing — maybe even to the point of derailing her train of thought — how incredibly good-looking he is. Showing the heroine responding so viscerally to the hero is a big clue that they're meant to be.

Digging deep

Give him moral, intellectual, and emotional strength. Remember the literal meaning of the word *hero.* Your hero has to be more than a male protagonist. He has to embody all the virtues the heroine deserves in a partner.

He needs to be honest and live by a strong moral code that is present in everything he does, even if he's overcoming a difficult past or makes mistakes in the present. He needs to be intelligent; no empty-headed pretty boys need apply for *this* position. And last (but far from least) he needs to be emotionally strong and reliable — and faithful, not necessarily from the beginning (although the reader doesn't want to see him sleeping around, even if the romantic relationship hasn't been solidified yet), but definitely by the end of the book. The reader needs to close the book knowing that these two people can be happy together forever, which means knowing his love for her is strong and true.

Creating conflict from character

Because the best conflict is emotional and is generated directly from your characters, your hero, just like your heroine, needs to have internal issues that drive him and contribute to the tensions separating him from the heroine. Like your heroine, your hero shouldn't be perfect, or he won't be interesting and won't have any room to develop as the book progresses; it's from his flaws and insecurities that his conflict will come. (For more on the subject of creating emotional conflict, see Chapter 5.)

Making things equal

Show him as the heroine's equal. Whether they're exchanging barbed remarks at a boring dinner party where the hostess seated them next to each other, not realizing they are both lawyers on opposite sides of a custody battle, or fighting their way to freedom side by side after being taken hostage by rebel forces during a luxury tour of the Amazon, don't let the heroine dominate or be dominated by the hero. If she's so strong or witty that she makes him look weak or stupid, or if he's superior and demeaning and undercuts her strengths (and by proxy the reader's), then they're not going to make a lasting match, because no one can be happy spending life in a one-down position. But if they're equals, the reader sees their potential as a match because they can go through life enjoying each other's company and meeting challenges together.

Shining but not outshining

Give your hero strengths that differ from but also complement the heroine's. Just as, in real life, good couples need each other, your hero and heroine should also need each other to feel complete. Maybe your couple is taken hostage by South American rebels and meet during an escape attempt. He's the tough guy who fights past the guards, and she's the clever one who talks their way onto a boat so they can escape (or vice versa!). They both shine, but neither outshines the other, because they're not competing in the same arenas.

Revealing his softer side

Let the hero's inner soft side be visible to your heroine. Maybe he and your heroine first encounter each other across the bargaining table during a hostile corporate takeover. She's about to lose the family firm to him, which really hurts, because her employees are like family to her and he has a reputation for being ruthless to his staff. Just when the situation is tensest, his young daughter, who's escaped from her nanny, runs in and turns the place upside down. Suddenly the heroine sees the hero's human side as he hugs his daughter, smiles, and forgets all about what's going on around him so he can hear about her first day of kindergarten. The heroine melts, and after that she never quite sees him as the bad guy again, no matter how much she tries.

Laughing it up

Never forget the power of humor. Laughter is sexy. Studies show that couples who laugh together have stronger relationships, so if your hero makes your heroine laugh, it's a good sign for their future. The hero and heroine's meeting may be difficult or awkward: They're playing lovers in a movie, and on the first day of shooting they have a sexy kissing scene. She's uncomfortable, not just because of the situation, but because he's her ex-husband, and all she can remember is how much it hurt when they separated. He senses her nervousness and decides to put her at ease, so he pratfalls out of bed, and suddenly she's laughing and remembering all the times they laughed together, not to mention wishing their kissing scene were for real, not just for the cameras. The key is to make sure the humor is character-driven, not slapstick, and that it's appropriate to their ages and situations.

Holding out for a hero: Alphas and others

REMEMBER

Not every hero is the same, but certain *types* of heroes exist that writers, editors, and, often, readers recognize. Each type of hero has his own appeal. Of course, you can combine attributes of the various types as you create your own hero, which allows you to craft just the right guy for your heroine *and* make a hero who's memorable to readers.

Any discussion of types of heroes is meant only as a starting point, because your goal is to always make your hero (like your heroine and your secondary characters) feel real. The tension between your couple needs to arise from the people they are, not from a contrived meeting of a stereotypical hero and heroine — so make your hero your own. As a basis for understanding heroes, here's some info on the kinds of men readers are used to falling for.

WARNING

Just as relationships depicted in romance novels don't mirror real-life relationships, the heroes also aren't like the men that women are looking to get involved with in real life. Romance novels are full of tension and drama, and romance heroes do their part to contribute. A perfect real-life boyfriend has no problem showing his feelings, and an imperfect real-life guy never figures out that he has any. Either way, these real-life boyfriends don't work as the hero of a romance novel. Real-life men and relationships are wonderful and fulfilling, but they lack the drama to power a compelling novel and keep readers turning pages. Be sure to avoid the true boy-next-door hero.

Leading the pack: The alpha hero

Have you ever heard of the alpha wolf? He's the leader of the pack. The one all the other wolves defer to. He is the wolf with all the power, and he takes his position for granted. An alpha hero is a lot like that wolf, except he wears a suit and tie, or maybe jeans and a leather jacket. Occasionally he even wears the human equivalent of sheep's clothing, but underneath, he's still all alpha. Here are the basic alpha traits:

>> An alpha hero takes charge of situations and people the minute he enters the room. To others, particularly the heroine, he generally seems dictatorial, rigid, even a big pain in the butt who needs to be taken down a peg. (Part of the heroine's conflict is almost always butting heads with an alpha guy to establish her own strength.)

>> An alpha hero is often a loner, and he usually works in an appropriately alpha job: corporate CEO, rancher, spy, policeman, fighter pilot. He's unlikely to be a teacher, and when he is, he's probably assuming the role for a reason. (Think Arnold Schwarzenegger in the movie *Kindergarten Cop,* but not played for comedy.) In his job, being tough is an asset; being tough helped him get to the top and stay there.

>> An alpha hero can make decisions and implement them in a second, and frequently the welfare of others — sometimes economically, sometimes their lives — depends on him. He's not used to thinking about feelings, his or anyone else's, and often women are eye- and arm-candy, because he doesn't let anyone get close — until he encounters the heroine.

>> An alpha hero appeals to the heroine (and the reader) because she gets to him as no woman ever has before. He may have been involved or even married before, but chances are his relationship broke up because of his alpha inability to let her in. Or maybe the relationship ended because she used him for his position and power (reinforcing his inability to trust a woman) or because she was a more traditional, submissive partner who died and provides a real contrast with the heroine. The heroine, however, is ultimately as strong as the alpha hero and breaks through his defenses. She makes him feel, and she gives as good as she gets, because she's his equal, which makes the two of them a match.

Years ago, every hero was an alpha, and a wide gap usually existed between him and the heroine in every way — age-wise, financially, and in career and social position. Throughout the book, he kept her in a one-down position, even though she did her best to combat him, and he never let on that she was getting to him. At the very end, he confessed his feelings for her and let her know how much she mattered to him.

These days, alpha heroes have a lot more range. Some still follow that classic pattern (particularly in historical romances, where that kind of relationship is more accurate for the time period, and in some series romances), but in most cases, the alpha hero is more complex. For example, including his point of view lets the reader see what the heroine can't: that he's feeling something for her beyond sexual attraction, and that he's often exaggerating his alpha tendencies to keep her from knowing how much she means to him.

TIP

As I discuss in the "Introducing imperfection" section earlier in the chapter, perfect characters aren't very interesting. An alpha guy may look perfect, but if he really were perfect, what would he need the heroine for? By giving him flaws and vulnerabilities, you also give the heroine a way into his life and his heart. Maybe he's suddenly presented with a 3-year-old daughter, the result of a long-ago one-night stand, and has no idea how to deal with the upheaval. Maybe he has demanding, disapproving parents, and envies the heroine's boisterous, loving family, and her own open, outgoing nature. Using such elements, you create chinks in his alpha armor, giving the heroine a way to reach him and the reader a reason to love him.

Opening up (but slowly): The beta hero

The beta hero is so-called simply because he provides a contrast to the alpha hero. The beta hero is still a true hero, but he's not as tough and unbending as an alpha hero. A beta hero interacts more with the heroine instead of just barking out orders, but he's no pushover — strong tension still needs to exist between them. Here are the beta basics:

>> A beta hero can be in pretty much any profession. He can excel at an alpha-style job, but he can also do jobs that don't come as naturally to an alpha, such as a teacher, doctor, writer, or scientist.

>> A beta hero is more likely to be a family man who has important relationships with his children, parents, or siblings, and he often has close friends as well. Unlike the loner alpha, a beta has a support system, and sometimes the heroine envies *his* good relationships. If a beta has a relationship in his past, it was quite possibly a good one, where he and his wife were a great couple, and either she died or the relationship ended in a more real-world way, like two nice people who just grew in different directions and divorced.

>> A beta hero's emotional issues are likely to be out on the table. Whereas an alpha hero refuses to acknowledge his issues with the heroine, the beta hero gets them out in the open piece by piece throughout the book. For example, if he has trouble trusting women, he won't hide that inside but will find ways to let her know he's not sure he can trust her, either — even though his attraction to her is clear. A beta hero comes with baggage, but he hasn't been as extremely affected by it as an alpha, even when their issues are the same. A beta hero's easier for the heroine — and the reader — to understand.

REMEMBER

Just because the issues are discussed doesn't mean he and the heroine discuss them calmly and rationally. (Where's the tension in that?) The issues between them are obvious to both of them — and to the reader — even if they seem unlikely to find a way to sort things out.

Breaking the rules: The bad-boy hero

The bad-boy hero is more accurately the reformed bad boy. When he was young, he was the town bad boy, the tough kid who scared the locals with his swagger, his hot car, and his I-don't-give-a-damn approach to the rules. He usually came from the wrong side of the tracks and often wasn't half as bad as the locals thought. And if he *was* bad, he wasn't bad in a big way, although that may not have saved him from taking the rap for anything from theft to rape to murder. Despite everything, he was usually irresistible to the local girls — or one local girl, in particular, who turns out to be the heroine.

The bad boy's transformation from outcast to hero can take various forms. Sometimes he stayed in town all along, possibly overcoming the stigma of his past and winning the locals' respect. Sometimes he lives on the fringes, the victim of whispers and finger-pointing. Sometimes he's just come back to town, possibly looking for revenge after a stint in prison for a crime he didn't commit, or maybe to show everyone he's made something of himself.

The bad boy's appeal lies in the old Beauty-and-the-Beast fantasy. Something's appealing about the edge of danger he carries, and something's seductive about being the one woman to tame him. In the end, he turns out to have all the essential heroic qualities, and his bad-boy persona becomes a thing of the past.

Feeling the pain: The tortured hero

The tortured hero hasn't been literally tortured, although it *is* a possibility, depending on the past you invent for him. Rather, he's emotionally tortured by something in his past, and that something causes him to put up barriers between himself and emotional intimacy.

Perhaps he's a former cop, and his wife and child were killed by a car bomb intended for him. Now he's tortured by guilt and never wants to get close to anyone again, because he can't bear the thought of putting anyone else at risk or of feeling the grief of such loss again. Maybe he had a terrible childhood that left him believing he's simply not capable of love. Maybe he's a vampire in love with a woman and is tormented that his only choices are to watch her wither and die of old age or to turn her into an immortal yet hunted creature like himself.

So what's the appeal of the tortured hero? Psychologists say that women are nurturers; they like to fix people and relationships. So a tortured hero is the ultimate challenge. In reality, this kind of guy is probably damaged goods and a bad bet for a relationship. But in a romance novel, he's a perfect romantic fantasy — a prize worth winning because the heroine alone can heal him.

Living and loving in style: The playboy hero

This type of hero is especially suited to a sexy romp or a battle of the sexes. He's the irresistible guy who has a woman — or two, or three — in every port. He loves women — all women. But settling down with just one isn't on his agenda. A playboy hero may know that he's using his attraction to all women as a form of self-protection, a method of making sure he isn't attracted to just one woman, thereby leaving himself vulnerable. Or he may genuinely think he's happy without strong emotional ties, because he hasn't seen love and marriage work. Maybe he became a playboy in response to a relationship gone wrong, or maybe he's a natural flirt who's just taking the path of least resistance through life and love.

Whatever made him a playboy, one thing is guaranteed: His world is rocked when he meets the heroine. Suddenly all other women lose their appeal — something that radically alters his self-image and makes him very unhappy at first. Almost always, his tension comes from that unhappiness when he realizes that he's been blindsided by love. But by the end of the book, he's very grateful for that emotional accident.

The hero is the prize the heroine wins, and a playboy can be thought of as the ultimate prize. The heroine becomes, in a sense, the world's most successful woman, the one who makes all other women fade to nothing in the eyes of the ultimate connoisseur of the female sex. Talk about the perfect couple!

Looking for love in all the wrong places

WARNING

Some kinds of heroes are a proven hard sell. I'm not saying it's impossible for you to find success with these heroes, because specific books with "problematic" heroes *have* sold — and very well. As the writer, you need to decide whether or not to let this information influence your decisions:

>> **Locales:** I don't always understand why readers dislike certain things, but I know that they've made certain dislikes clear. For whatever reason, heroes from certain locales (or whose names indicate a connection with those locales) tend not to be popular. Heroes from Germany, Scandinavia, and Russia have all proven a difficult sell. But keep an eye on the market. One breakout book can change the landscape.

>> **Job descriptions:** Unless you're a superstar author whose books sell on your name alone, back-cover copy is crucial in getting the reader to buy your book. One of the key pieces of information that back-cover copy conveys and that readers respond to is your hero's occupation. For the readers, certain jobs are shorthand for masculine: cowboy, spy, soldier, CEO, and cop. Other occupations indicate just the opposite and can negatively affect sales: playwright, dancer, sculptor, and painter.

TIP

If you choose a known unpopular element, you need to give your readers plenty of compelling emotional conflict (see Chapter 5) so the back-cover copy (and the book) can focus on what the readers want, not what they don't.

Hello, my name is . . .

REMEMBER

Just as the heroine's name is a crucial part of how the reader sees her, the hero's name says a lot about who he is, and it also needs to be chosen carefully. A reader needs to recognize your hero the minute he shows up on the page, and the right name tells her immediately that she's found her man. Listen to your instincts when naming your hero. Always be aware of the name you choose and how to make it work for you.

Strong men need strong names

You're probably not going to call your hero Casper Milquetoast, a name that screams — no, make that mumbles — weeniness. But you still have to be careful and avoid choosing a name that has connotations that work against the character you're creating.

TIP

In general, short names sound masculine and strong: Rafe, Gabe, and Jake. They're not fussy sounding, and heroes aren't fussy guys. Of course, longer names can work, too, as long as they sound masculine, like Rafael, Gabriel, and Jacob. They carry a certain weight and have a certain history to them, and their connotations work to your advantage. Active names, like Chase, sound strong and heroic, and hard sounds — Cord, Kyle, and Rick — also indicate strength and masculinity. Compare those names to Myron or Frances, which are generally considered geeky or weak sounding.

Avoiding childish nicknames

WARNING

Charlie and Stevie are fine nicknames for little boys, but remember that your hero's a man. He may be a Charles or a Steven, even a Steve, but if you give him a cute, little-boy nickname, the reader's likely to think of him as *her* little boy, and you want her to see him as the man she's falling in love with.

Hitting your mark: Accuracy counts

Being accurate when naming your hero is important. If your book is a historical romance, make his name specific to the time period. Seth and Caleb both have a strong sense of history to them that Pierce and Keshawn lack. If he comes from a particular country or region, give him a name that also comes from that area. Miguel works if he's Hispanic, for example, or Jean Paul if he's French. Names can even feel job-specific, in a way. For example, you're more likely to find a cowboy named Rafe than a corporate CEO.

WARNING

Native American heroes are particularly popular in historical and contemporary romances, which has led to an extra challenge: finding a name that indicates the hero's background without sounding phony or clichéd. I've lost count of how many characters named Hawk I've seen, so even if you use Hawk as part of his name, know that you need to work hard to make him stand out as an individual.

Switching order: Last names as first names

In romance novels (and often in real life), men are frequently referred to by their last names. Alex Chance may become Chance, while Keith McCord may become McCord or Mac. For this reason, you may want to give extra thought to your hero's surname.

Keepin' It Real: Secondary Characters

Although the hero and heroine are the key characters in any romance, they don't live in a vacuum. Like all of us, they have family, friends, and co-workers. These supporting characters are called *secondary characters.* Secondary characters range from parents, children, best friends, and bosses to villains and romantic rivals who create a sense of threat, to waitresses or mechanics who may have only a line or two of dialogue or description. Pay plenty of attention to them (even though you may not give them a lot of space), and you maximize your chances of creating a world that feels real.

REMEMBER

Secondary characters can be harder to create than your hero and heroine, because you use fewer words and pages to describe them.

Remembering their roles

In most cases, secondary characters exist because they play a specific role in the plot (this is especially true of villains and romantic rivals). They do the following:

>> **Provide a sense of place and reality.** Secondary characters make your hero and heroine's world feel full and real. With names, voices, and behavior, secondary characters give a sense of where and when things are happening, saving you from relying on narrative to get everything across.

>> **Parallel or contrast with the hero and heroine's relationship.** Using secondary characters in this way allows you to shed more light on the main characters' romance. A secondary couple may act as an example of two people who overcame issues similar to those that the hero and heroine face. Or they can serve as a cautionary tale, as an example of what the hero and heroine want to avoid. A secondary character who's open about wanting to find love can also provide a good contrast to a hero or heroine who's determined to avoid emotional entanglements and the risk of ending up unhappy.

>> **Help move the plot forward.** Your hero and heroine shouldn't — and probably can't — do everything for themselves. A villain or romantic rival plays a role no hero or heroine can, but sometimes a secondary character's role is less dramatic or obvious. You may just need someone to get hurt or trapped so your hero or heroine can demonstrate his or her skills; it can be something as mundane as fixing a car or as dramatic as making a critical scientific discovery — whatever your story needs.

- >> **Provide crucial information.** Secondary characters are helpful in providing two types of information:

  - **Factual information:** A secondary character may know something the hero and heroine don't, whether it's a clue to solving a mystery, how to break a horse, or how to negotiate a contract.

  - **Emotional information:** Secondary characters may also know pieces of emotional information. The hero and heroine can't sit down and discuss their feelings with each other, but they can talk about those feelings (the heroine, especially) with *other* characters. Conversations with friends and family are a good opportunity to let your hero and heroine start to express and understand their feelings about each other.

REMEMBER

Don't let your secondary characters take over the story. Remember that the role of a secondary character is one of support. Their lives and stories aren't important by themselves; they're important for the ways that they illuminate the central characters and their romance.

Avoiding stereotypes

WARNING

You have to watch out for stereotypes in all aspects of your novel. Falling into the trap of using types instead of individuals for your secondary characters is *very* easy. Avoid relying on the supportive best friend, the nit-picking boss, the leering villain, or the overprotective older brother.

You can give recognizable characteristics to secondary characters because you don't have the time or space to develop them in as much detail as your hero and heroine; however, they still must resonate as individuals. Be selective in the descriptions you include, so your secondary characters feel real, mixing unique details with broader brushstrokes.

Speaking up

Voices count. You don't want every character in your book, no matter how minor, to have such a quirky way of speaking that your novel sounds like lunchtime at the Tower of Babel. You can use voice to quickly and easily define your most important secondary characters: For example, older characters probably talk with more formality than a 30-something or a slang-slinging teen; someone from the South may speak with a relaxed cadence; and a non-native's accent may come across through syntax. Also, don't let your own speech and vocabulary come from every character's mouth, or all your characters will sound the same in such an obvious way that they won't seem real. (For specifics on creating and using your characters' voices, see Chapter 9.)

Naming the baby (and everyone else)

What's in a name? More than you might think. For better or worse, people often draw conclusions based on names, so use that to your advantage when you're creating your secondary characters because you don't have a lot of room to develop them. When someone's heritage — national, regional, or racial — is important, choose a name that conveys it. Keep names consistent with their generations, too.

For example, old-fashioned names usually indicate grandparents. Some brand names, like Mercedes or Zara, have a younger feel to them. Names in a historical romance must fit the period. Also, don't use too many similar names, because the reader becomes confused instead of being able to distinguish your characters from each other. For the same reason, don't start too many names with the same letter, and keep a running list to be sure you don't give two (or more!) characters the same last name. Keeping your main characters' names straight is easy, but not confusing all the minor characters' names is more difficult.

Factoring in the future

You may set up a secondary character to be the hero or heroine of a future connected book. In this case, focus on that character just a little more than you normally would and raise an unanswered question or two about them. The unanswered questions are a cue to the reader that she can expect to see that character again in a starring role.

WARNING

Just don't pay too much attention to this character by explaining and focusing on them too often in *this* book. If you start telling their story, it will compete with your hero and heroine's romance.

Also, be very sparing and discriminating when you use secondary characters' points of view. As a general rule, including secondary characters' points of view isn't only unnecessary, it's often a problem because it diffuses the focus of the book.

Laying Concrete Strategies for Creating Characters

You need to know your characters, including your secondary characters, inside and out. In the end, you'll know far more about their backstories than you ever tell your readers. The fact that you created your characters so completely helps them come across as real people. Here are some strategies for making them real in your own mind so they also feel real to your readers:

>> **Find pictures that look like your characters.** Whether you use movie-star photos or stock images, find pictures of people who look like your characters and hang them up in your workspace or keep them in your Scrivener file (see Chapter 3) to help you visualize them and keep the details in your mind as you write. Especially find pictures for your hero and heroine, but don't be afraid to add pictures that represent your secondary characters.

>> **Know your characters' voices.** You should hear your characters in your head as you write. If their voices are specific actors' or singers' voices, you can listen to them by playing a movie or some music in the background (if you're not distracted by it).

>> **Create a character board.** Whether you use index cards on a corkboard, sticky notes on the wall, or use Plottr or Scrivener (see Chapter 3), keep a file on every character that tells you everything you need to know about that character. You need to know every detail of their appearance; job; romantic history; family and educational backgrounds; favorite color, music, TV shows, and movies; how they dress; and whether they like animals, staying up late, getting up early, or sleeping away the weekend. Know the nuances of your characters' personalities and lives as well as you know your own or your best friend's.

>> **Run role-playing exercises for your characters.** Doing role-playing exercises is useful, especially when you're developing your hero and heroine. You need to know how they respond in all kinds of situations so their actions feel natural and believable when you commit them to the page. Before you start writing, give some thought to role playing. Think up situations your characters may face together and individually; then, based on everything you've decided about them, come up with their logical actions and responses. You can use everyday situations — like getting a flat tire on the way to a job interview — and extreme possibilities — like being carjacked on the way home from the grocery store. Writing your book is easier when you know how your characters will react in different situations, because as they face each new plot twist, their responses are second nature to you.

Chapter **5**

Crucial Ingredients for Every Plot: Conflict, Climax, and Resolution

P lot isn't just the heart of your story, it literally *is* your story. Your plot provides the context in which your hero and heroine's romance unfolds, but it's more than just the framework for that romantic picture. A plot moves, just as your romance moves. Ultimately, the plot and the romance should be like two completely entangled strands: Neither one can exist or make sense without the other. Plot brings your hero and heroine together, and then their romance moves the plot forward. Their decisions affect what happens, and what happens affects their future decisions. This chain of events doesn't end until happily ever after.

All romance plots consist of a number of key structural components — suspense, conflict, climax, and resolution. Suspense keeps the reader turning the pages and creates her need to know what happens next. Conflict gets your readers as emotionally involved in the story as the characters are and propels your plot forward. And finally, climax and resolution provide the grand finale — everything your plot has been building toward.

In this chapter, I explain how to create each piece of the plot puzzle and the ways in which they work together. Along the way, I unravel the plot and romance connections to help you discover how to seamlessly weave these elements together in your work. Because you can't fill in plot particulars until you have an idea for a story, I begin by providing suggestions on how you can generate ideas for your novel.

You Can't Have a Novel without a Plot

To be more accurate, maybe I should say that you can't have a romance novel (or any piece of popular fiction) without a plot. There are literary novels and examples of experimental fiction that don't have what's conventionally defined as a plot, but we're talking about romance novels, so plots are definitely on the agenda.

Every successful romance novel has a plot. In its simplest form, a *plot* is a series of interconnected events that progress through three stages:

>> A beginning, where the story is set in motion

>> A middle, where the bulk of the action takes place

>> An ending, where everything is resolved, the loose ends are tied up, and a satisfactory conclusion is reached

The beginning of a book is crucial. So crucial, in fact, that I devote Chapter 12 to the mechanics of creating a great beginning and *how* to start your story. In this chapter, I focus on the *what* of your story — the process of conceptualizing the story you want to tell, starting with the idea.

Where do ideas come from?

I wish I had a simple answer to this question — and so do the many published authors who hear "Where do you get your ideas?" all the time. Many of those authors are so instinctively attuned to the storytelling process that they aren't even conscious of where their ideas come from. For writers like this, their subconscious does the work for them, so by the time an idea hits their conscious mind, it seems to have sprung full-blown out of nowhere.

You may never have ideas without any conscious effort on your part, but you can teach yourself to find ideas when and where you need them. The real question isn't really "Where do ideas come from?" as much as "How do I recognize an idea?" There's no such thing as an idea store, even though Ideas Express would make our jobs as writers and editors much easier. Instead, the entire world is your idea store. Ideas are literally everywhere. You just need to train yourself to recognize them.

Approaching the world from different angles

You can begin your quest for the elusive idea in any number of ways, but in general, I see two perspectives from which you can approach this task:

>> **Emotional:** With this approach, you're examining the world for an idea that will drive the romantic, personal aspects of your story. For example, your starting point may be how a formerly abused woman learns to trust (and love) again, or how a lone-wolf hero finds his defenses penetrated by a bubbly 6-year-old blonde and her warm-hearted mother. Because romance novels are all about emotion, starting from this perspective works well, because you develop the key element first. Think of it as working from the inside out. After you have an idea in place, you can then move beyond the characters' personal concerns to construct the larger, external events around your emotional core.

>> **Intellectual:** This approach is like working from the outside in. You look for your ideas in larger-scale events (a scientific discovery, a paranormal event, a study on why marriages failed), rather than on the personal level. This approach can be trickier, because your job then is to insert the key ingredient — the romance — into this larger external plot.

TIP

How you get your ideas doesn't matter — what matters is simply that you get them. You can even develop your own approach that's unrelated to anything I suggest. The keys are to find a way to recognize ideas and capitalize on them, and to develop the emotional core that will drive your story before you start writing.

Finding ideas around every corner

REMEMBER

You probably move so quickly through life, juggling family, friends, work, and everything else, that you don't give yourself time to recognize all the ideas that are begging for your attention. Even so, we see and hear things every day that catch our imaginations. As a storyteller, you just need to take the next step and give yourself permission to notice and explore those promising ideas, with the thought of turning them into the basis for a romance. Ask yourself questions, the most effective of which usually start with "What if?" Questioning yourself is a great way to brainstorm and take your ideas to the next level, turning them into a story, and then populating that story with characters your readers will enjoy knowing.

Ideas are in the news, on the TV, in a local church bulletin, in gossip you overhear in line at the grocery store, on social media, in a story Uncle Ed tells at the family Thanksgiving dinner . . . anywhere and everywhere you find yourself interacting with the world.

TIP

Here are some examples of situations you run into every day, some of which are likely to catch your attention emotionally, others intellectually, and all of which give rise to the kinds of what-if situations that form the basis of a romance novel:

>> **The Internet is full of an especially juicy piece of romantic celebrity gossip.** Celebrities have chosen careers that lead to fame. What if someone who has no desire to live in the public eye, who even has good reason (like being in Witness Protection) to feel threatened by it, falls in love with someone who's chosen to live the celebrity life, and then is catapulted into that world herself?

>> **Scientists discover a promising new treatment for childhood leukemia.** What if a scientist is focused on finding a cure for leukemia because his sister died of the disease, but now the big drug interests are threatening to sideline his research in favor of another approach they think is more promising (and potentially profitable)? What if he must convince — by any means necessary — the beautiful but by-the-numbers corporate accountant to loosen the purse strings?

>> **Archeologists dig up a trove of Viking gold in a field in England.** How did the gold get there? What if a British maiden fell in love with a Viking warrior? Did he steal the gold from his lord and bury it, so he could run away with his true love and start a life with her? Why was he unable to retrieve the gold? What course did their love follow?

Anything you hear or see that interests you may potentially be an idea for your romance novel. Tune in your radar to the world around you, and don't let anything pass by — big or small, a human-interest story or a breaking headline — without turning it over in your mind, looking at it from all angles, and deciding whether there's something there that you can use.

At first, you may have to make an effort to tune in to the world around you. You may have to consciously tell yourself to pay attention and think more deeply about things. But eventually, there's a good chance that tuning yourself in will become a learned behavior. If you're lucky, it can become second nature, letting you go from worrying that you may never have an idea to having so many that you can't find time to write all of them.

Keep an idea file. Whether it's a manila envelope stuffed with clippings and notes or a Word document, save your ideas for future use and look through them periodically to give your subconscious something to work with. Another benefit to saving articles is that you already have a starting point for doing research later.

Asking questions develops your characters and plot

No matter how you're initially drawn to your idea, by the time you're ready to work with it, you should be looking at it in emotional terms, thinking of the ways in which your characters are going to respond and react, both intellectually and emotionally, because their reactions help drive your story forward. Ultimately, your entire book is based on the answers to the "What if?" questions you've asked yourself.

Frame your questions in emotional terms. Make them complex enough so that answering them takes a while; otherwise, you're not going to have enough story to tell. One of the most important interviewing rules is to never ask questions with yes and no answers, or else you can end up with the shortest, most boring interview on record. Instead, ask leading questions. For example, don't ask, "Mrs. Smith, did winning the lottery change your life?" Instead, ask, "Mrs. Smith, how did winning the lottery change your life?" Apply this strategy to shape the idea that will begin your book. Your initial "What if?" should be open-ended and/or complex enough that the answer spawns an entire scenario, allowing you to develop your characters and propel the plot. Essentially, your characters act out the scenario your "What if?" gives rise to, and that's your story.

Ask questions that require your characters to grow, change, and explore their emotions. Ask questions that push their buttons and their boundaries. Don't ask, "Would falling in love with a movie star change my heroine's life?" Instead, ask, "How would falling in love with a movie star change my heroine's life?" It's in describing the "how" that you find your story. By phrasing your question not in terms of *whether* but in terms of *how*, you ensure that the answer is in the form of a story and you focus the story on character experience and growth, a crucial element to all romances.

Letting your characters drive the plot

Although other types of popular fiction can be — and often are — plot-driven, romances are character-driven. A romance novel is based on emotional conflict, which is part of who your characters are and determines how they respond to each other and how they operate in tandem with the plot you create. By setting up a story that focuses on character growth, you set up a story that, as long as you emotionally challenge your hero and heroine, is automatically based on emotional conflict.

Throughout the course of your book, your characters' actions — which you've made the central focus of the story — are driven by their emotions, because emotion is the key motivating force in a romance novel. Your characters, their decisions, actions, and responses, propel and control the plot, keeping your reader interested — all because you knew how to spot an idea and think about it the right way.

TIP

You should be able to describe the setup of your book for anyone who asks. A *setup* is a brief (that's key) explanation of what will drive your story and make it interesting to a reader. The best setups contain everything a writer or an editor needs to know in as few words as possible. I sometimes half-jokingly say that I work with authors who could write me one line on a cocktail napkin and, based on that, I would trust them to write an entire book. I say that because, in just a line or two, the right setup can contain enough information to make the characters and their conflict vivid and complex, which is a signal that the author has the basis for an entire book.

Here's a sample setup, presented as briefly as possible:

> An heiress who (thinks she) doesn't like kids runs away from an arranged marriage and finds herself masquerading as a nanny to the 3-year-old twin sons of a rancher who's sworn off love.

In that one sentence, you get an immediate sense of who the characters are, where they're likely to butt heads, and even where some of the plot details are likely to come from: different worlds (big bucks versus the ranch life). Try writing your own setup in a line or two and see if you can include the key information that tells an editor you have a story to tell.

Suspense: Every Story Has It

A good idea is a necessary starting point, but you need more than that to have a successful book. You also have to execute it well. Two writers starting with the same potential-filled premise will write two entirely different books. The one who understands suspense will write a page-turner; the one who doesn't will write the cure for insomnia.

REMEMBER

In your romance, a reader cares about what's happening because of two reasons: her interest in and identification with your characters (see Chapter 4), and the emotional conflict inherent in your setup. After you've created compelling characters and an emotionally intriguing idea to hook your reader's interest, you can move on to maintaining her interest by creating suspense and using it to your advantage.

When I talk about suspense in storytelling, I'm not talking about the kind of suspense that involves dark alleys, dead bodies, and smoking guns. Those elements *are* one definition of the word, and a very legitimate one. As I discuss in Chapter 2, romantic suspense novels are one of the most successful romantic subgenres. But dark-and-dangerous suspense isn't the only kind. All good storytelling involves suspense in a more general form. In a broad sense, readers are prey to suspense when they care about what's going to happen to a particular character or in a particular situation and then have to wait to find out. Their desire to know more is what keeps them turning pages.

A writer who knows how to handle suspense understands that to keep her reader reading, she has to do two things: Make her reader care about what's happening in the story, and create suspense by doling out information — the payoff — in increments, withholding the most important pieces until the end. Every scene not only moves the story and the romance forward, but it also leaves the reader wanting, needing, to know more. Whether the scene ends on a cliffhanger or simply raises a new complication that's followed up on later, the reader is left in suspense, and that leads her to read the next scene, and the next, in hope of getting the answers she wants.

Using romance to create suspense

Working with suspense is a bit like mimicking the rise and fall of the sea. First you rev your reader's interest to a high pitch, then you drop back without completely satisfying her, and then you do it again. You work incrementally, getting a little closer to fulfillment — for your characters and your reader — with every scene, but you always stop short of giving them everything they want.

REMEMBER

In a romance novel, the reader's main interest is in the relationship's progress, so your most effective strategy for building suspense is through that relationship. Your reader wants to see the relationship deepen in two areas as the romance develops:

>> **Physical intimacy:** Anything from a kiss to full-on lovemaking

>> **Emotional intimacy:** The final payoff

TIP

When you're building suspense, don't develop these two types of intimacies in tandem. They work most effectively when developed independently of each other. In a real-world romance, physical and emotional intimacy tend to develop at a matching pace. As a couple grows closer emotionally, their physical relationship deepens. (Not that a proposal is always a prerequisite for lovemaking, but both people usually sense that the relationship has potential.) This scenario is wonderful in the real world, but it doesn't have enough suspense to support a romance novel.

In a romance novel, the reader doesn't want the course of the relationship to run smoothly; if it does, she gets bored. She wants to worry that your hero and heroine won't end up together — even though she knows they belong together and that the very fact she's reading a romance novel means they will be together in the end. But she pretends she doesn't know, and you let her. That's where suspense comes into play. Whether you use the characters' own emotional issues or a clever plot twist to keep them from being a happy couple, by depriving them of ultimate romantic satisfaction you're also depriving the reader — and keeping her in suspense as she waits for that happiness. See the "Taking two steps forward and one step back" section later in this chapter for information on just how to do this.

Other ways of creating twists and turns

Even though your reader's main interest and your most effective tool for creating suspense is the central romance, it's not the only tool you have available. You can also use both plot-related twists and your secondary characters to keep readers guessing.

REMEMBER

One advantage to both of these *secondary suspense* tools, which form a helpful backup to your primary source of suspense — what will happen with the hero and heroine's relationship? — is that you can pay them off as you go along, giving your reader satisfaction on one level while still withholding the ultimate payoff of the romance.

Working your plot

Plot elements can be interesting in their own right. Even though the reader picks up the book for the romance, plot elements work on a subsidiary level, and the desire to see how they turn out is another factor that keeps her reading. Will the serial killer be caught? Where's the deadly formula? How will the custody battle be resolved? If you pose the question intriguingly enough, your reader will definitely want to know the answer.

Plot developments that are also closely tied to the progress of the romance are the strongest source of secondary suspense. For example, is the missing formula hidden — unknown to her — in the heroine's purse? Is the hero actually an undercover operative sent to retrieve it? After she discovers who he really is, her immediate response is likely to be that he's been romancing her not out of genuine interest, but because she has something that he wants. Plot affects emotion, and the relationship is in trouble again. Every plot offers opportunities to affect your characters' emotions, and the more closely you intertwine the plot with the characters' emotional lives (something I discuss later in this chapter, in the "Letting conflict complicate your plot" section), the more frequent and effective those opportunities will be.

TIP

The more you make your hero and heroine care about the outcome of any plot-related question, the more your reader will care about it, too.

Using secondary characters

Secondary characters can also provide a secondary source of suspense. Although their fates shouldn't rival the hero and heroine's relationship, their stories can still capture and hold your reader's interest. Secondary characters' plotlines often exist to parallel or illuminate the central romance, which gives them added interest. Will a secondary character have a healthy baby, find his missing son, or recover from her heart surgery? The answers aren't earth-shattering, but they *will* matter to your reader, so use them to your advantage.

Making Sense Matters

Your hero and heroine's emotional conflict, which works to keep them apart even when they want to be together, is the single most important factor in driving your plot and creating your reader's need to finish the book. But your plot still has to make sense, so making the elements in your story move logically is crucial.

Every plot dictates its own internal logic. You must follow the logic you set up in your story line. A romantic suspense plot requires careful fact- and timeline-checking to make sure you're not creating a large hole in the plot. A marriage-of-convenience plot is simpler, but still requires you to move the book along in a believable time frame and not change the rules midstream.

REMEMBER

It can be easy to get so caught up in your characters' emotions that you forget to keep an eye on the outside world. But without acknowledging how things work in real life, the plot falls apart before it's even begun. Readers keep track of how the book's moving on every level, and if you get the mechanics wrong, they'll notice.

Major mistakes in anything from the timeline to the topography pull your reader out of the story. Hiring a good content editor can help you keep things on track.

WARNING

I could give you a lot of examples, but the following mistake is obvious enough to make my point. I've seen this mistake a number of times, and it undercuts a book so thoroughly from the beginning that it doesn't matter how well-drawn the hero and heroine's emotions are, because the book will never make sense.

The heroine comes home to find her apartment ransacked. Upset, she runs next door, where the handsome hero (who has probably just moved in) is waiting to help and offer support. They go back to her place to see what they can figure out and spend the rest of the book solving the mystery and falling in love (in spite of the requisite emotional suspense and conflict, of course). The problem? The hero and heroine don't call the police anywhere along the way, and no official crime scene investigation ever occurs. On top of that problem, in most cases, neither the hero nor the heroine has the skills or expertise to solve the case, which makes the reader skeptical about the plot's plausibility.

The problem isn't that the basic plot setup can't work — the author just has to acknowledge how things happen in the real world first. She can do so in plenty of ways:

>> **Have the characters call the police.** Let the police start an official investigation. If they're not taking it as seriously or being as thorough as the hero and heroine would like, they can still investigate on the side.

>> **Give the heroine a good reason for not contacting the police.** Her ex-husband is a cop and she doesn't want to give him a way back into her life. Her three overprotective older brothers are all cops and will use the break-in as an excuse to pressure her to get married, move back home, and so on. If she's not being physically threatened by what happened (and what's likely to happen next), you can get away with an explanation like this, so long as you acknowledge that calling the police would be the logical response and come up with a reason for her not to.

>> **Give the hero or heroine the expertise to deal with the problem.** In the circumstances I lay out, the hero is likely to be a cop, ex-cop, private investigator, and so on. Either way, the decision to go it alone makes much more sense if one of them has the skills to investigate.

REMEMBER

Your characters' actions always need to be believable and believably motivated, both emotionally and in terms of real-world logic.

Creating Emotional Conflict and Tension

The conflict, or tension, between your hero and heroine should always drive your plot. Your novel should also have a certain story-related momentum, but the key factor that keeps your reader turning pages is the progress of the romance, which is driven by the conflict between the hero and heroine.

REMEMBER

You can use different techniques and combinations of techniques to create conflict between your hero and heroine. However you craft that conflict, though, one point is key: You need to create a source of emotional conflict and tension for your hero and heroine — something that exists separately from the specifics of the plot, something inside each of them that would create a problem whether they met in Maine or on the moon, though the problem certainly should be exacerbated by their situation.

After you decide where the emotional tension comes from, you can create and complicate it at will. By manipulating that emotional tension, you're better able to keep your reader involved and happy from start to finish.

Emotional versus intellectual conflict

Without the surrounding context of a plot, the distinction between emotional and intellectual conflict is easy to make, yet writers continually struggle with it in their manuscripts. Simply put, an *intellectual conflict* is a conflict of ideas, while an *emotional conflict* is one that grows from feelings.

The temptation to use an intellectual conflict — and even to mistake it for an emotional one — is understandable, because intellectual conflicts are obvious — and everywhere, and many are fascinating. The morning paper and the news are full of debates over important concerns like foreign and domestic policy, the economy, and the environment, and smaller issues, like uniforms in public schools and lawn-watering restrictions.

What makes a conflict intellectual is the fact that it starts out in the mind. People's feelings about an issue can be very strong, and arguing them into seeing another point of view may be impossible; but even so, every argument has two sides, and intelligent people can make a case for either side. Intellectual conflicts can be interesting, but in the context of a romance novel — where the intent is to engage the reader's heart, not her head — they're counterproductive if they appear front and center.

Emotions, unlike opinions, don't need to have a logical basis and can't be reasoned away. They come from inside and simply *are.* They're not up for discussion or argument. Your emotions are an intrinsic part of who you are. They're not something you decided on one day after you took a course, read a book, or saw a news special; they come from your genetic makeup, the way you were raised, and your experiences in life and love. They affect how you see yourself, your family and friends, and — maybe most of all — who and how you love.

Highlighting emotional conflict

You can't build every plot completely around the emotional conflict, but every plot needs to highlight that conflict whenever possible. The more complicated your plot is, the more threads you have going on at once; however, emotional tension should underlie everything that's happening. The emotional conflict should always be in the characters' and the readers' minds. Here are a couple of sample heroines and scenarios that show you how to create an emotional conflict for each of them:

>> **Heroine 1:** Born to a single mother, abandoned to the foster-care system, and shuttled from family to family, she's likely to be self-contained, independent, distrustful, wary of forming close bonds, lacking self-esteem, and practically incapable of believing that she deserves love.

>> **Heroine 2:** Raised in a large, tight-knit family, the only girl among six children, doted on and cherished, encouraged in safe directions but protected — even overprotected — from risk, she's likely to have a bright, open personality and to make friends easily. She's just as likely to doubt her ability to operate independently and fear being smothered by love, especially romantic love.

Intellectually, in a debate over cocktails, these heroines may be identical, but in every way that counts, they're polar opposites and always will be. They approach life in completely different ways. Both may be wary of love, but for totally different reasons, which means their emotional hot buttons are different. They're also drawn to and wary of completely different characteristics in men.

Their choices in life are driven by their inner selves, the emotional human beings that they are:

>> **Heroine 1** may choose a way of life that lets her remain aloof from others — maybe as a researcher in a high-tech lab or a computer programmer — because that's how she protects her tender emotional core, the part that's always felt abandoned and is afraid to love because she's sure she'll only be abandoned again.

>> **Heroine 2** may be busy making her way in the police department, proving to her big, overprotective family (and, not incidentally, herself) that she can go it alone and cut it as a beat cop in a tough neighborhood.

Enter the hero, a police detective working on a case. He shares the same views on politics, religion, and all the rest, so he can't argue with either woman on that score. Like Heroine 1, he was raised in foster care, but he had a younger sister who was raised with him, and from the time he was a little kid, he's been her protector. He joined the force to protect even more people. Plus, when his parents died, he was old enough to remember what being part of a loving family was like, and he wants that again.

Both heroines see a murder take place and need to be put into protective custody until the killer's apprehended, tried, and — with the benefit of their testimonies — sent away for life. One of the heroines lucks out and gets the hero as her watchdog at the safe house. The story plays out differently depending on which heroine the hero is assigned to:

>> **Heroine 1:** If she gets the hero as her protector, she's going to resent him spending the long hours they're confined together trying to connect with her on the subject of their shared backgrounds, because she doesn't want to bring up all those painful memories. And she certainly doesn't want to find herself hooked on this incredible guy who can — even in her present scary situation — make her laugh, get her talking about everything under the sun, even when she keeps telling herself to shut up, and who's sexy beyond belief, besides.

For the hero, it makes him nuts that she continues shutting him down and withdrawing just when he thinks he's getting close to her. Even though he knows keeping his heart uninvolved would be smart, he can't help being drawn to her, so much so that he has to remind himself that he's on the job and pull back — just as he's about to kiss her. She feels rejected, all the old hurts of her childhood rise up, and they're on the outs with each other and neither one knows why. As simple as that, I've set up an emotional conflict without any effort beyond creating complex characters and letting them react believably.

>> **Heroine 2:** If she gets locked away with the hero, she's going to react differently for different reasons. She's going to bridle at his protective side, point out that she's a cop, too, and is more than capable of taking care of herself. She will think his fantasy of having a big, happy family would make her crazy, because she'd end up lost in the ruckus, taking care of everyone in that traditionally female way that she's sworn isn't for her.

He can't believe she doesn't understand the value of family and is fighting to break away from hers. He respects her professional abilities plenty, but in the circumstances, she *does* need to be protected, and why can't she see that he's just the guy to do it? They keep butting heads, but they're also attracted, challenged, and in no way ready to write each other off.

Plot — the need to lock the hero and heroine together in a safe house — puts them together but doesn't provide the conflict. Plot gives the hero and heroine the opportunity to be in conflict, but the conflict itself is emotional. It comes from within, from a clash between who they are, not what they think.

TIP

In any romance novel, the emotional conflict needs to affect the hero and heroine's relationship, to have romantic ramifications, so that they're irresistibly drawn toward each other, while simultaneously feeling that a relationship can't possibly work between them.

Taking care with intellectual conflict

WARNING

You can use elements of intellectual conflict in your book, too, but you have to be careful. Keep these two tips in mind:

>> Intellectual conflict can never be substituted for emotional conflict.

>> Relate any elements of intellectual conflict to the characters' emotional conflict as much as possible.

To clarify the second bullet point, here's an example to demonstrate this strategy. He's a developer; she's an environmentalist. He wants to use a piece of property to build housing; she wants to preserve it to save the rare spotted squirrel. Arguments about the housing needs of people versus the need to preserve the environment ensue. Any reader who's stayed awake long enough to make it to the end finds out that they compromise and build cluster housing on one section of the property and maintain the rest as legally protected woodland. The characters thought their way to a mutually acceptable solution. Everybody wins, and now the two of them can act on their mutual attraction. As a plot, it's an exercise in mental gymnastics and nothing more. The story has no heart.

However, the story could have heart. Maybe the hero's not just an in-it-for-the-money developer but is someone who has a mission: providing reasonably priced housing for people who may otherwise never get to own a nice home in a place where they can raise their families. Perhaps he was raised by a hard-working single mother who barely made the rent on a cheap apartment, and this is his way of giving back to the world in her memory. The heroine was raised in the inner city, and the only time she ever saw the country was on a city-sponsored summer program. She's determined to save a little piece of the wild within spitting distance of the city so less fortunate kids will always have a place they can get away to and meet nature.

This plot isn't the most compelling one on the planet, but at least now it has an emotional component, and you can see how the two types of conflict can work together. I'm not recommending this approach — taking an intellectual conflict and adding an emotional element to make it a book — because it works backward. By the time you start writing, your idea should already be an emotional one, even if it started from an intellectual point.

Internal versus external conflict

Another (and related) way to look at conflict is as internal versus external. *Internal conflict* comes from the characters themselves; it's whatever they bring to the story, both emotionally and intellectually. *External conflict* comes from the plot and circumstances, or is created by other characters.

Emotional conflict is always internal. This kind of conflict finds a way to manifest itself whatever the circumstances are. Going back to my example of the heroine from the big family and the protective hero, these two people are going to have issues no matter how or where they meet, simply because of who they are.

An example of external conflict is your hero and heroine arguing over the best way to handle the case. Any two cops — including two men or two women — can do that. You can't substitute external conflicts for internal ones, but you can enhance emotional conflicts by using externals to provide a context that gives your hero and heroine a chance to be together and seemingly at odds against one thing (how to handle the case, in the example above) while what they're *really* arguing over is something else entirely, in this case his tendency to protect — or overprotect, as she sees it — her.

Your hero and heroine can't spend the entire book talking about their emotional conflicts, otherwise your story ends up reading like a long session at a psychotherapist's office. An external conflict lets your characters talk about something concrete with their emotional issues as a subtext — a subtext that you can clarify by getting into their heads for a point-of-view look at what's going on, which I talk about in Chapter 9.

Personal versus situational conflict

One final way to talk about conflict is as personal versus situational. *Personal conflicts* are conflicts that grow from the innate issues and insecurities that everyone has. You carry around certain feelings inside yourself that are personal to you. In most of your day-to-day relationships, they don't raise their heads, but with the people who matter most, your personal issues are important. Your family and friends — these are the people whose opinions count and who have the ability to make you feel great or horrible. Those people who are close to you matter on a personal level, and with them, your deepest feelings come into play. This situation is the same with your hero and heroine; they can touch each other on the deepest, most personal levels.

A *situational conflict* arises from place and plot. In the earlier safe-house example, the situational conflict comes from locking the hero and heroine up where they can't get away from each other, which forces them to deal with their internal, emotional issues or else spend the entire book in separate rooms. As with intellectual and external conflicts, situational conflict can work with the key emotional tension your hero and heroine have to deal with, but situational conflict can never substitute for emotional conflict. Situational conflict can provide the hothouse atmosphere where tension can grow, but the novel's deeper issues are always the characters' personal and emotional conflicts.

TIP

The best romances are built around a complex emotional conflict that's played out in an equally interesting and tightly connected context — one that forces the characters to deal with each other and their issues.

Handling Conflict Effectively

Coming up with the right idea and creating characters whose emotional makeup allows for conflict isn't enough. You still need to use that conflict to drive your story. Your idea and the basis of the tension between your hero and heroine form the beginning of the story. Working with that tension drives your story through the middle and on to the end.

Keeping them together

Your plot is your best tool for keeping your hero and heroine together, which gives them the opportunity to focus on their emotional issues. Your hero and heroine need to be physically together for the bulk of your book, which may seem obvious, but I long ago lost count of the number of manuscripts I've seen where the hero and heroine don't even meet until the end of the first chapter or later. Or where they're apart for 20 pages as the book progresses, going about their solitary, even if somewhat related, business.

REMEMBER

A strong romance plot puts the hero and heroine together early on and, no matter how much difficulty they may be having connecting emotionally, the plot physically separates them as infrequently as possible. Close proximity allows the characters an opportunity to externalize their internal, emotional conflicts. Here are some of the most common issues romance characters face:

>> **Trust issues:** What if a cop hero has problems trusting women? Maybe he messed up on a case because he fell for a witness who wasn't as innocent as she pretended to be. Now he's falling into that nightmare all over again, investigating the heroine, who's under suspicion of murdering her husband. She insists she didn't do it, and the hero believes her. But why? Because she really *is* innocent, or just because he wants her to be? Either way, he's putting his entire career at risk by falling for her. The investigation keeps them together and gives them something to talk about while they work out their emotional issues, which provide the subtext for every conversation.

>> **Control issues:** What if your heroine comes from a wealthy, pampered, but ultimately confining, background? She's worked hard to prove herself, to get out from under her tycoon father's thumb and build her own business from the ground up. She's not about to give up calling the shots — and then along comes the hero, who engineers a hostile takeover of her company. The battle of wills has begun. The overt fight is for control of the company, but the real fight is for control of her heart.

>> **Self-image issues:** What if your heroine, despite being the youngest daughter of an earl, was always gawky, awkward, and more at home in the stables than learning to paint delicate watercolors? She still dresses in drab colors and oversized dresses, and now her father has offered her in marriage to a duke — the most handsome man she's ever seen, and one who deserves a beautiful wife. She can't believe she's grown into a woman who could catch his eye, so when they argue over her preference for horseback riding over hosting tea parties, what they're really talking about is her inability to believe he could possibly love someone like her.

WARNING

One of the major pitfalls I see with new romance writers is to attempt a plot in which the heroine and hero are physically apart for much of the book. This can be difficult to pull off in a romance novel and takes a great amount of skill. If you're new to romance writing, I recommend sticking with the general rule that your two main characters should be together for the majority of the book.

Letting conflict complicate your plot

Just as your plot offers the context for the romance to play out, the romance and the conflict that complicates it should drive the plot forward, creating an inseparable whole. Take, for example, the cop hero from the previous section, who has trust issues because he was burned after falling for a woman who was involved in a case he was investigating, and now finds himself drawn to the heroine, a suspect in the murder of her husband.

Logic demands that an investigation occur and that clues be followed up on, but the developing relationship and the tension between the hero and heroine should motivate as much of the action as possible. The hero hopes that the heroine is innocent, and maybe even sits on evidence that seems to indict her (difficult divorce proceedings, for example, that would have left her with very little, but now she stands to inherit quite a lot) while he looks for information to clear her. All the while he's furious with himself for falling for another woman who's undoubtedly only using him.

The heroine is covering for a younger brother who she's afraid has followed up his spoiled childhood by getting mixed up with embezzlers, ending up involved in her estranged husband's death. By nature, the heroine's open and honest, but she has to fight these natural inclinations and lie to the hero, putting her reputation and freedom at risk — even though she's attracted to him and wants to level with him and see where the attraction might go.

With both the hero and heroine drawn to, but also distrustful of, each other, their decisions are based not just on logic and a desire to get at the truth, but also on emotion and a desire to figure out the dynamics of the romance.

REMEMBER

Basing key decisions on the characters' emotions and not just on logic is a tactic that works with any story line and is the key to creating a compelling romance novel. And convincing emotional motivations are an outgrowth of believable, complex characters.

Taking two steps forward and one step back

Timing plays a key role in the tension of your novel. In real life, as I point out in the "Using romance to create suspense" section earlier in this chapter, relationships tend to run smoothly, with emotional and physical intimacy building on each other. Couples have setbacks along the way, but they usually talk things out and keep going, moving along the path together — ideally until they realize they want to spend their lives together. Romance novels build toward that same happy ending, but they follow a much rockier road.

TIP

The progress of the romance, in terms of both emotional and physical intimacy, creates the suspense necessary to hold your reader's attention. Instead of progressing smoothly, move your romance like a dance: two steps forward and one step back. Your hero and heroine should always be making progress, but slowly, and far from easily. Here are two tips you can use when you move your romance two steps forward and one step back:

>> **Follow every success with a reversal.** The key is in not letting an exchange of confidences and intimacy lead to more closeness. There will be times in the book when the characters will grow closer emotionally, when they'll trust each other, maybe confide in each other, and when they'll also get closer physically. But when they're done talking, when the embrace is over or when they wake up in each other's arms after a night of blissful lovemaking, make their relationship take a backward step. Going back to the cop/suspect example, maybe the hero pushes what he sees as his advantage after a night of lovemaking, asking her for information, proof that he can use to clear her or knowledge that may lead him to the real killer. Suddenly realizing how close she's come to giving up her brother, she withdraws emotionally, refuses to say anything more about the case, and maybe even leads him to believe she made love to him only to secure his sympathies. He feels he's been used again, and he's angrier with himself than he is with her.

>> **Play the scene from another angle.** You could play that same scene from the other character's perspective. You could make the heroine realize that she's let herself be seduced — literally — by the hero, and recognize how easily she could let herself rely on him, love him, and just tell him the truth. Then she could help her brother through the investigation and trial with the financial resources she inherits. But she stops herself, feeling selfish and disloyal to her brother, and immediately treats the hero coldly. Once again, the hero feels used and betrayed.

Both scenarios work, and both have the same result: The hero and heroine are left in conflict, unable to trust each other and follow up on their attraction. Yet neither of them is able to forget their moments of intimacy and honesty on every level, and those memories underlie all their future interactions. They've tasted what could have been, and they've had to back off, wanting more and yet feeling that a relationship is impossible.

Repeat that pattern of progress followed by a step back throughout the course of your novel, each time making staying apart harder for your hero and heroine. The closer they get, the more they long to stay close. Each conversation, kiss, and time they make love is a reminder of what they want and can't have, because each intimacy is followed by a reversal.

The wedges you use to drive your couple apart must be as believable as their growing feelings for each other. Years ago, heroes and heroines of romance novels were driven apart by misunderstandings more often than anything concrete and believable (see the "Cutting the Other Woman out of the picture" sidebar), but readers these days expect real conflict, not something that could be solved with one simple conversation.

CUTTING THE OTHER WOMAN OUT OF THE PICTURE

Not too many years ago, simple misunderstandings were a common tool to create conflict, and none was more common than the Other Woman. A sample scenario: The heroine would call the hero while he was away, and the Other Woman, who was really only his assistant, would answer the phone. (The Other Woman and Other Man were such common character types that they were always capitalized and rarely had much personality beyond being unpleasantly clichéd.) But the Other Woman wanted to be more. While the hero was otherwise engaged and didn't know the heroine had even called, the Other Woman would imply that all sorts of intimacies were going on and that he was right there and unwilling to waste time talking to the heroine.

The heroine, instead of reaming the hero out the next time she saw him and asking just what game he was playing, immediately and without a word packed a suitcase (always including one uncrushable evening gown, just in case) and ran off to the Outback or somewhere else suitably remote. Or she simply refused to talk to the hero, and the two of them shared smoldering looks and angry remarks but no actual conversation, because if they'd actually talked, the truth would have come out and the book would have been over.

I'm glad to say that those days are over. Neither heroines nor readers are satisfied with such transparent plotting and meatless conflicts. A modern heroine, even in a historical romance, has too much backbone to avoid confrontation. Current readers are looking for much more convincing and interesting plotting, so steer clear of using simple misunderstandings.

Using sexual tension to deepen conflict

Both emotional and physical intimacy can help you create and work with conflict, but sexual tension lends itself to additional discussion and strategies. Sexual tension begins the moment your hero and heroine lay eyes on each other, and it continues throughout the manuscript, whether they never share so much as a chaste kiss or engage in sexual athletics to rival those in any adult film. Sexual tension comes from sexual longing and, at least in the world of romance novels, sexual longing never wanes when a couple is truly meant to be together.

Simply by its existence, sexual attraction and the struggle that comes from the couple's inability to satisfy their desire (no matter how often they indulge in it) adds to the effect of the emotional tension. Friends can share all kinds of confidences, but physical intimacy is reserved for a lover or a spouse. Physical intimacy is what sets a couple's intimacy apart from everything else. It's the ultimate prize.

The hero and heroine's sexual longing reminds them of what they want and can't have — what they're being deprived of by their inability to sort out their emotions: true emotional intimacy.

Because their emotional issues threaten to separate them at any point, their love-making feels all the more poignant, because each time may be their last. For more on using love scenes — and the different ways men and women react to physical intimacy — to create tension, check out Chapter 11.

Dreaming of love

Your reader should long for the love scenes just as much as the hero and heroine, and one trick for satisfying her and increasing her longing (as well as at least one of the character's) is through a dream. The hero and heroine may not be able to make love in actuality for plenty of reasons. For example:

>> **Physical impossibility:** Your plot may have a point that dictates your couple be in separate places (but not too often). Or one of them could be ill or injured, so they can't follow up on their desires. These obstacles can help build sexual tension, so long as you make sure they're in each other's minds even when they can't be in each other's arms.

>> **Emotional separation:** As the conflict waxes and wanes, your plot likely has points where, no matter how physically attracted your hero and heroine are to one another, they're so upset with each other that lovemaking would be a betrayal of their own feelings and integrity.

>> **Timing:** The timing may be too early in the relationship — particularly in a historical romance, where social mores dictate the behavior of the sexes — for the couple to physically get together without undercutting them as characters.

>> **Subgenre restrictions:** In some romance series, as well as the entire inspirational romance subgenre, showing the characters making love or, in the latter case, being sexually intimate at all, is inappropriate. With certain caveats, though, a dream sequence can be an allowable way of making the reader feel the characters' romantic longing for each other, though without getting graphic.

In any of these circumstances, a dream can help build the sexual tension and add dimension to the conflict. In all but the last instance, a dream allows your hero, heroine, and reader to indulge in essentially guilt- and tension-free sexual enjoyment, fulfilling the need for them to get together and providing a hint of what their relationship *could* be like. At the same time, because their lovemaking was just a dream, you increase the reader's desire for the characters to make love for real — not to mention the characters' own desire. Lastly, a dream adds an edge to all their future encounters, because whichever character had the dream feels an awareness, even embarrassment, and a sense of intimacy that's simultaneously both real and imaginary, but still powerful.

REMEMBER

If you face subgenre restrictions, you need to make the dream far less explicit. In the case of an inspirational or sweet romance, the dream can't be explicit at all; stop it with a kiss, at most, and include few details. The characters' longings, and the subsequent dream, need to be more romantic than sexual. The dream may involve a wedding ceremony, and then stop at the bedroom door on the wedding night. Or it may feature the hero and heroine as a married couple sharing breakfast, with a warm, satisfied look and the touch of one hand on another. These dreams imply sexual fulfillment in an acceptable context — marriage — but the terms are entirely emotional and romantic.

Saving "I love you" for the right moment

REMEMBER

The quickest way you can diffuse both sexual tension and the power of your emotional conflict is to have your hero and/or your heroine confess their love. From then on, all suspense is gone. Your reader's wish is fulfilled, and all that's left is for the hero and heroine to talk out their problems in a rational (read: boring) way — and your reader's not interested in that conversation.

Part of maintaining emotional tension throughout the book, even if the characters make love, is withholding those three longed-for words: I love you. However, the hero and heroine can separately realize how they feel, and the reader can be privy to their thoughts. So long as you maintain the fiction that your hero and heroine won't be able to overcome their problems, you add tension to the story, because readers know how much is at stake: real love that may never be given a chance to flourish.

TIP

Every rule has an exception. In some successful romance novels, the hero and heroine confess their love early, and then face legitimate obstacles before they can fulfill that love. This trick is difficult to pull off, however. I see far more writers who try this plot fail than succeed. So my advice — especially when you're still perfecting your craft — is to follow the usual path of saving the confession of love for the climax and resolution.

WARNING

If you make sure your hero and heroine don't suspect each other's feelings, they're free to recognize their own feelings at any point in the book. Making their feelings believable is important. Let the reader see the characters' feelings develop in the course of the story, and they become part of the development and step-by-step solution of the emotional conflict. I see two main mistakes that writers make:

>> **The unmotivated realization of love:** Too often I see characters who realize out of the blue that they love each other. Up to that point, they've done nothing but argue and feel a strong attraction, but they haven't been growing closer or felt genuine emotional longing as they dealt with their issues. Love that comes out of nowhere isn't believable. You need to build up to love in ways that let the reader, and sometimes even other characters, recognize it before the hero or heroine does.

>> **The unmarked realization of love:** In an unmarked realization of love, the heroine realizes that she loves the hero (or vice versa), and then just moves on with whatever thought she was having, not even noticing that she's just reached a milestone. Whether she tries to talk herself out of the feeling, is amazed that she feels so much for such an unexpected person, or is thrilled, or whatever it is that she feels, she needs to react. The hero, too, needs to react when he first realizes he loves the heroine. This moment is key and can't pass unnoticed.

And They Lived Happily Ever After

REMEMBER

The words "happily ever after" rarely (if ever) appear in romance novels anymore, but they're still a powerful force in the characters' and the reader's minds. Happily ever after represents the ideal end to every romance — in real life as well as fiction. The biggest difference between the two worlds is that in a well-constructed romance novel, the promise of happily ever after is fulfilled, unlike real life, where 50 percent of marriages end in divorce.

Every romance exists to fulfill the reader's expectations (see Chapter 2). The final expectation every reader has when reading a romance novel is that it will end with the hero and heroine expecting to spend their lives together and face any future trials as one. Timing is the key to making your reader believe in your hero and heroine's happily ever after. How you build up to the climax and the mutual confession of love, and the support you give to the resolution, determine whether your reader believes in your happily-ever-after ending.

TIP

Not every romance novel needs to end with the actual marriage or even a formal proposal. (The one exception is when you're writing an inspirational or Christian romance, where the explicit commitment to marriage is crucial.) In some romances, the author shoehorns those proposal and/or marriage scenes into the final chapter or adds them as an unnecessary epilogue. My recommendation is to cut them, because they make the storytelling feel awkward or drag the book on past the natural finale. Assuring the reader that the couple is emotionally committed to each other is what's important. Without that assurance, you may have a wonderful piece of women's fiction, but you don't have a romance novel.

Making your reader believe

REMEMBER

As you build toward resolution and happily ever after, you need to be sure to bring your reader along with you. At this final stage of the book, every single element comes together. Any flaw can draw your reader out of your novel's world and back into the real world. Once the fantasy is broken, you may lose her forever — not just for this book, but for every book you ever write.

When you hit this final stage, you've written the bulk of the book, and you're down to the last chapter or two. Your reader ought to be turning pages more quickly than ever at this point, being carried along by:

>> **Your reader's belief in your characters:** The belief in your characters is probably the single biggest factor in your reader's enjoyment and the biggest motivator in getting them to turn the pages. At this point, because of their identification with the heroine, your reader should feel that their own happiness depends on the couple finally overcoming your carefully built tension and confessing their feelings.

>> **Your reader feeling that the tension has reached a make-or-break point:** Your reader should feel this way for two reasons. The first is simply that they realize the book doesn't have many pages left, so if the conflicts aren't resolved now, they never will be. The second reason is that if you've effectively built the tension by moving forward, backward, and then forward again, your characters are at a point where they don't have any options left except solving their problems or watching the entire relationship end.

>> **Your pacing:** As you build toward the climax and resolution, speed up your pacing using short, intercut scenes, mini-cliffhangers, and active prose to carry the reader forward. (Read Chapter 10 for tips on all these pacing techniques.) Don't use long, leisurely descriptions at the end of your novel; instead, use broad brushstrokes that tell the reader what they have to know and keep them moving forward.

With these elements working together, you're ready to take your characters and your reader through to the climax. Then you can move on to the resolution, so your hero and heroine can get on with living happily ever after.

Dark moment: Where all is lost

Most romance novels have a dark moment. This is where the mounting tension gets to be too much for your characters and they have to step back — emotionally and sometimes physically — from each other. But it's in this dark moment (and moving into the climax) that your characters realize the growth they've had throughout the book.

At this point in the book, your characters may feel like there's no way for them to make their relationship work. This part of the book is where they are in the most agony, pulled apart from the one they love the most. They struggle with this, and it is gut-wrenching for them. If they are not physically pulled apart, they are emotionally apart, which is tearing their hearts out.

It's hard for writers to see their characters in torment, but try not to rush the dark moment. I've seen books where the dark moment happens in one sentence, and then the characters move on from that. It's not going to be satisfying for the reader if you don't show how your characters are longing for each other. They need to finally admit that they will do anything to repair the damage that's been done. They need to feel heartache in order to experience that last bit of growth and finally overcome whatever it is that has kept them apart physically or emotionally.

Climax: Timing is everything

REMEMBER

In a novel, the climax is the moment when everything comes to a head. The climax always comes right before the end of the book: All the threads of the story combine to reach a make-or-break point. The tension — on all levels — is at its highest peak, and it's now or never for finding a solution or giving up in defeat. If you're into diagramming your story, it's the top of the tension mountain. The climax is the characters' last chance to solve everything — not just the emotional tension (so the romance is free to go on unencumbered), but also any remaining external, intellectual, and situational tension, and any plot issues.

Real-world relationships frequently develop without drama and major confrontation. But a romance novel needs to build to a dramatic payoff. It's part of the promise of a romance novel, and it paves the way for the happily ever after. Your reader expects it, so building up to it is crucial.

At that climactic moment, the characters break through their emotional walls. Even if they don't have a chance to admit how they feel and that they're committed to making things work between them, the reader's left in no doubt that the moment's coming — and usually the characters are pretty sure of it, too. They may sort out some of the specifics, or they may save those for the resolution, which follows closely — sometimes so closely that it's really part of the same scene.

The *resolution* is characterized by an easing back of tension that comes from knowing everything's going to be okay, and it's the scene where everything gets figured out. The climax is often over quickly — especially in books with a lot of action or suspense, where events are moving as quickly as emotions and there's no time for a lot of talk. The resolution is the characters' chance to figure out details, tie up loose ends in the plot and their emotional conflict, and talk about the future they plan to share. As its name implies, the resolution resolves whatever's left to be resolved.

TIP

Don't get too hung up worrying about where your climax ends and your resolution begins, or exactly what plot point or revelation goes where. The line between them is often so blurred that they end up being the same thing. They're really only points on a continuum, and so long as a reader feels like she got everything she wanted from your book, she's not going to care how the scenes were broken down.

After the reader has read the climax, she will breathe a huge sigh of relief (even if only metaphorically). If your hero and heroine haven't out and out admitted their love yet, your reader knows that they will, and any major plot difficulties that were hanging over their heads have also been dealt with. That leads you to the final stage of your novel: the resolution.

Resolution: Endings made easy

Underestimating the importance of the resolution is easy to do, and I often see authors rush through it or even leave it out altogether, thinking that the climax takes care of everything. But that thinking is just not true. In fact, the resolution is crucial in sending the reader off feeling satisfied and eager to see more of your work.

The climax often passes by in a rush. The hero and heroine may not have time to do more than acknowledge their feelings. In a romantic suspense novel, the action may be so intense that the characters don't even get that satisfaction, especially if one of them gets hurt. In a case like that, your use of point of view tells the reader how they feel, but they aren't able to tell each other, so the resolution is even more crucial to your story.

REMEMBER

The resolution can be an extension of the climactic scene or it can be a separate scene, but the function of the resolution is always the same: to provide the couple with a chance to talk out their emotional conflict in light of the fact that they've finally mutually confessed their love. In some cases, the resolution is also the scene that first lets them voice their feelings.

Real emotional issues don't go away just because two people fall in love. That holds true in real life, and it's also true in your romance. If you've created complex characters and a complex source of emotional tension, that tension isn't going to go away as if it never existed, so you need to give your hero and heroine a chance to confront their remaining issues.

WARNING

Don't devote pages to a detailed psychological discussion of where their issues came from and how they're going to cure each other. For one thing, you will have dealt with some of those issues incrementally in the course of the book, as you let your characters move two steps forward and one step back. In addition, a long discussion would just get boring.

Letting your hero and heroine talk in emotional terms is important. They've finally admitted their feelings for each other, and new love is a heady thing. You want to cover just enough territory to let the reader know that they recognize what their issues have been, and that they're more than capable of dealing with them.

Epilogue

Not every romance has an epilogue; however, I've noticed that readers really love them, and it gives you a chance to tie up loose ends, let your reader see your happy couple in their new life, and resolve any issues with secondary characters. If you feel as if your book was sufficiently resolved with the last chapter, you can skip the epilogue, just be aware that readers sometimes expect an epilogue that shows the happy couple.

One trend I've seen work well in recent years is presenting the epilogue in the point of view of one of the secondary characters, a character who is going to be a main character in the next book. This can excite the reader and prepare them for this secondary character's story, while simultaneously tying up loose ends. If you're planning a series, this tactic might work well for you.

Chapter **6**

Setting the Scene

Have you heard that the three most important things to think about when you're buying a house are location, location, location? Well, location may not be the *most* important thing to think about when you're writing a romance novel, but it definitely counts for a lot. The right setting can tempt readers to buy your book, while the wrong one can turn them off. The locale that you choose can show off your characters' best traits or provide a challenge that brings out their undiscovered strengths. You can use place to prime your characters — and your readers — to feel romantic or to keep them on edge and looking over their shoulders.

Your romance novel isn't only set in a particular place; it's also set in a particular time. The term *setting* refers to both the place and time in which your story takes place. You may be writing a book set in what I call the *eternal present,* which makes the reader feel as if she's reading a book that could be happening at that very moment. Or you may choose a particular period in history: the Regency period, the Gold Rush, World War II, or the Vietnam era. The *when* of your book is just as important as the *where* in terms of determining what the world is like and how your characters fit into it.

Before you start writing, take some time to think about where and when your story's going to take place and how you can use your setting as you write — it definitely makes the novel-writing process smoother.

Sometimes you just know, without even thinking, where you want to set your novel. Your decision may be based on the simple fact that you grew up on a ranch in Montana, so Montana ranch life is what you want to write about. Maybe you've always harbored a secret wish that you'd been born in medieval England, so you naturally gravitate toward that period for your romance.

If you already have your setting in mind, you're lucky, because you've already made an important decision. If this is the case, keep reading to see what you still have to think about in order to effectively use your setting. If you don't already have a setting in mind, you need to make a conscious decision, and this chapter can help. Here I talk about how to choose your where and when, and how to use both to your best advantage.

Deciding Where Your Story Takes Place

Just as having a romance without a hero and heroine is impossible, so is telling their story without knowing where the action is taking place. Readers want to know where things are happening, just as a matter of curiosity. More importantly, the setting has implications for your characters and plot.

Your setting can set your plot apart from similar story lines. The same basic plot — a marriage of convenience, for example — looks very different set in a small European principality versus small-town U.S.A. Some plots only work in certain settings. For example, stranding your heroine with a stranger in the middle of a crowded city is pretty difficult to pull off, but stranding her with a stranger in the Rocky Mountains is relatively easy. The same principle holds true when you're talking about characters. A cop hero comes across one way in a small midwestern town and quite another in New York City.

Following the lead of your characters and plot

Most of the time, before you start looking for a setting, you already have either your hero and heroine or your basic plot in mind — and sometimes both. (Check out Chapter 4 for the ins and outs of character development and Chapter 5 for the essentials of constructing a plot.) Look at what you know about your characters and plot, and use that information as your starting point for deciding where you want your story to take place.

>> **Characters:** If you've chosen a cowboy hero, you're most likely thinking of using a western setting, while a hard-driven CEO heroine may have you thinking more of a big city.

>> **Plot:** If you have a particular plot in mind, certain settings lend themselves naturally. Corporate espionage is more likely to have a city setting, and a hunt to save the world from a deadly terrorist could easily be set overseas against an international background.

You may have multiple location possibilities open to you. For example, a runaway princess story may have you thinking of settings as diverse as the Australian Outback, a small town in Kansas, or Los Angeles, simply because she could get lost in any of them.

After you consider basic character and plot implications, you can start to narrow down the geography and choose a specific locale, not just the Midwest but Chicago or Peoria; not just Europe but London, Paris, or the Spanish countryside.

Narrowing down the geography

With a general idea of your setting in mind, ask yourself questions to help narrow down your options until you know exactly where you want to set your romance. The following are some sample scenarios that show you how to zero in on a setting. In each case, the more questions you ask, the closer you get to figuring out your ultimate answer — where you want to set your book.

>> **Western:** You know you'd like to write a western, so the setting has to be (you guessed it) out West. Your story could take place anywhere from downtown Denver to a pueblo in New Mexico to a reservation in North Dakota to a ranch in Wyoming, Montana, Texas, or several other states to the slopes of the Rocky Mountains. Is your hero a cowboy and your heroine the sheriff who's investigating cattle rustling on his land? Then you may want to set it in Colorado.

Is your hero or heroine Native American? If not, think twice about selecting the pueblo or the reservation. A ranch with a nearby town or a small city (for the heroine's base of operations) sounds like what you need. So what state? Have you recently read an article on cattle rustling out West? Where was it taking place? That may be a good state to use. Or are you already familiar with a particular state? Are you interested in finding out more? The answer to that question could solve your problem. If you've read a dozen books about ranches in Texas but none set in Wyoming, why not choose Wyoming and stand out?

>> **International intrigue:** Your plot description already tells you to set all or most of your book outside the United States. Are you looking for a plot ripped straight from the headlines? In that case, the news of the day is your map to an answer. Are you interested in a mystery with its roots in World War II, a Cold War conspiracy, or a palace intrigue among the British royal family? Are you a Francophile who takes any excuse to discover more about Paris, your favorite city? Is your plot about money laundering? (If so, the Cayman Islands are known as banking havens.)

Digging even deeper

Every book takes place in a country, a state, a city or town, or a jungle, a desert, or any other climatic region you can think of — but your setting isn't only a particular geographic point. If you're writing a medical romance, your setting is also a hospital, a free clinic, or a doctor's office. Perhaps your setting is a ranch, the headquarters of a multinational conglomerate, a haunted house, or a tropical resort.

TIP

Give as much thought to creating and describing the immediate environs as you do to the larger world around them. But keep in mind that some books are set in such a limited locale — in a hospital or mountain cabin or on a cruise ship — that the big-picture geographical setting, although mentioned, is less important and needs less attention than the immediate environs.

Joining the real world or living in your imagination

Most romance novels are set in real places, at least as far as countries go. And so far, I've never seen anyone make up a 51st state. But you may find it easier to make up a town rather than choosing a real one simply based on the amount of information available for your research:

>> When you're looking for a big city, finding information on a real city like Chicago, London, or Sydney is easy, and each one lends its own cachet and personality to your work.

>> If you choose a real small town, getting accurate information is often hard, and there's no excitement boost from choosing Grants, New Mexico, or Homer, New York, because most readers haven't heard of them before.

REMEMBER

With small-town settings, choosing a real place provides a few advantages, like getting local support, but you get one huge advantage from creating a fictional locale: complete control. You can design the town to be exactly what you need it to be, and that aspect can be a big help as you write. You can place buildings where you need them to be and set your town alongside a lake or in the mountains or wherever you want, even if a real town isn't anywhere nearby.

Sometimes creating an entire country even makes sense. Fictional countries let you avoid the following:

>> **Alienating readers due to political or ideological differences:** If you want to set a book in a place that is considered a political hot spot, you run the risk of alienating some of your potential readers because of differing political sympathies. If your story requires that all readers share a certain point of

view, you may find it easiest to create a country so you can stack the deck in your favor.

>> **The research hassles that complex royal lineages present:** If you want to deal with royal characters — not just duchesses and earls, but kings, queens, princes, and princesses — creating your own kingdom and monarchy is almost certainly easier. Not only does it give you complete control of your characters and the specifics of their rule, but it also lets you create whatever lineage best serves your story.

Keeping your setting in check

Setting is important; however, it's not the point of your book. Travel guides are popular, but for entirely different reasons.

REMEMBER

Romances are about people, not places. Your setting's role is to provide a context for the central romance. A well-chosen setting can enhance the romance, and a poorly chosen one can detract from it. Never let your setting take precedence over your characters. Too much time spent on setting means too little time spent on characters. (There are some exceptions to this general rule; see the last section, "Making your setting a character," for more.) Here are some tips for choosing your setting:

>> **Be sparing and sporadic.** Instead of writing large chunks of description about your setting and dropping them into your text almost as interruptions to your story, work in a sentence here and a sentence there. Mingle the description of your setting with the rest of your text so it feels like a natural part of the novel, not a digression.

>> **Don't fall in love with your setting.** No matter how much you love the setting that you've chosen, save your emotional energy for your characters. Wax rhapsodic about the beauty of your heroine, not the beauty of the tropics. Be descriptive without being doting.

>> **Choose telling details.** Tell the reader what she needs to know to get a clear picture of the setting; then go on to include only details that enhance the story, relate to the characters' experiences, move the story forward in some way, or are otherwise germane. Don't waste time on the area's history, a tour of Main Street, or anything else that doesn't have direct relevance to your characters and plot.

>> **Let your characters do the work.** Whenever the opportunity presents itself, use your characters' points of view, their reactions, and even dialogue (as long as it sounds natural), to describe your setting. Because the description comes from the characters, the reader will feel more interested in it than if it comes via straight narration.

Telling Time

Contemporary or historical, the time period you choose for your manuscript is part of your setting, too. However, because your reader is living in the same time period as a contemporary, she tends not to think of it as an era in the same way she thinks of a Regency, medieval, or World War II romance. In a contemporary romance, your reader doesn't have to wonder how people dress or get around, or what the social mores are, because they're second nature. You don't need to explain anything extra about the period. But in a historical romance, you need to think more consciously about the when of your story and its importance for the characters, as well as what you need to tell the reader about the period.

REMEMBER

Just as you need to define and describe the physical setting of your story for the reader, when you're writing a historical romance, you need to define and describe the era of history as well. The guidelines used to describe an era are pretty much the same as those you use to keep yourself in check when you talk about the physical setting because, just as a romance novel shouldn't become a travel guide, it also shouldn't become a history text or even a historical novel (which places much more emphasis on the history than is necessary in a historical romance). Here are some tips to keep in mind when determining the amount of history to include:

- » **Remember that you're writing a romance.** All sorts of fascinating and historically important things may have gone on during the period: the Napoleonic Wars, the Industrial Revolution, or the Gold Rush. But don't inundate your reader with history. Mention events to indicate the time period and create a sense of the societal concerns and tensions your characters are living with. Keep the reader's attention on your characters, and work in the historical details when and where they're important to the characters or necessary to the reader's understanding of the story. As you begin the book, use period details as background, not as ends in themselves. As the story progresses, don't remind the reader with every sentence that she's reading about the past.

- » **Don't become enamored with history.** As you research, you find out all kinds of fascinating things, and often times you feel tempted to drop them into your novel so the readers can share them, but you need to resist this temptation. Unless you can justify including a piece of information based purely on storytelling grounds, leave it out. History isn't the story, it's part of the context for your story. Remember, more character and more story is always better than more history.

- » **Use your characters to weave in historical details.** Keep your characters at the forefront from the very beginning, and work in the historical details through their experiences and points of view. Don't just describe a muddy street, the sound of carriage wheels and the squawking of geese being carted to market; instead, describe your heroine as she holds up the hem of her dress to keep it out of the mud, dodges to avoid the wheels of a rich man's carriage, and thinks the squawking of the geese is making her pounding headache even worse. That way you're getting across your characters and the reality of their world at the same time — and in a way that's the most effective and interesting for your reader.

On a related note, you also have to make sure you keep you characters consistent with the times. Everything about them — the way they dress, act, think, speak, and so on — must mesh with the era. Check out chapters 4 and 9 for more information.

Using Your Setting to the Fullest

In some ways, setting is the unsung hero of your book. If you use it well, the reader will hardly even notice, and she almost certainly won't comment. (If you don't, trust me, she'll say something.) Your setting can very effectively help the reader understand your characters and sometimes even operate as a character of sorts itself. The key is knowing how — and when — to make that happen.

Illuminating your characters

If you were to see me working at home, you would see my laid-back nature. I like to be comfortable while still getting the job done. My couch reclines, and this is where I do most of my typing, keeping my water bottle full and my snacks handy. I frequently get up and walk as I take breaks, and I usually brainstorm while staring at the wall or out the window. If you stick around, you'd see me interacting with my family, changing into Mom mode when dealing with my kids. If you were to meet me at a conference, you'd see the professional side of me. At home, I'm quiet and often working by myself. At a conference, I talk to people. I like to get to know others even though I'm a natural introvert. Your characters will also carry a range of personal preferences.

REMEMBER

Your setting can offer your characters the same opportunities to express the different sides of themselves, to face and master a variety of challenges. You can use setting to illuminate and enhance your characters in three key ways. Use one, two, or even all three of the strategies I provide in the following three subsections in every book you write and in relation to both your hero and your heroine. In every case, a change of scene leads to a new challenge and/or a fresh success — and, of course, romance.

TIP

To decide the best strategy (or strategies) for using setting to deepen your characters, ask yourself these key questions:

1. **What do I want the reader to know about my character?**

2. **How can my setting help the reader better understand the character?**

Demonstrating competence

Showing that your hero and heroine are strong and capable is important, because that's what makes them admirable and worthy of their roles. One simple way you can demonstrate these qualities is by showing your characters operating successfully in their natural settings. For example:

» **Show your heroine, a successful pediatrician, deftly handling an office full of patients.** Calm, cool, and collected in the face of crying kids and nervous parents, she has an especially powerful effect on the good-looking single father whose little girl has taken a bad spill off her bike. Of course, his subsequent dinner invitation is only to thank her for how well she soothed and treated his daughter, right?

» **Show your cowboy hero sitting tall in the saddle while cutting an unruly cow from the herd.** Whether your heroine is an expert horsewoman herself or a total greenhorn, she's going to feel her heart beat a little faster at the sight of this ruggedly handsome man handling his horse as if born to the saddle.

» **Let your fireman hero pull a child from a burning school.** Meanwhile, let the news photographer heroine document the rescue. Better yet, let him pull *her* child from the flames, and then finish the scene with a hug that starts from relief and gratitude but ends with a frisson of physical awareness.

REMEMBER

By showing your characters at their best in their normal settings, you let your readers see how the characters' strengths can be admirable and complementary, and sometimes sexy and emotionally stirring, as well.

Uncovering vulnerabilities

Characters need strengths, but your hero and heroine also need to be flawed, to have normal human vulnerabilities (see Chapter 4). Setting can also help bring those vulnerabilities to the surface.

Suppose your heroine is cool, calm, and collected as she goes about her day running one of North America's most successful jewelry websites. The way she can fire an employee without batting an eye convinces everyone that her heart's made out of the same cubic zirconia that her company sells so successfully. It's not true, of course, and you need to convince your reader of that before she decides the heroine is someone she can't possibly identify with. Simple: Take her out of her office, where everything's under control, and put her somewhere where she's not in control and her vulnerabilities can come through. For example:

>> **A wilderness survival program for CEOs:** She could agree to do the program for publicity, but suddenly she's the lone woman, and everyone seems to know more than she does about everything from building a fire to pitching a tent. The hero could be a rival businessman whose company is trying to take over hers, but in this new setting they must become temporary allies. Now that he's seen her at what she considers her worst, that experience changes everything when they're back across the negotiating table from each other.

>> **A family reunion on a cruise ship:** If your business-savvy heroine has to spend a week with family instead of employees, she can be thrown off-kilter. Just what is a driven CEO — who normally has every minute scheduled and the phone glued to her ear — supposed to do lying on the lido deck out of cell range? Suddenly she has time to think, to inventory what's missing in her life — like the kind of life her sister has with her husband and kids. Even so, she's not really thinking seriously about the handsome, witty, single dad who's brought his kids on the cruise to take their minds off the anniversary of their mother's death. Or is she?

>> **A hospital bed:** She's worked herself right into a bad case of walking pneumonia, so bad that she's not even up and walking anymore — she's in a hospital bed. Not only is she unable to give anyone orders, but she also has to take them from other people every minute of the day. Her brain feels fuzzy, she's sick and unhappy and knows she looks awful — and here comes Dr. Gorgeous.

In each case, taking the heroine out of her everyday setting and putting her in a new setting — or a new role in that setting — catches her off guard and makes her think about things she normally ignores. It showcases her weaknesses instead of her strengths, and lets people — hero and reader alike — see past her carefully constructed in-charge persona, which helps make her into the imperfectly perfect heroine I describe in Chapter 4.

Bringing out the best

One way to let your characters grow is to challenge them and let them rise to those challenges. Your setting can be a key part of that process. After you've used the setting to demonstrate your hero or heroine's flaws, show them standing up to whatever difficulties have been thrown in their way. For example:

>> **Strand your hero and heroine in a mountain cabin when a mudslide closes the road.** She's a city girl all the way, so the prospect of spending some

indeterminate amount of time without electricity or (gasp!) indoor plumbing doesn't fill her with happiness, to say the least. The hero, a rancher who ended up taking shelter in the same cabin, can't believe he's going to have to put up with Miss Priss for who knows how long.

Things don't start off well, but before too long her natural optimism has reasserted itself and she's pulling pictures out of an old magazine and nailing them to the wall for décor, mixing up an improbable combination of canned goods from the cupboards to create a surprisingly tasty meal to cook over the fire the hero set, and tempting a lost puppy out of the woods with the leftovers. As much as he doesn't want to get involved with a woman whose normal life is so different from his, the hero soon finds her impossible to resist.

» **A tough-talking CEO is forced to take time off to play Mr. Mom when he takes over the care of his late sister's baby.** No more boardroom table and contentious shareholders' meetings. Now it's nursery furniture and a fussy newborn for this hero, and he couldn't feel any less competent if he tried. Stuck at home with a baby whose idea of communication is crying loud, louder, and loudest, he can't change a diaper to save his life. Mixing formula means mixing a mess, and every time he tries to bathe the baby, he's the one who gets wet. Being stuck inside the house is making him crazy.

He doesn't know what to do, other than thank heaven for the single mom next door who takes him under her wing and teaches him that parenthood can be paradise. Before long, even midnight feedings don't faze him, although he likes daytime better — when his neighbor's around. But just so he can get advice, or so he tells himself.

» **Put your ranch-bred tomboy heroine in silk or satin and watch for sparks.** As a working rancher, she's as at home on horseback as any cowboy, but she's definitely out of her element when she has to dress up and play hostess for the nearest town's annual Christmas fundraising dance. She has trouble keeping her balance in heels, keeps tugging at her skirt and wishing she were wearing denim, and the makeup she let herself get talked into wearing feels like a Halloween mask. So why does that gorgeous guy keep staring at her from across the room?

She has no idea that he's a Dallas tycoon looking to buy a ranch-country getaway and that he thinks she's a wonderful contrast to all the sophisticated, even jaded, women he deals with all the time. He can't help admiring the way she has a smile and a cheerful word for everyone, even though she obviously wishes her dress weren't so mouth-wateringly tight or her heels so high. He thinks that more women should have her selflessness and her ability to laugh it off when they can't manage a two-step in three-inch heels. Right there and then, he vows that this is a woman he has to get to know better.

Making your setting a character

Most of the time, you won't need to (and shouldn't) use the suggestions in this section because, most of the time, you won't want to (and shouldn't) draw a ton of attention to setting. You won't have a reason to make setting function as a secondary character.

That said, you may face occasions when atmosphere is *so* crucial that the setting takes on added importance and functions almost like a character, with its influence directly felt. Usually this occurs when you want your setting to indicate menace and a sense of deepening threat. Sometimes you only need that added effect for a scene or two; other times you want to keep the feeling through the book. Here are a few examples where setting takes on added importance:

>> Your story is a suspenseful one, so as the villains close in on your hero and heroine, every shadow, cracking twig, or rustling of leaves sounds like a threat.

>> You're writing a Gothic romance or a romance set in a haunted house, in which case the house itself is part of the threat.

TIP

Whatever the reason, here are some tactics you can utilize to milk your setting for extra effect:

>> **Take more time describing your setting.** Don't simply use longer chunks of narration; a subtle interweaving is still the most effective road to take, just do so more often and in more detail. Don't say it's a moonlit night in the woods and leave it at that. Take time to describe the way the moon casts shadows, and, later, comment on the way the light shifts when a cloud crosses the face of the moon. Does the sky look darker and the stars brighter when the moon is full? Do sounds from the forest seem scary in the strange brightness of the night? Mention those details, too. The ongoing accumulation of detail builds atmosphere and starts to draw the reader's attention to the setting. The extra attention you pay to setting indicates its importance.

>> **Use more adjectives.** Ordinarily, you should use a minimal number of adjectives to describe your setting — just enough to get the job done. When you want to give your setting a more active role, use more adjectives than usual to help draw attention to it. For example, don't just say "moonlight," say "a cold light" or "a pale, thin light." Adjectives add personality to a place, just as they do to a character.

>> **Use loaded words.** Pick words for their effects; choose words that convey and evoke emotion. Mountains aren't just high; they loom threateningly. An old house doesn't just creak; it groans like an animal in pain. Choose words that don't just tell the reader something factual, but instead make her feel

their effects. A house isn't just deserted; its windows stare out like animal eyes seeking prey in the forest. Again, you're personalizing your setting, treating it like a character, so it affects your heroine, hero, and reader just as another character would.

>> **Have characters react to setting as they would to another person.** If your characters — especially your hero and heroine — react to your setting as if it's a character (getting spooked, feeling as if they're being watched, even just jumping at an unexpected noise), your reader will react right along with them. Let your characters attribute personality to the setting, even let them comment on it, and it takes on added meaning for the reader, as well.

REMEMBER

In some cases, setting *can* become like a supporting character and add depth and impact to your book, but be careful not to let the setting take over from the characters.

TRAVELING THE WRONG WAY DOWN A ONE-WAY STREET

Even though 99 percent of the time your setting will literally be kept in the background, if you make a mistake, someone will catch it. If you write about New York City, where most avenues and streets are one way, be sure you have traffic running in the correct direction. If your heroine drives from Los Angeles to San Diego, be sure it takes the correct amount of time. If your couple embraces passionately while watching the sunset, be sure they're somewhere that faces west. In other words, do your research, even on the smallest details. We live in a day and age where information is available at the tips of our fingers, but make sure the information you're getting is accurate. Double check your facts on reliable websites, and if possible, talk to someone who has been to the location you're writing about.

Chapter **7**

Outlining versus Discovery Writing

There is no one "right" way to write a book. Whatever way works for you is the right way. If you've been struggling to follow a specific method — forcing yourself to work in one particular way because that's what you've been told was "correct" — stop! Instead, do what works for you. If you're not sure what that is, this chapter helps you figure that out.

The best way to uncover your writing process is to dig in and try different things. In this chapter I talk about different ways to write and what has worked well for other writers. Try the ones that sound the best to you. In the end, you may come up with your own way of doing it, and that's okay, too.

Identifying What Kind of Writer You Are

If you've written a few books already, you might already know your particular writing process. In general, there are two approaches that most writers fall into: outlining and discovery writing. If you're not sure what these styles are, or if you're just starting out writing a novel, you may need help figuring out what works well for you.

Outlining is when you figure out all your major plot points, or what happens in your story, before you sit down to write. Outlining is great for writers who want to map out their story before they begin to fill in those small details, like conversations and internal monologue. Outlining helps you figure out where your story needs to go, so when you sit down to write you can be more effective. An outline can also help you through writer's block if you are struggling with what to write next.

Discovery writing is when you simply sit down and start writing without figuring out where the story is going. It's uncovering the story as you go, as if you were a sculptor and you're chiseling away at a block of stone. As you write, the story unfolds before you, sometimes taking you in a direction you didn't see coming.

Both methods are valid, and there are famous authors in both camps. The important thing is to discover which way you work best with, and how your creativity is unlocked. If you find a method that combines the two, that's fantastic. You do you.

TIP

The best way to find what works for you is to dig in and try different methods. Try outlining your novel and see if it makes you excited to write it. For me, outlining was not a natural fit. No matter what method of outlining I tried, I couldn't come up with great ideas. I found that great ideas came more freely when I was in the middle of a scene and immersed in story, dialogue, inner thought, and emotion. The point is that every writer is different.

Outlining methods

To help you figure out if you work better with an outline, try some of these outlining methods to see if any work well for you:

>> **Write a synopsis of each chapter, plotting what will happen.** This can be as detailed or as simplified as you'd like. I know one author who writes pages and pages of her outline longhand in a notebook, because that's what helps her think best. Another author friend writes shorter outlines, just getting the bones of the story down.

>> **Write scene ideas on sticky notes or notecards.** This method is great if you like to shuffle your scenes around, putting them in different ways to figure out which works best. You can move them where you want, add scenes, or even discard them altogether. I've seen authors use different colors to indicate different points of view to keep them straight.

>> **Use a storyboard with the three-act structure laid out, adding scenes where they would fall in each act.** This can help you with your story arc if you often have trouble with a saggy middle, or a flat ending.

>> **Use software such as Scrivener or Plottr to help you plot your novel.** The perks with using software are cool, allowing you to use a virtual corkboard, move things around virtually, color code your scenes, or add photos to your notes.

>> **Instead of outlining your entire novel, try outlining one chapter at a time.** Having a sharper plan can help you get your daily work done faster because you know what your scene will look like before you write it. But it also allows for the flexibility of the story to form as you go and is a hybrid form of discovery writing in that regard.

Try some of these methods and see if outlining helps you write. If it helps you focus and collect your thoughts, then you are an outline writer. If you freeze up when outlining, or if it causes you to lose interest in writing, then maybe you're a discovery writer, or "pantser," as some people fondly call it, meaning you write by the seat of your pants.

Discovery writing methods

If you think you discovery writing might be a better fit for you, here are some tips to try it out and help you decide:

>> **Try starting with a scene.** Put your characters in a difficult situation and see how they would handle it. You may find that your characters' personalities come out as you're writing, as you force them into a conflict. The higher the tension, the better.

>> **Write the bones first.** If you're unsure where you want your scene to go, write the bones of the scene first, with setting and dialogue, and fill in the details later. Starting with the dialogue can sometimes help you figure out what your characters are doing and feeling, and those actions and thoughts can be layered in after you have the skeleton of the scene down.

>> **Write the "candy bar" scenes first.** These are the scenes you are so excited to write that they almost write themselves, and often have the most tension and conflict. These are the scenes that may have been percolating through your mind — the ones that made you excited to write the book in the first place.

>> **Write what comes into your mind.** Start with one sentence, and then another. Keep going, writing whatever comes into your mind. You may not even use it in your book, but keep going to discover what your story is about. Discovery writers thrive on story, and do their best work when they are immersed in scene and dialogue.

>> **Don't look at the blank page as a stumbling block.** I like to look at a blank page as having unlimited possibilities. Anything can happen next, so it becomes exciting for me rather than daunting.

Outlining: Mapping Out Your Story

Many authors find that an outline is a helpful road map to use. Just as you would use a road map to plan your route from New York City to Los Angeles, you use your outline to map out your novel from beginning to end. Your outline is a document in progress that you can revise as often as you need to.

Your outline helps you keep your focus and makes you think about what's most important about your characters, your plot, and the emotional development of the relationship, which is key in writing a romance.

REMEMBER

The great thing about writing a romance is that you always know how the book is going to end — with a happily ever after. Figuring out the ending can be one of the most difficult things in writing, so having this expectation from readers will help you as you outline. You are working toward your couple being happy, in love, and together in the end.

What can an outline do for you?

There are a lot of advantages to figuring out as much of your story as you can ahead of time. Having an outline helps you:

>> **Streamline the writing process.** Nothing can ever make writing a book easy. Writing a book can be time-consuming, draining, and difficult, and writing a romance, especially, lays all your emotions bare. Starting with an outline can help you write faster because you'll know where the story is going, and it identifies your goals for each chapter.

>> **Pitch a project.** If your goal is to traditionally publish (see Chapter 17), your outline can help you present your book in a professional and succinct way. Conferences provide great opportunities to pitch, as well as talk about your book with other authors. If you have an outline, you already have an answer to "What are you writing?" Instead of stuttering your way through a disjointed series of scenes, you have a coherent — even intriguing — story to talk about.

>> **Guesstimate your manuscript's length.** After you have an idea of your story, you can get a general sense of how long your finished book will be.

If you have a complicated plot with lots of twists and turns, your book will naturally be longer. If your goal is to write for a traditional publishing line, you may need to trim the page count to fit their guidelines. If you're planning on a 100,000-word mainstream romance but have a relatively straightforward plot, your outline can tell you that you need to aim for a shorter format or build in some additional complications.

REMEMBER

Your outline is for you and no one else. It should help you write, not hinder you. It can be whatever you need it to be to help you get the job done. If it does the opposite and stunts your creativity, stop doing it. Try something else.

What belongs in an outline?

Ultimately, the answer to this question is "Anything that will help you write your book." Because no one else ever has to see it, your outline can be as detailed, as messy, or as idiosyncratic as you want. It's a tool to help you, and you can custom-design it. There are certain basics, though, that you should think your way through before you sit down to do any actual writing. Here are some questions to consider answering in your outline if you are working with one:

>> **Who are your hero and heroine, and what's the basis of their emotional conflict?** The answers to these questions are crucial to the setup and development of both the romance and the plot, so get a handle on those answers from the get-go. The emotional conflict is what will drive your entire plot forward, and this is usually what I start with when writing a new book. I find that looking at *tropes* — popular plot devices — is very helpful when trying to figure out the driving force of my conflict because the popular tropes naturally carry with them a high level of conflict. (See Chapter 19 for ten popular tropes in romance writing.) Outlining this can help you keep track of the various conflict stages.

>> **Where — and how — will your book begin?** Chances are you're going to know a lot of background information on your characters and their story that won't end up in your novel, so you need to decide what goes on page one and how it will all unfold from there. If you choose the most effective beginning for your book ahead of time (see Chapter 12 for hints on knowing where to start), you can save yourself a lot of time, because you won't have to go back and rewrite when you realize that you've made the common error of starting in the wrong place. Outlining can help you find the best place to begin your novel.

>> **How will the big events of the story progress and fit together?** Instead of writing yourself into a corner where nothing makes sense and you have to go back and rethink your whole story, outline your way from point to point,

making sure your story line is logical. The more complicated your story line is — and especially if you're incorporating suspense into your plot — the more crucial this is.

>> **How will the characters' developing relationship affect the story line and vice versa?** The emotional logic of your story has to work just as much as the plot-based logic does. By outlining, you get to work through your characters' emotional issues and make sure their behavior makes sense — and also that it makes sense when considered alongside the plot. Don't forget to include the repercussions of your hero and heroine's developing physical intimacy, too.

TIP

Outlining can happen at any point in the writing process. You don't always have to outline before you start writing the book. Some authors find it's helpful to write a chapter or two first — even though those chapters may ultimately be discarded — just to get to know the characters better and get a sense of where the characters are driving the story. Once you get more familiar with your ideas, then an outline can serve to round them out.

Start your outline at whatever point is most helpful for you. Your outline exists specifically for your own benefit. If you need to write your way through lengthy pieces of background information on your characters, their situations, or anything else to get into your story and your characters' heads, do it. Just be aware of the point where the manuscript itself will begin.

REMEMBER

Think of the big events in the book — both the major plot points and the key moments in the relationship — as *milestones.* They should stand out as destination points on your outline, and the rest of your story involves moving from one to the next in believable, interesting ways. In fact, one way to begin writing your outline is to start by laying out the milestone events. Then you can figure out the details of moving from one to the next. That way you never lose sight of your interim goals as your characters move from point to point in the story. (Check out Chapter 10 for a full discussion of these milestones as they relate to pacing.)

Using your outline effectively

After you've created your outline, the next step is to move forward with your writing, remembering that your outline is there to help you, not hinder you, both as you write and once you've finished your manuscript. You can use your outline to help you craft a query letter, for example, if you are trying to traditionally publish. Your outline might also help you distill down your plot so you can write an effective blurb.

Listening to your creativity

Talking about listening to your creativity in a chapter on outlining may seem odd, but an outline truly gives you a framework where your creativity can flourish. It frees you from thinking about the mundane details, so you can focus on characterization and emotion, without stressing over the basic logic of your plot.

Because you aren't worrying about plot mechanics, you're able to get deeply into developing your characters, giving them the freedom to take over and make your book stronger because the emotions are so genuine (the key drawing card for the reader). The trickiest or most unique plot in the world means nothing if your characters and their romance don't resonate with readers. Your outline lets the creativity in your writing shine through.

Before you write a chapter, take a moment to sit with your outline and think about what you're going to put into the next scene. Get to know your goals for the chapter, and where the tension will come from. Tension is what moves every story forward, so if there isn't enough tension in the next scene, create some. I know as authors we adore the characters we create, but happy people living happy lives is boring — and unrealistic. Give them trials and challenges that readers can identify with.

Lastly, if your characters take you away from your outline, don't panic. Follow the path that leads to the best story. Most often the best story will be the one with the greatest amount of emotion and tension. Let that emotion drive your story forward and don't be afraid to revise your outline if needed.

Discovery Writing: Letting Your Story Unfold

If you find that outlining stifles your creativity, try discovery writing. This basically means you sit down to write your book without an outline. You start by writing the first scene that comes to your mind, and you keep going. That doesn't mean you don't have to plot — it just means you plot as you write, checking your story to make sure the structure is there after the fact.

Many discovery writers do a lot of rewriting because they are discovering who their characters are and what the plot of the book is as they write, and sometimes that means fixing things along the way. Discovery writers also usually end up checking on their plot points as they write, making sure their pressure points and plot twists, those parts of the story that add conflict and tension, come at the right points in the story. For example, at the midpoint in your book you usually will have something happen that changes the relationship between your two characters. If you're an outliner, this is plotted out beforehand. But a discovery writer will often not even know what the midpoint plot turn will be, they will just intuitively write one in as they are nearing that middle point in the book.

TIP

I've read quite a few books on the craft of writing, and many of them agree that story is something that is engrained in the human mind. We naturally gravitate to the same structure as we tell a story. It feels comfortable to us. So don't be intimidated to feel your way through your story. We are often intuitive enough to be able to let the story have some autonomy and free flow from our imagination. Trust your instincts. If your gut is telling you that you need a plot twist to make things more interesting, go ahead and write one in.

When I was writing my first book I was surprised at how well I could visualize the scene I was writing, even though I couldn't see much further ahead. I remember telling my mother how I felt like writing this book was like walking in the woods at night with a flashlight. I could clearly see the ground I was walking on, and maybe a few steps ahead, but everything beyond that was dark. I was afraid that I would write a few paragraphs and then get stuck. But as soon as I took two or three steps forward, more of the plot would unfold before my eyes. The process fascinated me.

WARNING

Discovery writing doesn't give you the complete and total freedom to write whatever you want. You still need to stay within the confines of the genre you're writing in. There are reader expectations you need to fulfill. Your plot still needs to make sense, and your characters' motivations need to be coherent. Keep in mind that while discovery writing does give you the freedom to explore new ideas as you write, which can be exciting, it can also be a bit daunting if you find yourself with more ideas than you know what to do with.

Letting the characters guide you

One of the best things about discovery writing is the ability to allow your characters to take control. This means as you're writing, your character might say something you weren't expecting, or do something you hadn't planned. This can be brilliant, but it can also end up causing you to veer off track, even writing yourself out of the genre you want to write, which is romance. Here are some tips for keeping yourself on track:

>> **Remember the internal conflict.** No matter how your characters begin to form, make sure your story's core tension is coming from their internal struggles, and that those struggles make sense. Be sure to adapt the plot to fit how your characters are developing.

Let's say you had planned to write about an arrogant alpha male who butts heads with his assistant. But as his character develops, you find that he's coming out with more heart and depth. You decide not to force the plot to fit your original idea. If a conflict is forced between him and his assistant, readers will see right through it. Instead of them butting heads over his arrogance, you choose to pull in more tension from his newly formed personality. Maybe an option could be to change the plot so he's grieving the loss of his fiancée, and that's why he's struggling to accept his attraction to his new assistant and is coming across as arrogant.

>> **Use rising tension.** As you write, keep the rising tension in mind. Your characters can guide the story, but be sure to place them in situations that will raise the stakes and increase the conflict. For example, if your hero asks your heroine out, you might have her refuse, with a good reason why she won't go out with him. There is no tension in a happy couple going on a date. Try to think of ways to increase the tension rather than allowing your characters to date and always have a lovely time.

>> **Use your plot to force your characters together.** More than half your book should have your characters on the page together. However, if you're creating the correct inner conflict, your characters may not want to be together, at least initially, so you'll need to use the plot to put them in a situation where they have to be together. Trap them in a storm, force them into a pretend relationship, or give her a promotion so she becomes his boss and they have to work together.

Plotting as you go

As you write your story, keep the structure of a romance in mind. You can use any type of story structure; it doesn't matter as long as you've got the basics down.

For example, when I write I use the three-act structure split into four parts:

>> The first quarter is act one, where I introduce characters, plot threads, and set things up.

>> The second quarter moves us into act two, where I spend time deepening the main relationship and moving my plot threads along. The midpoint brings a change to the hero and heroine's relationship.

>> The third quarter is spent heightening emotions, pulling and pushing my characters together and apart.

>> The last quarter is where I move into the third act and where everything culminates. The dark moment happens, the climax, and finally the resolution.

Let's look at a practical application of this. If your goal is to reach 50,000 words, keep that word count in mind as you write. The first quarter of your novel will be filled with scenes that introduce new plot threads which, for your word count goal, is the first 12,500 words. (This is simply a goal. It doesn't mean you can't introduce a new plot thread after 12,500 words. It's just something to keep in mind as you're writing.)

The first quarter

Here are some things you should include in the first quarter of your book:

- **The introduction:** Introduce your main characters, their goals, and all of the things that are stopping them from reaching their goals.

- **The inciting incident:** Make something happen to change things, and start the story in motion. Often with a romance it's where the two main characters meet for the first time. If they already know each other, it's often a situation that changes their relationship. For example, she gets fired and is no longer his boss.

- **The adhesion setup:** Create a plot that places your two main characters together for most or all of the book. Whatever it is, this must force the two characters to be in the same place at the same time. This is usually an external plot force, like an arranged marriage in historical romance.

- **The repelling force:** Set up what pulls your characters apart. Whatever repels the two of them, it must be good enough to repel them until the climax of the book. This is usually an inner conflict instead of an outside force. I often layer several things together that repel them, so as they overcome some of those forces, something else takes the forefront. For example, the heroine dislikes the hero because his father put her father out of business, but now they are stuck together in an arranged marriage and forced to be together.

- **The subplot setup:** Introduce secondary characters and the things that are going on in their lives. (Be careful not to let your subplots take over the book, which can happen especially to discovery writers.) When crafting subplots, try to think of things that can help force your characters together. For example, the heroine's mother could have an illness, which is why she pressured her daughter to get married. This subplot explains why they had to fake a marriage and pushes the two of them to spend time together, as she sees her mother every weekend for family dinner.

- **The flaws:** Both your hero and heroine need to have flaws. Yes, you want your characters to be likeable, but you also need to show their human side. Give them flaws your readers can relate to, such as stubbornness or a quick temper.

>> **The attraction:** Your characters should start feeling attracted to each other in the first quarter of your story. If you're writing a sweet romance, this attraction starts out small. Try not to overdo this in the first quarter. You want to hint at the sparks that will fly. If you're writing a steamier romance, you can make the attraction stronger, just leave yourself room for it to grow as the book progresses.

The second quarter

The second quarter of your novel is filled with deepening relationships and starting down those subplots you've introduced. By this time the adhesion is set up and doing its job of putting the two main characters together on the page. The repelling force is also set up, making it so your characters have all kinds of reasons why they don't want to spend time together. They don't want to fall in love, despite their attraction.

When you reach about 25,000 words — half of your target word count for purposes of this example — you need some kind of midpoint. This is usually something that changes the couple's relationship somehow. Maybe they kiss for the first time, or have an emotional scene where some revelation comes out that changes the dynamic between them in some way. Whatever you do for your midpoint, just know that you're using this to show the way their developing relationship is changing them. This is part of their character arc.

The third quarter

The third quarter of your novel is spent heightening emotions. This is where you can really let your characters' romance shine and allow them to fall in love, and fall hard. At the same time they are struggling with their inner conflict, not yet allowing themselves to embrace that love. They take steps forward to further the relationship, and then take steps back. By the end of the third quarter, they should be an emotional mess!

The fourth quarter

The fourth quarter is where you can begin leading up to the dark moment where everything falls apart. If I'm going to do something to break my character, this is where it happens. My dark moment is where I usually have my characters finally realize that love is more important than anything. They finally can overcome their fear, their past pain, or their insecurities. Whatever was keeping them from a happy ending must be resolved before you move into the climax and finally the resolution. All of these things, along with the epilogue, happen in your fourth quarter.

Getting stuck in the rewriting trap

As a writer, you must be open to rewriting, doing several drafts, then polishing and getting things right. However, rewriting the same passages repeatedly, or the entire book over and over, can be a delaying tactic — a way of keeping yourself safe by not sending your book out into the world, where rejection is a definite possibility.

You can get caught in the rewriting trap without even realizing it, because every time you go over your manuscript, you *will* find something — even if it's only a typo or a missing comma — to fix. Or maybe you realize how crucial it is to get your opening just right, so you can't let go of Chapter 1, because another approach may make it just a teensy bit more compelling. Don't get caught in this trap.

How do you know if you're stuck in a rewriting trap? As yourself these questions:

>> **Are you still working on the same manuscript for the last ten years?** Yes, it can take more than a year to finish a book. My first book took four years. But I was rewriting large chunks of the book. If you're continuing to work on that same manuscript you "finished" ten years ago, you may be stuck in a rewriting trap.

>> **Do you find yourself moving commas around?** If you're on your 18 draft and you're playing around with miniscule things, it's time to get that manuscript to an editor and out of the drafting rut you're in.

>> **Is your story mental cement?** If you came up with this story concept years ago and it's just not working no matter how much you fuss with it, it's possible that your story concept is too hardened into something inflexible to craft into a working story arc. Sometimes a story idea just doesn't work for one reason or another. It's okay to let it go and come up with something new and fresh.

Rewriting doesn't improve your writing in the way that writing a new book will. If you're stuck in this trap, set aside your manuscript and start something new. Often, after you've written a new book, you can more easily go back and see what might not be working in an older manuscript.

3

Putting Pen to Paper

Use your authorial voice to write effective descriptions and keep your story moving.

Let your characters speak and give each a distinctive voice.

Learn the secrets of great writing: pacing and plotting.

Write compelling love scenes, from sweet to sexy.

Chapter **8**

Finding Your Own Voice

I n a romance novel, the characters' voices — especially the hero and heroine's — are key, because it's their relationship that the reader is interested in. But, as the author, your voice matters, too. The way you tell the story is as important as the story you tell, even though, if you do your job right, the reader may never even notice your style and voice, because she's paying attention to the characters and events. A reader doesn't pick up a romance to marvel at a pretty turn of phrase or to compliment the author's use of metaphor. A reader picks up a romance novel for the emotional fulfillment that comes from seeing two right-for-each-other people get together. Everything you do as a writer should illuminate that romance and its emotional conclusion, not draw attention to your own abilities. In this chapter, I talk about what to do and what *not* to do, so that the *telling* part of *storytelling* leaves plenty of room for your *story*.

Speaking Up for Yourself

You probably don't plan out every sentence before speaking or listen closely to yourself when you're telling your husband or best friend what went on at work or the funny thing that happened when you were walking the dog. But the truth is, we're all natural storytellers, and we practice our craft every day when we tell the people in our lives what we've been doing. We talk about not only *what* happened, but also *who* was involved, *what* they did, *what* they said, *where* the event took place, and *how* it ended up. We talk our way through what happened, and our audience laughs, groans, cries, or offers us hugs when we tell our stories well. As you write your romance novel, you want your story to have the same effect.

REMEMBER

You need to tell your story in a way that makes your reader react the way you want her to. You need to write effectively without calling attention to the writing itself. If your reader pauses to admire your prose, then you've pulled her out of your story and away from your characters. Everything you do as a writer needs to keep the reader intrigued and foster her identification with the characters, because that keeps her turning pages. Successfully using author voice can help you in these areas. Finding your *author voice* involves recognizing and going with your own natural bent — whether that's to be funny, dramatic, atmospheric, or anything else — and then developing an awareness of your own language, rhythms, and vocabulary. As a writer, you need to find your own voice, and then keep yourself from taking too loudly.

TIP

The most effective author voice serves the story, not the other way around. Keep that tip in mind as you work, and your own voice will become stronger and more effective.

Revealing where readers hear your voice

Asking where readers hear your voice is a natural question because, technically, you're writing the whole book. But a large part of what the author does (as I discuss in Chapter 9) is give voices to their characters, creating the illusion that they're speaking for themselves. Your voice comes into play in between the characters' conversations and thoughts.

Romances are sometimes written in *first person,* especially in romantic comedy (in which case, the entire book reflects a single character's voice), but the majority of category romances are written in *third person* (with the focus moving from character to character but staying mostly on the heroine and, secondarily, the hero). A romance novel rarely uses true *omniscient narration,* a literary device in which the narrator is a separate voice, divorced from any character's thoughts and feelings, that often delivers information no character is capable of knowing.

WARNING

Because romance novels are all about emotion, which is entirely personal, the impersonal omniscient viewpoint, even if used only as an occasional interjection, works against the book's nature. Likewise, avoid foreshadowing: Let your reader experience events as they occur, because they'll have much more impact. Don't interrupt the flow of the story with an omniscient aside like "If she'd only known what the morning would bring, she wouldn't have fallen asleep with a smile on her lips."

You should tell every scene in a romance from a particular character's point of view, though not every element of the scene involves dialogue or directly reported thoughts, both of which showcase the characters' voices. The other elements — description and narration — showcase the author's voice.

>> **Description:** Descriptions, whether of a person, place, or thing, are rarely done in dialogue because they usually sound awkward — sort of like those ridiculous soap opera scenes where two characters sit down over coffee to rehash the history of a relationship they both know very well. They're talking about it for the viewers' benefit, which makes the scene artificial. The same thing happens in a book when dialogue is the outlet for description. For example, one character is unlikely to describe to another the office where they're meeting or the local landscape surrounding the ranch where the story takes place.

Descriptions give you a chance to use your authorial voice to show the reader where the characters are and what's going on. Also, use your own voice when describing a character. Even if your heroine describes the hero to a friend, she's going to do it in normal conversational terms. His hair is merely black, not jet black, for example, and she won't hit on every detail of his appearance. By using your own voice, you can go further with your description, making it more effective and complete, while still making the heroine's feelings about him clear.

>> **Narration:** In every romance novel, there are times when you need to tell the readers what someone is doing and why they're doing it. Keep such sections brief and interspersed with "personalizing" elements. For example, if you have your hero climbing a sheer cliff face in search of the heroine, who's trapped on a ledge above, you need to tell readers something about the mechanics of how he makes it up the cliff. You can mingle the "right hand here, left foot there" bits with his feelings about what he's doing: fear that he's too late, determination to make the climb despite fatigue and pain, and fantasies of what they can do after they're safely at the bottom.

For the purposes of this chapter, and to differentiate the description of actions and thoughts from the description of a person, place, or thing, I use the term *narration,* not only to refer to the complete act of telling a story, but also to the ways you describe the characters' *actions,* or the things that your characters do. A related term, one that groups description and narration together to include everything that's not dialogue or a character's direct thoughts, is *narrative,* and I use this term frequently in Chapter 9, when I discuss your characters' voices.

I provide all kinds of additional information on description and narration later in this chapter (see the sections "Putting the Show in Show and Tell" and "Telling It Like It Is").

Your voice and your characters' voices often intertwine in everything except dialogue. Don't try too hard to separate your voice from the other voices. Concentrate on telling your story in the most effective manner, and don't get lost in analyzing your prose.

Making the language your own

The first thing every romance writer needs to do is tell a story their own way, which means finding a personal way of handling language. The good news is, you've already done most of the work: We're all storytellers every day; all you need to do is listen to yourself and discover the storytelling style you've developed over your lifetime. Then adapt your own natural conversational style and make it the basis of your writing style. You don't need to start from scratch, just take what you already know and do, and build on it.

Do you like to make people laugh? Or are you in your element creating drama in the everyday? When you talk about what happened at work, do you put words into people's mouths and act out each person's part? Or do you love to delve into the nuances of description, creating a sense of atmosphere so your listeners feel as if they're in the middle of the scene? How you answer these questions will help you decide not only what kind of story to tell (a humorous or a dramatic one, for example) but also how to tell it.

We all overuse certain words, like a piece of current slang, an all-purpose response ("Brilliant!"), or a favorite descriptor ("beautiful"). As a writer, you need to be the most articulate version of yourself, and you can do that by varying your word choices. Not only does it get boring, even irritating, to hear the same words — especially adjectives — used over and over again, but they also stop having any meaning and they interrupt the flow of the story. If everything's beautiful or big or great, how can any one person or peril stand out?

If you're most comfortable using dialogue, don't make yourself crazy trying to write long, beautiful descriptions. Instead, stick to the basics and be straightforward, without getting lost in long metaphors. On the other hand, if you love to create an atmosphere with long descriptions, use your skill, but don't go on too long before allowing your characters to speak, too.

If you're a plain speaker, not given to lots of adjectives and adverbs, nothing's wrong with being a plain writer, too — just not *too* plain. Readers need details about people and places, but don't feel you have to describe every little thing. Decide what's truly important and spend extra time and words on that subject only. The very fact that you've spent extra time on a detail will stand out to the reader and emphasize its importance.

Choosing your words wisely

As an author, the decisions you make affect how your reader sees your characters and their story. The words you choose provide the reader's only knowledge of what's happening, where, and to whom, so choose them wisely.

You can't write clear descriptions and narration (and make your reader see what you want her to see) without using adjectives and, to a lesser extent, adverbs. For example, a house, a big house, and a mansion are vastly different. And not all mansions are created equal. Is your hero's mansion made of glass walls and angular rooflines, modern and stark? Or does he live in an ivy-covered, centuries-old manor that's foreboding and gray?

Characters going up a hill can trudge along breathing hard, or sprint quickly to the top. A soldier walking wearily up the path toward home after a year fighting with the Confederacy is very different from a soldier, shiny in his new uniform, jaunting up the path to his girlfriend's house to propose before shipping out to a distant land.

REMEMBER

Effective prose doesn't shout, "Look at me! Look at me!" Effective prose does its job without attracting the reader's attention, whether because something's wrong *or* something's right.

Too many adjectives and adverbs can get in the way of what counts: your characters and their romance. Keep the phrase "less is more" in mind when you write. Too much of a good thing is still too much, and overwriting is a far worse thing than underwriting. I've read manuscripts where even the adjectives had adjectives, and no character just walked without doing so arrogantly, stiffly, or primly. Most of the time you just want to move someone from one place to another, and how they get there doesn't really matter. You don't want the reader to wonder how many more ways you can describe walking and forget all about what the characters are feeling.

And although the reader may care how the heroine's dressed, getting down the details of every character's wardrobe probably isn't important. Use a general phrase whenever one will serve, such as "well-dressed" or "sloppy." If you do describe something in more detail, don't go overboard. The heroine's dress can be silky, ankle-length, with flowing lines, and in an emerald shade that reflects the color of her eyes. But don't describe it in such detail that a reader's eyes glaze over and you sound like you're quoting a fashion column: ankle-length, cut on the bias, with sleeves ending 3 inches above the wrists, and a skirt that moves with her but is narrow enough to make climbing stairs a challenge, and a shade of green that's like a deep emerald crossed with the shade of a forest in full sunlight, and on and on. Your reader will lose interest and move on.

Mixing what you say with what your characters know

Your authorial voice is filtered through a character's point of view, usually the hero or heroine's. What you're really doing when you describe a character or place, for example, is describing what your heroine sees and, often, personalizing it with her reactions. Her thoughts and feelings are threaded through your description. When writing, be sure that the tone of your description is in keeping with who she is and what she knows, which can be a very fine line to walk.

Here's an example: Your hero is a cutting-edge physicist and your heroine is meeting him for the first time in his lab to ask him to participate in a local bachelor auction. In this case, you need to describe the hero and the lab. But because the heroine isn't a scientist herself, she's not going to know what all the equipment is, so be careful that you don't describe it all by name, which implies that she does.

> Leah took a look around the room. Easily the most noticeable thing in it was the man himself. Marcus Whitford was 6'2", at least, and as far from the stereotypical science nerd as a man could be. His thick, mink-brown hair made her long to reach out and touch it, and his whiskey-colored eyes held both intelligence and humor. Afraid she was staring, she looked away and noticed that an Amegamagmamometer stood next to a stainless steel apoplectimeter, and a gleaming countertop held a minimicrotiptopper.

Nothing is wrong with the first part of the previous paragraph, which shows you how to mix your voice with the heroine's reactions. But you lose your reader with the last sentence. They know that your heroine has no way of knowing what all that equipment is, so your reader loses her connection to your character and your story. In these situations, generalities can serve you well: Your heroine can simply notice all the equipment and how impressive it looks, even though she has no idea what any of it does. You can also use dialogue so the hero can explain some of the equipment to her, although you can run into pitfalls here (see Chapter 9 for more on dialogue).

Use the same caution in narration, as well, and don't let your characters demonstrate more knowledge than they can believably possess. For example, your heroine may get a chance to watch the hero work in his lab, in which case, unless he tells her about the process he's demonstrating, she's not going to know exactly what he's doing, just that it's complicated, time-consuming, and other nonspecific things.

Putting the Show in Show and Tell

Readers hear the author's voice the most in descriptions, mainly because descriptions are usually presented in chunks, without being broken up by a lot of dialogue or action. As long as your descriptions are presented effectively and don't go on too long, they don't stop the reader in her tracks, or pull her attention away from the world of your story and back to the real world. In this section, I give you a few key points to remember when you're writing descriptions (in addition to the general rules of good writing that I discuss in the "Speaking Up for Yourself" section earlier in this chapter).

Knowing what you need to say, and then saying it

You need to know going into a description what information is important and what's not. Knowing what you want to say keeps you from getting carried away by how clearly you see the scene in your mind and how much you enjoy writing about it. You may be tempted to fill in every detail, to paint as complete a picture as possible. However, you need to avoid this temptation.

WARNING

In writing, the medium is linear, and your reader's progress is dictated by the words you choose and the order in which you present them. You're never able to describe every detail, and attempting to gets in the way of your real goals. This is what is meant by "telling." Instead, focus on different ways you can weave details into the action. This is what is meant by "showing."

Avoiding lost readers

If your description goes on too long and is too complex, your reader just gets lost. As you write, you see the scene in your head, so the details are all clear to you. But the reader's trying to paint the picture as she reads, and the perfect description quickly turns into a confused scribble when there are too many details to focus on.

REMEMBER

Only details that either provide a sense of the overall picture or play a role later in the novel matter, so focus on them and let the others go unspoken.

Preventing boredom

Descriptions that go on too long make your book drag. Slow pacing (as I discuss in Chapter 10) is a problem that can literally put your reader to sleep. Keep your descriptions to a paragraph or two, not drawn out into something you can count in pages — which means you should focus on only what the reader needs to know.

Often, you get a chance to fill in more details later in the book, creating your description piece by piece, rather than in one hard-to-digest chunk.

For example, if you're writing a Regency romance, your hero probably lives in a manor house, which the reader needs to be able to visualize. As your heroine's carriage drives up the tree-lined approach, your reader sees the house for the first time, so start your description with the stately façade and a general sense of the landscaping, perhaps mentioning the terrace and garden bordering the east side of the house, the gazebo on the small rise to the west, or how the property slopes to meet the sea to the south. As the heroine walks inside, you can describe the foyer and perhaps the bedroom that she's led to.

Instead of giving the heroine and the reader a room-by-room tour of the house, end your description there, let the book move on, and describe other rooms later, when the action takes the characters into them. And if the heroine never sees all the rooms — the kitchens, for example — your reader never needs to see them, either, even if they're mentioned at some point in the book.

As for the garden, the gazebo, or the sea, you may not need to describe them further, unless they become key to the action. If the hero dances the heroine out onto the terrace and then leads her into the garden to steal a kiss, that's the time to talk about statuary and the romantic scent of roses by moonlight.

Speaking metaphorically

Use metaphors in moderation. Incorporating a lot of metaphors in your descriptions can be tempting, because they give you a chance to be creative and stretch your skills. Do your best to resist the temptation, though. Too many metaphors — just like too many adjectives — get in the way of your real goal: involving the reader in your characters' relationship. When used sparingly, metaphors add to a description; each time you're tempted to add one, make sure that it contributes to the overall impact of your story. If you're just showcasing your own skills, cut it. For example, it's difficult to get through a paragraph like this:

> She stood, her anger about to bubble over. He was handsome, but he reeked of presumption. How dare he? Silence blanketed the area. She shot daggers at him. The fire between them cooled.

Any one of these metaphors could be used once with great effect, but used all together, it's too much.

Describing your characters

Character descriptions are subject to the same cautions as all descriptions (see the "Choosing your words wisely" section earlier in this chapter). You want to give a complete and compelling picture of your hero and heroine, and your major supporting players also require enough description to make them individuals in the reader's mind — just not so much that they rival your main characters in importance. Describe minor characters fully enough to fulfill the reader's need for information, but no more.

TIP

The amount of time spent describing a character is a signal to the reader about how important the character is, so keep the amount of detail appropriate to the role.

Making every word count

Choose loaded words, not neutral ones, so that every word counts. As much as possible, use words that do more than describe the basics. Use words — or add extra, if the payoff's great enough — that convey feeling and affect your reader. A canyon isn't just deep, it's dizzying. A mountainside isn't just rocky, it's jagged. Your heroine's hair isn't just soft, it's silken. A sideboard isn't just loaded with serving dishes, it's groaning under the weight of them. The air isn't just thick, it's swirling with dank tendrils of mist. Know what effect you want to create and choose the most effective words. One well-chosen word is worth more than a dozen that don't quite hit your mark.

TIP

Don't get lost in your thesaurus. A thesaurus can be a great tool when used sparingly and with knowledge. It can also mark a writer as a rank amateur who hasn't mastered either vocabulary or the tenets of good writing. (For more on the problems presented by overusing a thesaurus, see Chapter 14.)

Talking too much

Make sure that you don't talk too much, whether in your description or narration. This idea is key and is really an extension of knowing what you need to say. Describe something because, and only because, the reader needs that knowledge to fully enjoy your book. As the author, your job is always to give the reader what they want, and what they want is interaction between the hero and heroine and their eventual happy (and romantic) ending.

REMEMBER

To keep the reader happy, you need to keep the book moving. To keep the book moving, you have to keep your descriptive passages to a minimum and make them as brief as possible (see the "Moving right along" section later in this chapter). Don't describe things that are interesting but unimportant. Even if your reader shares your interest, the book ultimately loses its ability to compel her to turn the pages, because you're taking too many side trips into territory that isn't directly related to the events in your story. She may finish the novel, but she's unlikely to look for more of your books in the future. Those readers who don't find your digressions interesting lose patience even sooner and put the book down for good.

WARNING

Don't use your book as a soapbox. Romance novels are popular because they entertain readers and offer an escape from real life into a world of romantic fantasy. Don't use your book as a pulpit from which to preach your views on politics, world peace, ecology, the economy, or anything else. Your characters are welcome to have opinions of their own, but when you forget the rules of good characterization and put your own opinions into your characters' mouths, or slip them into your descriptive or narrative passages, the reader knows you are preaching to her — and she'll disconnect.

Telling It Like It Is

Much of the action in any book can easily be described in minor phrases, often interspersed with dialogue. For example, the heroine walks across a room while talking to her best friend, or the hero shuffles papers on his desk while talking on the phone to the heroine. Similarly, just a few straightforward lines are enough to explain a character's actions: The hero saddles a horse and rides off across the pasture, or the heroine puts a pie in the oven and then sits down to read while it bakes. The tips in this section can apply to these minor examples, but they're most impactful when you need to spend an extended amount of time talking about what a character is doing, and you don't want to confuse your reader or slow down your story.

Keeping your writing clear

One advantage that the movies have over books is in clarity. Watching something happen on-screen is the easiest way to understand what's going on and what even a complex process entails. In the absence of visuals, authors have to describe what are sometimes complicated actions so the reader understands what's occurring. The following tips can help you maintain clarity:

>> **Simplify, simplify, simplify.** The more complicated the action is, the more confusing it is for the reader. Simplify as much as you can. For example, if your hero's a doctor and your heroine's a nurse, and you have a key scene set in the operating room, focus on the interaction between the two of them — which is what the reader really wants to see — and not the by-the-book

details of the operation. Tell the reader enough so she can follow how the operation is progressing, paralleling the progress of the operation with what the characters are *really* thinking about, but not so much that she feels like she is performing the operation and doesn't have time to worry about a romance going on in the background.

» **Keep the tech talk to a minimum.** Every profession and hobby has a specialized vocabulary. Used judiciously, pieces of that vocabulary can give your book the ring of authenticity. But when you load a scene with too many specialized words that most readers don't understand, you confuse people, slow the book down, and even cause some readers to put your book down in frustration.

As you describe what the characters are doing, choose words with meanings that are clear from the context so the reader doesn't feel like she's missing something by not knowing a definition. If your heroine is getting her horse ready to ride, say that she bridles her horse. Don't complicate the process by saying that she slips the egg-butt snaffle into the horse's mouth, adjusts the martingale, and tightens the throat latch.

» **Summarize when you can.** If your hero and heroine are in a car, racing through the narrow streets of a small Italian village with a killer on their tail, don't map out every twist and turn of the route. Use a sentence or two to say that they're going at a breakneck pace, sending pets and pedestrians scattering, passing the small hotel where the heroine stayed, and blindly rounding corners. Spend the rest of the scene on what counts: their conversation and how they feel about what's going on.

TIP

You can use these same techniques to get across accurate information that you turned up in your research. Stick to what the reader needs to know, break the information into manageable chunks and insert it as necessary. Mix the chunks of information with action, and remember to be as clear as you can. You want to teach the reader what she needs to know without her realizing she's just gone back to school.

Moving right along

Don't get so caught up describing what the characters are doing that you lose track of the emotional side of your story or slow your pacing. Being clear and concise always helps maintain your story's emotion and pacing, but the following strategies can also help keep things rolling.

Mixing action with dialogue or thoughts

A step-by-step explanation of what's going on can be dry and unemotional, and your reader isn't looking for an instruction manual or a textbook. If you mix dialogue or a character's inner responses with the more cut-and-dried description of unfolding events, you not only break up the potentially dry part into easier-to-digest pieces, but you also add emotional resonance to it. If you have your couple investigating a case, examining reports and clues, let the heroine notice the concentration in the hero's eyes as he reads through the case reports. Let the hero see how vulnerable she looks when he asks her about her missing sister. Intersperse their reactions to each other with the action, and the action automatically becomes more interesting to the reader.

Writing prose that moves

Some scenes move quickly just because of what's happening. A car chase has its own momentum, and a life-and-death operation keeps people reading quickly so they can discover the outcome. But what if your characters are mucking out stalls? That's not a dramatic activity and certainly isn't an intrinsically romantic one.

TIP

If you have a scene that feels clunky, try combining some sentences to move the prose along more efficiently. Notice the difference between the following two paragraphs. Nothing different happens in the second paragraph than in the first, but the prose moves more quickly in the second paragraph because the sentences run longer and are more active, so the reader isn't constantly being pulled up short.

> *Rick lifted a forkful of manure. He tossed it into the wheelbarrow, and then looked over at Melanie. She had almost finished the first stall. She didn't look happy, though. He hoisted another forkful of dirty straw, then another. Soon he had filled the wheelbarrow. He would have to pass by her on his way to the manure pile. He hoped she wouldn't toss a barbed remark — or worse — his way.*

versus

> *As he tossed a forkful of manure into the wheelbarrow, Rick looked over at Melanie. Despite having almost finished the first stall, she looked anything but happy. He went back to heaving dirty straw, and soon he'd filled the wheelbarrow. As he wheeled it past her, he found himself hoping she wouldn't be tossing any barbed remarks — or worse — in his direction.*

TIP

Another part of writing prose that moves is using contractions; for example, "he'd" instead of "he had" in the previous paragraph. Romances are popular fiction, and even the narrative passages should feel informal and move quickly. That means contractions aren't only fine, they're preferable.

Making life interesting

Make sure that something interesting — emotionally, plotwise, or both — is happening. You may have your characters mucking out stalls for a good plot-related reason — maybe someone's been doping racehorses and the heroine's about to uncover a syringe in the straw — but the scene always moves faster when something emotionally important is also hanging in the balance. Maybe the hero's trying to figure out how to ask the heroine on a date, but first her bad mood gets in the way, followed by the discovery of the syringe. He's lost his chance, but your reader hasn't lost a step, because so much has happened that she hasn't had time to be bored by the characters mucking out stalls.

Breaking up the action

Breaking up the action is a technique that works well when you need to talk about something that's not very exciting (like mucking out stalls). The technique works even better when you're talking about something that *is* exciting. Start the action, and then cut away to something else — like a scene that's occurring simultane-ously elsewhere, or a flashback, a memory, or a daydream. If the action you're leaving isn't exciting by its own nature, then your reader will enjoy the break. And if the action you're leaving *is* exciting, she'll read quickly so she can get back and see what happens. Essentially, you'll have built a mini-cliffhanger into the mid-dle of your scene. Chapter 12 gives you more information on starting and stopping the action.

Chapter 9

Letting Your Characters Speak

There are two kinds of voices in a romance novel, and both are important. The first is your own author voice, which I discuss in Chapter 8. You develop your author voice after writing a few manuscripts. The second — your characters' voices — is the subject of this chapter. Character voices develop over time as well, as you get to know your characters.

Your voice should, for the most part, go unnoticed. Your reader *should* hear your characters' voices and feel that your characters are the ones actually carrying the story. In your reader's mind, real voices make for real people, and real people create the kind of identification and emotional involvement that make a reader happy with your book and can propel you to the top of her must-read list.

You have three techniques at your disposal for conveying your characters' voices — dialogue, point of view, and internal monologue. Once you master these three techniques, you can feel confident that you're doing all you can to let your characters carry the story and, in the process, deepen your reader's involvement in what's going on. In this chapter, I talk about using all three of these approaches to give your characters their own voices, as well as how to navigate around some traps that writers often fall into, so you can make your book and your characters strong and compelling.

Giving Your Characters Voices

The best possible thing that can happen to you as an author is for your characters to become so real in your own mind that writing dialogue feels almost like taking dictation. Their voices should become so real that the reader feels like she's eavesdropping on their lives.

REMEMBER

Your characters' voices come across most noticeably in dialogue, which is literally their chance to speak. But the totality of any character's voice is a conglomeration of dialogue with their personalized thoughts and feelings. The role of character voice is to present a particular character's words, thoughts, and feelings, allowing the reader to always recognize that character.

Making every character unique (and real)

Just as you wouldn't make two characters look the same (unless they're twins or your plot depends on the similarity in their looks), you don't want to make any two characters sound exactly the same, either. Even though people from the same part of the country, or members of the same family, may sound a lot alike (sharing speech patterns, vocabulary, and even expressions), they don't usually sound identical to each other, and neither should your fictional characters.

In order for your reader to connect with your characters, your characters must feel real. To make every character, even the secondary ones, feel real, you have to give each one a voice of their own. (For all the ins and outs of characterization, see Chapter 4; also see the "Meeting the secondary-character challenge" section later in this chapter.) There are plenty of tools and tips to make every character sound unique. Here are a few to consider.

Reining in your own voice

Don't let your own voice come through for every character. Your heroine, especially in your first book, may sound a lot like you. That's okay — just be sure every heroine you ever write doesn't also sound like you, because you don't want readers to think you can't actually create a character. Even if your heroine sounds like you, make sure nobody else in the book does, otherwise all of your characters will end up sounding like the same person.

TIP

It can be hard to listening to your own voice objectively and then avoid replicating it, but you can do two things to help yourself:

>> Compare your speech patterns to those of other people (friends and family who live far away included, to account for regionalisms) and see whether you

have certain words or phrases you use constantly that others don't. Then avoid having all your characters use those phrases.

» Make a conscious effort to create unique voices for your characters, comparing their speech patterns to each other and varying them.

Bringing up backgrounds

A character from the South talks differently than one from New England, not to mention one from Merry *Olde* England. Don't go overboard highlighting regional differences, but don't ignore them, either. Education and social standing also affect the way people, including your characters, speak. Word order, cadences and pronunciation, and colloquialisms can help differentiate characters' voices.

Separating the sexes

Men and women talk differently. Women are more likely to focus on feelings, and men on problem solving. It's a cliché, but it's true, so don't make your men — especially your hero — too sensitive and self-aware. Your hero shouldn't be a caveman, but he should be a *man.*

TIP

If your hero's dialogue seems to be having a gender-identity problem, pay attention to how men talk to each other in movies and television. You'll learn more from paying attention to how dialogue is written for other male characters than you will from real-life people.

If you do try and get ideas from listening to real-life conversations, remember that writing dialogue is very different from dictating what people say. In real life, people interject a lot of "um's" and "ah's," and they often make small talk. Try not to have your characters ask something banal like "How was your day?" or talk about the weather.

A strong, proactive heroine should still sound like a woman, not one of the guys. If circumstances demand that she talk tough — for example, if she's in the military and giving orders to a bunch of hard cases who can't believe their commanding officer is a woman — be sure you use her point of view to counter the impression her words give. (For tips on that, check out the "Point of View: How to Choose and How to Use" section later in this chapter.)

Avoiding clichés

Not every waitress snaps gum while she talks, and not all single women in their 30s are bitter about men. Even if a character shares an aspect of the cliché, that aspect shouldn't be the sum total of their personality, so don't make that

30-something friend drag her bad experiences with men into every conversation. Let her talk about other things, too.

Spoken clichés can be just as off-putting. Unless it's part of someone's character to always reel off a cliché at any difficult moment, try not to use more than a few and make sure that you use them effectively — as a way for your hero to avoid revealing his real emotions, for example. But don't let clichés substitute for a character's real voice.

Speaking up

Remember that dialogue represents spoken English. People speak informally — sometimes even ungrammatically, depending on their backgrounds — so don't let your characters sound like examples from a grammar text. Even if speaking in perfect English informs your character, be sure they still sound like a person, even if an uptight, snobby, or pretentious one. And don't make everyone informal in the exact same way.

To see just how real your dialogue sounds, read it aloud. Read it into a voice recorder, if possible, and then play it back. Even the act of reading it aloud will tell you a lot about the dialogue's quality. Do the words flow easily, or have you placed them awkwardly, so that they trip you up? Are your sentences so long that you can't even complete them without pausing for a breath? Are there so many asides that you forget where you are? Is figuring out where to pause or what to empha-size impossible? If you answer "yes" to any of these questions, go back and rework the dialogue until it sounds like spoken, not written, English.

Working out the quirks

Use quirks sparingly. You can set someone's dialogue apart by giving them a verbal quirk or a difficulty in pronunciation: a tendency to pause a lot, to cut themselves off and correct themselves as they go, a lisp, or a stutter. Used spar-ingly, such a noticeable speech pattern can help to create a character's voice, but remember that a little goes a long way. Don't insert the quirk into that character's every line. Use (or mention) it often enough to let the reader know it exists, but don't bash her senseless by emphasizing it. You also shouldn't give every character a quirk or a problem, and you probably want to steer clear of giving them to your hero and heroine at all. They're on the page most of the time, and you can drive yourself — and your reader — nuts if you have to work something so noticeable into the bulk of their dialogue.

Giving every character a consistent voice

After you create a unique voice for each character, you need to keep that voice consistent and not let one character's speech patterns start leaching into another's. Depending on your own writing preferences and how real each character has become to you, you may find that keeping voices unique is easy to do. Character voice will be one of the aspects of your proofreading process. It's a good idea to pay special attention to voices during one of your later reads of the story.

TIP

Devoting one proofing pass solely to looking at dialogue helps catch a lot of problems. Think about the voice you intended to create for each character and make sure you stayed true to your vision all the way through. Consistency is the key to keeping the reader's attention and involvement. Make sure you aren't overusing certain words or expressions, putting them in everyone's mouth. Make sure a character who normally speaks in short, declarative sentences doesn't suddenly launch into a long, self-involved soliloquy (unless that dramatic change is important to your story). Make sure a character who's not too bright and never graduated high school doesn't suddenly start using the word "soliloquy."

Meeting the secondary-character challenge

Usually, the task of writing dialogue is relatively easy with your hero and heroine, because they're your most fully realized characters, so you may not even have to think very hard about how they sound. In fact, if you're writing a contemporary romance, the heroine of your first book will quite often sound a lot like you, so she's very easy for you to create.

REMEMBER

It's often a trickier proposition to make the secondary characters sound unique, because they're not on stage as much — sometimes only for a single scene or a single line — so the temptation is to hurry through their bits, have them play their parts (giving information, acting as a sounding board for the hero or heroine, and so on), and then move on with your main story. As a result, they often sound like clichés: the supportive best friend, the hound-dog male co-worker who comments on every woman, the amusingly bitter single friend, the Cockney coachman.

Don't try so hard to make every character stand out as wise, exceptionally quick- or slow-witted, or anything else that can distract your reader from the central romance. Think of them in the Hollywood sense — they're characters, not extras, but they also have a specific job to do. They're meant to support your hero and heroine and *their* story, not shout, "Look at me!"

SPEAKING HISTORICALLY

If you're writing an historical romance, think about the vocabulary and speech patterns of the era you've chosen. At the same time, keep in mind you're writing for a contemporary audience, so make sure your reader can understand your dialogue. Avoid *anachronisms,* words and phrases (and facts) that are inappropriate to the time. To avoid using words that are too modern for your setting, use an etymological dictionary to tell you when a word came into general use in the English language. On the other hand, don't immerse yourself so deeply in the past that your reader doesn't understand anything your characters are saying.

Also avoid using stiffness and formality as a way to indicate that you're writing about the past, especially for lower-class characters in what was almost certainly an extremely class-conscious society. Historical dialogue still has to flow and sound smooth to a contemporary reader's ear; if the dialogue's too stiff, it won't sound natural, and the reader will lose interest in your characters and their story. Don't rely on words like *thee, hath,* and *canst* over and over. Don't use them at all unless they're appropriate for the particular period you've chosen. Even if these words are historically correct, don't load up every sentence with them, otherwise your dialogue gets in the way of readers actually getting to know and care about your characters as people.

You can also get trapped in writing secondary characters who don't have any personality at all, whose dialogue is so plain that a reader forgets about them as soon as she reads what they have to say. With truly minor characters, this trap is less problematic, even a potential positive, simply because they're less important. Just remember that for any character who has an actual role to play (as opposed to a minor character who says a line like "You can catch the 4:07 on platform nine if you hurry"), dialogue without a unique character voice leaves a vacuum in your book. Such a vacuum leaves the door open for your reader to lose interest and put your book down for good.

Writing Great Dialogue

No matter how beautifully you write *narrative* — which includes everything that represents your voice rather than your characters' voices — no matter how clever your plot, no matter how complex and interesting an emotional conflict you set up, if you can't write dialogue, you can't write a good romance. Dialogue makes your characters exist for the reader. They get to speak up, step off the page, and enter into the reader's mind and heart. Good dialogue is one of the make-or-break elements every editor looks for. I spend some time in this section giving you some dialogue ins and outs.

Using dialect and accents effectively

Part of creating unique character voices comes from knowing your characters' backgrounds and incorporating that knowledge into their dialogue. That often means writing dialect or an accent — one of the trickiest things to do right, and getting it wrong sends up a red flag to an editor, or your readers, telling them that you're not a pro.

REMEMBER

Here's the short and simple thing to remember: Whether you're dealing with your hero, heroine, or a secondary character, don't spell out dialects and accents phonetically. It looks ridiculous:

> *"Eeze zat true?" Pierre asked. "Eeze Emeelee really meesing?"*

or

> *"Ah juss doe know, shuguh," May-Ellen said. "Whah don' you go ask yer pappy?"*

This dialogue is hard to read, for one thing. So many words are misspelled, even if they're written out phonetically, that the reader gets pulled right out of the world of the book. The dialogue is also so self-conscious that it's laughable, which may be fine if you're writing romantic comedy and a character's overdoing things for effect, but if you're writing romantic suspense and trying to build up a menacing atmosphere, it isn't so great. Instead, follow this advice:

>> Use an occasional "misspelled" word and let that stand in for the rest, and occasionally describe the way the reader should be hearing the words. Definitely mention an accent the first time a character speaks, which is also a good time to misspell a word or two, and then remind the reader of the character's quirks every so often as you go on. Not every time the character speaks, though, otherwise the reader will feel like you're smacking her over the head with the info. This strategy also holds true if you want to indicate any kind of verbal quirk, such as speaking slowly, with frequent pauses. Inserting ellipses every few words looks awkward; an occasional reminder to the reader is much more effective.

>> Instead of writing *just* (or *juss*), write *jus'*, letting the apostrophe stand in for the missing letter. Although this rule seems to contradict the dialogue strategy I previously advise you on, using an apostrophe to indicate a dropped letter is one case where you should be consistent. If you drop the final *g* in a character's dialogue, do so each time they speak. If the character says *runnin'*, then they also say *goin'*, *smilin'*, and *sittin'*. Because the apostrophe makes for such an unmistakable visual, I recommend avoiding it in your hero and heroine's dialogue, because they'll be speaking so often during the course of your book. If you must have a character drop their final g, make it a secondary character who has very little dialogue in your book.

>> You can also use word order to indicate an accent. English *syntax* — the normal patterns of speech and sentence structure that govern the way nouns, verbs, and other parts of speech are organized — is different from the syntax of other languages, so use the character's native syntax, along with a mention of their accent, to tell the reader how to hear the character's speech. Be careful, though — don't jumble up the word order so thoroughly that sentences become impossible to follow. As with so many other things in written dialogue, a little goes a long way.

>> An occasional regionalism or tossed-in foreign word (one that the reader can easily understand in context) can also indicate where a character's from and give a unique edge to their dialogue without getting in the way. You want to flavor the dialogue without overwhelming the reader.

Keepin' it cool: A word about slang

You can use slang as a wonderful way to differentiate characters, to tell the young from the old, Yankees from Southern belles or from Aussie jackaroos. But a little goes a long way if you're writing for a general audience. (A hip-hop flavored romance is going to lean much more heavily on accurate and very specific slang, which will appeal to a narrower target audience.)

WARNING

Using slang has pitfalls, though, even when you don't overuse it. You need to be aware of these pitfalls so you can decide how to avoid them. By its very nature, slang ties itself to a specific time period — often a very brief one — and sometimes even to a specific place. If you get it wrong, you risk looking foolish and, worse, making your characters look foolish and turning off your reader. This risk isn't just a part of historical romances, where you don't want contemporary expressions like "bling," "it blew me away," or "lit" to intrude.

Don't use last year's slang in a contemporary romance, a book intended to take place in what I always call the *eternal present*, because your reader should feel that your story could be taking place that very minute, even though you may have written it a year or more ago. Passé slang makes your book sound dated, as does setting a book in the '90s and having your characters all speak like refugees from the '60s. Writing a book set in the '50s and using '60s slang isn't any better, because readers will certainly pick up on the inaccuracies.

TIP

Ultimately, you need to decide for yourself just how current and time-sensitive you want your language to be. When I am asked for advice, I always suggest keeping slang to a minimum (the youngest characters usually use the most slang in their speech, just like in real life) and steering clear of trendy phrases in favor of those phrases that have stood the test of time. *Cool* will probably be with us forever and, well, I'm cool with that.

Another reason to steer clear of too much slang is that slang makes translating your book for sale in foreign markets more difficult. Translation is generally more of an issue with series books, because so many of them are published overseas, than for all but the most popular mainstream authors. Because your goal is to be popular, sell a lot of copies, and be available all over the world, you may want to keep the slang issue in mind even if you're writing mainstream romances.

Using dialogue to convey information naturally

Most people don't lecture for a living, and the same is true of most characters. Even when your character's an expert in their field, putting long, fact-filled speeches in their mouth still doesn't read well. Having long passages of spoken explanation, monologues, or the recitation of endless facts plunked down in the middle of the story is simply a turn-off (and, generally, a real drag on pacing).

I'm not saying that you can't use your characters to convey necessary pieces of information, whether that info is a description of someone or somewhere, a plot twist, or details of your research, but I *am* saying that you need to be very careful in how you do it. As I discuss in Chapter 13, you have to first accept the fact that your research will uncover a lot more info than your reader needs or wants to know. Before anyone starts saying anything, pare down the information so that you know which bits need to go into the book and which bits don't. Apply this same strategy when you want to convey a detailed description of something or a complex piece of plotting. Dialogue may help you get the basics across, but it's not the place to put every detail or twist.

TIP

After you've decided what essential information you need to include, think about the best way to incorporate it. You may decide narrative is the way to go, in which case, take a look at the section in Chapter 8 where I talk about narrative writing. The techniques I discuss in Chapter 8 apply to conveying any kind of information. If you decide to let your characters get the information across for you, here are some tips to keep in mind:

>> **Break it up.** A long lecture really stops your story's momentum. Deal with the information piecemeal, letting your characters explain only what's necessary — and only *when* it's necessary.

>> **Use natural language.** Don't make a character who usually talks in a normal, realistic way suddenly get all stiff and formal, as if they're quoting an instruction manual or addressing a grad-school seminar (unless they actually are). Keep their speech patterns normal and avoid as many technical terms as you can.

- **Don't forget that you're writing a romance.** Along with conveying information, convey characterization, whether through tone of voice or the characters' behavior — for example, the hero's inability to focus fully on what the heroine's telling him because he can't stop looking at her lips, or the heroine momentarily losing her train of thought when she notices how handsome the hero looks when he's listening intently.

- **Use conversation.** Alternating between questions and answers lets you follow these tips simultaneously. It's especially helpful if you have a fair bit of information that you have to convey all at once. This technique breaks things up and gives everything a normal, conversational feel (if it's done right). Using conversation also lets you build your characters while you convey information, because you show them reacting to each other. You can even convey emotional subtext while your characters talk about whatever cold, hard facts you need to convey. Just don't let the Q & A session go on so long that it feels like an interview.

WARNING

Avoid having two characters talk about something they both know simply because the reader needs to know it. I see this mistake all the time. The reader gets irritated because the conversation feels so artificial. If you're in a position where you need to tell the reader something and the characters can't talk about it naturally, you can always drop into someone's point of view or use internal monologue, which I talk about later in this chapter.

Putting dialogue on paper

Writing good dialogue involves more than just knowing what your characters need to say and how they would go about saying it. You also need to know how to put it on the page so that it works for an editor as well as a reader. Some editors feel more strongly than others about various formatting points, but you can't go wrong if you take the following tips to heart:

- **Don't use semicolons or colons in dialogue.** Semicolons and colons are written punctuation. In speech, meaning dialogue, people either pause (a comma) or stop and start another sentence (a period). Punctuating your dialogue that way better reflects real speech and sounds more realistic in the reader's mind. Plus, the dialogue doesn't look so written, even though it is.

- **Don't use parentheses in dialogue.** Like semicolons and colons, parentheses are written punctuation. Set off an aside with dashes or ellipses, both of which reflect natural speech patterns.

- **Avoid exclamation points.** You don't need to avoid them all the time, just 99 percent of it. An exclamation point indicates that a character yells a piece of dialogue or speaks with strong emotion, and most people don't speak at the tops of their voices all the time. If you emphasize everything with an exclamation point, nothing stands out after a while. It's like the boy who cried wolf. When you finally really need to have someone shout something important, like yelling, *Get down!* When bullets start flying, the exclamation doesn't register on your reader as any more important than *I'm going to the store!* or *We're out of fabric softener!*

» **Use he said, she said.** You don't need to use characters' names all the time in dialogue attribution. After you establish who's speaking, you can use pronouns most, if not all, of the time. Text reads as self-conscious and awkward when you see names everywhere, and it feels repetitive in a way pronouns don't.

» **Be conservative with dialogue tags.** In an effort to sound different from everyone else or to clarify how a piece of dialogue should sound, authors sometimes ignore the perfectly serviceable (and usually preferable) *said* in favor of words like *groaned, hissed, chortled, cried, giggled, sighed, shouted, laughed,* and so on.

All of those descriptors are fine — occasionally (okay, except maybe *chortled,* which describes a sound that I just don't think most people make). Like exclamation points, save them for when you really need them. Most dialogue is simply spoken, and the words and context give all the necessary clues as to how it gets said. Save extraordinary tags for extraordinary circumstances. If every line has a unique tag attached to it, the tags start drawing attention to themselves at the expense of what your characters are actually saying.

» **Remember that a dialogue tag has to indicate sound.** You speak dialogue, so any tag attached to it has to involve noise. Dialogue can't be smiled or grinned or seethed, or, worse yet, acted out. For example, this sentence is wrong: *"Hi there," he walked across the room.* If you need to get across something beyond the sound of a line, go with something like:

- *"Hi there." He walked across the room.*

- *"Hello," he said with a smile.*

- *"I can't believe you did that," she said, seething internally.*

» **Don't hiss without an s.** Hissing, by definition, requires an *ess* sound. You can hiss *yes* or *I hate Christmas* (though only if you're very, very mean), but you can't hiss *no* or *I hate my birthday.* Unfortunately, I don't know of any way to describe that way of speaking that's a cross between a hiss and a whisper in a single word, so if you want a character to deliver a line in that unfortunately indescribable tone, you have to do your best to indicate it in some way other than calling it a hiss.

» **Be careful with unattributed dialogue.** If two characters are talking, you don't have to identify the speaker of each line, so long as the reader knows who's speaking. Pages and pages of unattributed dialogue will almost certainly confuse your reader, though, especially if the speeches are brief and don't give you a chance to use voice to establish character. I've been confused more than once, and I've counted speeches from the last attributed line and discovered that the author got confused, too, having the same person say something and then provide the response.

>> **Use extra care with three or more speakers.** You can't just say *he said* and *she said* when your conversation has three or more speakers, because you're going to have at least two characters of the same gender. That's the time to use names or descriptions (*the older woman, the heavyset man*) to identify the speaker. Never use unattributed dialogue in scenes with many characters.

>> **Apply the rules of logic.** In real life, conversations are often elliptical, and people answer questions or refer to things that someone said several sentences back. In written dialogue, though, responses need to follow logically on what was said immediately beforehand, not a line or three back. Written dialogue needs to feel real, rather than be real. Be sure that one character's response follows logically from the last thing the previous character said, and don't put too much narrative or description in between, diverting the reader's train of thought.

Choosing and Using Point of View

Even when your characters aren't speaking to each other, they can still speak to the reader via your use of point of view (or POV) and internal monologue (a way of revealing a character's innermost thoughts). Most popular fiction deals heavily in POV, but romance is especially reliant on it, because romances are all about emotion, and the best way to communicate emotion — or build a reader's identification with a character — is through POV.

REMEMBER

Point of view, as it's used in this book and in terms of popular fiction, generally means describing the action as a particular character experiences it, complete with thoughts, reactions, and emotional responses. Using a character's POV doesn't mean dropping into first person, though you can use first person for brief periods (usually only a line or two, as a character talks to themselves silently; see the "Is there a place for first person point of view?" sidebar later in this chapter).

What are they thinking?

Most of the time, you should use point of view in small doses — a line or two attached to a piece of dialogue or mixed in with the action of the book. As I say in

Chapter 8, your narrative voice and your characters' thoughts often become so intertwined that one can't even exist without the other, especially if you're writing in deep third person. Your voice tells the reader what's happening in terms of place and plot. Point of view lets you clarify what's going on inside your characters' minds, telling the reader what your characters can't tell each other, and clarifying why things are happening and what they really mean.

Articulating the attraction

Because a writer builds a romance around two characters falling in love but not being able to talk about it (as I discuss in Chapter 5), your characters very often say and do one thing while thinking something else entirely. Because of that, you need point of view to describe what's really going on. Otherwise, the reader can't understand your characters' inner lives, which are the most important sides of things in a book that's ultimately all about emotions.

Your hero and heroine may be having a knockdown, drag-out fight about something plot-related, and if the reader only sees their dialogue, she thinks they hate each other. By getting inside your characters' minds, you can give the reader the real story. You can show her that they're actually incredibly attracted to each other, even when they're making each other furious — that your heroine hates being at odds with your hero, that he loves to watch her eyes snap with anger and wonders if they'd spark equally hot with passion.

You can do the same thing during action scenes. Even as you put most of the focus on the externals, on what's happening, a few economical but well-placed lines of POV, even just a word or two, can keep the romance front and center in your reader's mind, adding emotional depth to the simplest actions.

Feeling the love

One of the most important places where your characters' thoughts can illuminate what's really going on is in your love scenes. Your characters can't let each other know how they feel before the climax of the story or it will destroy the tension, but your reader needs to know they're not just indulging in a purely physical one- (or two- or more) night stand, and that they're developing real feelings for each other. Point of view is crucial because it lets you make the characters' feelings, not just their actions, clear, and the reader cares about their feelings. Your characters' feelings make them come alive as sympathetic people deserving not only of expressing love but of feeling it.

Getting practical

Other times, you may need to drop from dialogue or action into a key character's point of view because it's the easiest way to convey a critical piece of information.

Having two characters discussing the details of something they both already know sometimes feels artificial, but you can use one character's POV to give the reader the information in a subtler, more natural way. Other times, you don't have anyone else on the scene, so your character's thoughts are the only way to get information to the reader and still keep the story moving forward.

Knowing whose voice to use

To use point of view effectively, you need to decide whose head to get into. *First person point of view,* usually told from the heroine's perspective (using the pronouns "I," "me," "we") has become more popular in romantic comedy, and even some mainstream romance. Category romances are mostly written in *third person point of view,* changing between the heroine's and hero's points of view (using the pronouns "she" and "he"). Before you decide which perspective is right for your book, you might try writing the first scene both ways and see which way you like better.

REMEMBER

Romances don't generally use a lot of points of view other than those of the two main characters. As a general rule, if the heroine or the hero is present, use one or both of their points of view, not the POV of any other characters on hand. Jumping into minor characters' heads simply because they're there is, at best, self-indulgent and, at worst, lazy and amateurish. You can't go wrong telling a romance only from the heroine and hero's points of view (or even just the heroine's, though keeping the reader in the dark as to the hero's thoughts can prove tricky in terms of building up understanding and empathy).

In romantic suspense, you may get the villain's point of view, and important secondary characters in any romance sometimes have points of view as well (mainly when they have crucial insights into the hero and heroine's relationship or when they're involved in a strong secondary romance).

Series romances limit the number of points of view more strictly than mainstream romances do, in large part because of the constraints of length. Knowing your market also helps you determine how free you can be in choosing point-of-view characters.

WARNING

Avoid using so many points of view that the book, and the reader, loses focus. A romance, by definition, tells the story of a single relationship that ends happily, and too many points of view get in the way of that, turning the book into women's fiction or a relationship novel, both of which are related to romance fiction but not synonymous with it.

Determining where to begin

I strongly recommend beginning with your heroine's point of view because the story is hers, and your reader needs to identify with her. But you can begin with the hero's thoughts, if you want, without too much worry, because your reader needs to fall in love with him, too, so the sooner the better, right?

Whichever POV you start with, be sure to get them together quickly (in the same scene, not necessarily emotionally) and make sure that they focus on each other, even though the tension between them should be quite high early on in your story. You definitely don't want to write a long excursion into one character's POV, focusing on all kinds of non-romance-related things, and then write a similar excursion into the other character's POV, before they finally start to think about what's supposed to be going on in the book — their relationship.

WARNING

Starting from a third character's point of view is tricky and usually ineffective, though a brief prologue that sets up the danger can sometimes be effective in romantic suspense. It helps, though, to include one of the main characters in such a prologue, either as part of the action or as the subject of the bad guy's (or gal's) plotting. (See Chapter 12 for more info on starting your novel effectively, including tips to keep in mind when using a prologue.)

Moving from scene to scene

As you continue with the book, tell every scene, to a greater or lesser degree, from one (or more) character's point of view, not from your own as the author. Sometimes choosing whose point of view to use is easy, because your scene features only your hero or heroine (or a key secondary character who can provide necessary information that the hero or heroine can't). But, in many cases, you can choose between at least two points of view — the heroine's *or* the hero's.

TIP

As with so many things, I'm not big on rules. I rarely analyze whether a book uses 50 percent or more of the heroine's POV as compared to the hero's or anyone else's. I'm more concerned with whether the book works, meaning whether the writer made the most effective choices for their characters, the story, and the intended readership. If you're aiming for a particular editor or a particular series, and they *do* have preferences, even requirements, regarding POV, listen to them and not me, because you have to give your particular editor what they want.

There are two schools of thought on using point of view within a scene:

>> **Single point of view:** This more formal school holds that you need to choose a character — for example, the heroine — and stick with her point of view for the duration of the scene or, at the very least, for a substantial portion of it. To switch POV, you need to insert a time or scene break. Editors who

subscribe to this outlook usually require writers to revise scenes that employ multiple points of view so that those scenes reflect only one POV.

>> **Multiple points of view:** This school says that moving back and forth between your characters' points of view within the scene is fine as long as the reader doesn't get confused as to whose head she's in at any given time. You'll often find bestselling mainstream romance authors (Nora Roberts is one) who do this in their work. If you study how they do this, they're usually using a method of pulling back the camera, so to speak, to a more general point of view before narrowing in on another character. This technique is easy to confuse with head hopping, which means you're abruptly changing from one character's point of view to another.

If you're gearing a book toward a particular editor, you may know how they feel about point of view, either because they've talked about it at a conference or in a newsletter interview, or because you can make an educated guess based on reading work by the authors you know they edit. The same holds true, at least to a certain extent, if you're aiming for a specific line of series romances. By reading books from that line — something you should be doing in any case — you can at least see what's generally allowed in the line, although you may not be able to gauge a specific editor's preferences.

If you're indie publishing, do what feels right to you, but be aware that it's more difficult to change point of view in the middle of a scene without confusing the reader. I usually suggest ending the scene before changing into another character's point of view, especially if you're new to writing. Plus, in my opinion, many instances of head hopping can easily be avoided by showing what a character is thinking through body language, which requires a little more thought but usually reads better in the end.

If you are switching between the hero and heroine's points of view, when you start a scene you will need to ground the reader in whose point of view they are in. I do this through describing my characters' actions and thoughts. You'll also need to decide which point of view is best to use for each scene. Ask yourself who — your hero or your heroine — has the most at stake, the most to learn, the most to tell the reader, or the most interesting take on things. Then choose his or her point of view for that scene. If you can't decide, opt for the heroine's POV, because she's your reader's way into the story.

Don't show the same scene twice, once from the heroine's point of view and again from the hero's. Too often, authors simply use this approach as a way, and an ineffective one, to lengthen a book that doesn't have enough going on. Sometimes, though, the characters see things in different ways, and you may need to show that to further your story. If you're not using multiple points of view, tell the scene from one character's point of view — say the heroine's — and then, later, let the hero reflect on that same scene. Don't retell the entire scene — just use a key moment to spur the hero to reflect on how he felt or to recall the key piece of information you need the reader to know.

Internal monologues and how to use them

An *internal monologue* is basically point of view writ large, or at least long. Most of the time, you convey your characters' thoughts and feelings in brief, even subtle, ways. But sometimes you need to stay inside someone's head longer to convey an important point. That extended trip is referred to as an internal monologue. No formula says that "If it's over *x* number of lines, it's an internal monologue." But trust me, you'll know one when you see one. Internal monologue isn't only help-ful, it's almost required, in two basic instances (both of which can recur in your book): times of emotional stress and personal revelation, and points when you need to convey a larger-than-usual amount of information.

IS THERE A PLACE FOR FIRST PERSON POINT OF VIEW?

More than half of all romance novels are written in third person point of view, but first person romances are becoming more popular. If you want to try first person POV, watch out for these pitfalls, and do your best to avoid them.

- **The me-me-me syndrome:** A lot of first person narration falls into the trap of sounding self-important or too self-involved. You may have trouble making some-one entirely sympathetic when she's spending several hundred pages essentially talking about herself, so think long and hard about whether you, and your heroine, are up to the challenge. The fact that she's the only point of view character puts extra pressure on her, because the reader gets no respite from her; so even if she's not actively ego-centric, you may want to put extra work into making sure that readers will find her interesting and appealing.

- **Limiting reader access:** Although you get to tell the reader everything your heroine knows, she's not going to know everything that's going on in her world, so getting across all the details of the plot can be tough. You will also have to con-vey the other characters' thoughts and feelings entirely through their words and behavior without the benefit of their POV insights. In other words, first person can be quite limiting in ways that many writers (and some readers) find frustrating.

The most important use of internal monologue is at moments of great emotional stress and revelation. I'm always amazed at how often I'm reading a manuscript, as caught up in the characters' difficult romance as any reader, and I finally reach the welcome point where one of them (usually the heroine first, and the hero later — maybe much later) realizes he or she loves the other. This revelation is huge. It's the key to everything else that will happen and yet the author simply mentions it as casually as if she were saying that the heroine loves fresh-baked chocolate chip cookies and then moves on.

A moment like that is the time for an internal monologue. The reader wants — *needs* — to know how the heroine feels about her sudden realization. Is she furious with herself for falling in love with someone who can never love her back? Furious with the hero for showing her his vulnerable side and making her fall for him, when he's the single most unsuitable man on the planet? Relieved to know she can feel love again, when she'd thought she was dead inside? Afraid, because she knows she and the hero can never work things out, so she's bound to get her heart broken in the end?

Whatever it is she is feeling, those feelings are dramatic, complicated, and fascinating. You need to spend some time inside her head in order to tell the reader all about them. Your heroine needs to marvel at her feelings, analyze them, and try to figure out what they mean for her future. Your reader needs and wants to see all of that, and you need to provide it by writing an internal monologue.

Your book has other emotional points when having your characters think about their feelings and the developing relationship makes sense, and you can also use an internal monologue in those places, too. Any situation where a real person would take a breather and ponder the big stuff going on in their life, or where some new development has just changed the picture and the character needs to do a little rethinking, lends itself to an internal monologue, even if it's only a paragraph long.

The second use for internal monologue is a more practical one. You can use an internal monologue to convey information — explaining how something works, what motivates a character, what a character thinks motivates someone else, or any other type of information that doesn't comfortably fit in conversation and needs more than a line or two of explanation or clarification.

Check out these tips for writing effective internal monologues:

>> **Remember your character's voice.** People think pretty much the same way they speak, so even if you're not using first person POV, you still need to keep your character's voice in mind and let it flavor their internal monologue. Internal monologue should feel conversational, even though no actual

conversation is going on. It also needs to stay true to the character as you've created them.

>> **Use action or dialogue when it can do the work.** Too often I see manuscripts where the characters spend a lot of time thinking about what happened between them, but the author never actually shows them together or doesn't show them together often enough. Internal monologues can show the reader important details, but she still wants to actually experience the action of the story, not just hear thoughts about it.

>> **Keep it short.** There's no hard-and-fast rule on lengths, but most of the time, devote only a page or two, maximum, to an internal monologue. Often you only need a paragraph or two. You may find an exception, but if your internal monologues go on for pages every time, you most likely have other problems going on. You're probably repeating yourself and can cut out a lot of what you've written. If you can't cut it down, find a way to break it up into smaller, more manageable pieces.

Chapter **10**

Pacing: The Secrets of Writing a Page-Turning Romance

A great story badly (especially boringly) told fails as a story. That's not a cliché, but it should be, because it's as true as any cliché I know. The best romances are constantly referred to as page-turners, and that term refers directly to pacing.

You probably know someone who can take the most interesting events and turn them into a foolproof cure for insomnia. Somewhere between "I was cashing my paycheck when two masked gunmen ran into the bank" and "Then the cute policeman asked me if I wanted to go to dinner" lies a wealth of boring detail ("It was 3:14 p.m., well, really 3:17 p.m., but my watch is slow") and digression ("I was wearing that great dress I bought when Lisa and I went shopping two weeks ago"). In real life, you can nudge your friend to keep the story moving, but in a book, your reader is pretty well stuck. She can skim, but the point of reading a romance is to immerse yourself in a world of emotion, not hunt for pieces of interesting information. If a reader ends up skimming big chunks of your book to get to the good parts, she's going to feel she didn't get her money's worth, and she's not going to waste time and money on you again.

Pacing — knowing what to say and when and how to say it — is what keeps your story moving and your reader engaged. Using the techniques in this chapter, you can tell your story in the best possible way.

TIP

I frame this discussion about pacing in terms of your entire book, but you need to think about how to pace individual scenes, especially key moments involving action and emotional revelations, and also love scenes, which can be slow and sensuous or intense and fast-paced. The general pacing techniques I provide for your manuscript are just as applicable to individual scenes.

Pacing Doesn't Mean Racing

Overall, you want your book to move along at a good clip, but that doesn't mean you have to race for the finish line (or the final page) or that every paragraph has to move quickly. For one thing, if your pacing is all the same — whether that's fast, slow, or somewhere in between — your book gets boring. To quote another applicable cliché, variety is the spice of life. Your book benefits if you vary the pace. Slow things down occasionally, not to a crawl or a dead stop, but just enough so that the reader feels the difference.

Nonstop excitement ends up feeling like the normal state of affairs, so eventually it's no longer exciting. If you slow things down to a more usual pace, your reader's adrenalin starts pumping again the next time the action and the emotion pick up.

You also need to give your reader an occasional breather, especially when you're writing action or adventure. If you have your characters perched on an emotional high wire, your reader needs a break occasionally. After you've revealed a key piece of information or allowed the characters a moment of emotional or physical closeness, let them, and the reader, enjoy that moment. Give them time to reflect on what it means and then move forward toward the next milestone. Just be sure you never bring the book to a halt. Vary the tempo, but don't stop it in its tracks.

Pacing and Plotting: Two Halves of a Whole

The first thing you need to know is that pacing and plotting go hand in hand. Your plot is concrete, made up of events that move in succession and create your story. *Pacing* is a key technique for both structuring those elements and writing about them. If you have a strong, interesting plot, the reader already wants to turn the pages. If you know the tricks of successful pacing, you can make her want to turn those pages even faster. First, you need to figure out how to recognize the key elements of your story (the plot), which are the building blocks you use to then create pacing that works.

TIP

Good pacing is more about structural decisions than about your actual writing. A lot of would-be authors don't know that. Now that you do, you're a step ahead because you can — and should — think about pacing from the moment you start conceptualizing your story's plot points.

Knowing what readers care about

If the only things that made readers turn pages were action, action, and more action, things would get really boring really quickly, because everything would be the same. Your characters don't need to be running around doing exciting things all the time in order for your book to move. Even if you do write a more action-oriented romance, you still need to break up that action.

Mystery, suspense, and adventure plots, or any kind of a search (for treasure, for the truth about someone's past or a child's parentage, for a cure or other scientific discovery, or for the answer to a secret) have a built-in momentum. To achieve effective pacing, you need more than an exciting plot. You have to be able to recognize the romance story beats, or the key plot points that need to happen in each romance, before you can use your action effectively.

Recognizing key plot points

Your plot should include certain key events, what I call *milestones*. With a few major exceptions, the specifics vary from book to book, because your story is never exactly like anyone else's. Those few exceptions are crucial, though, because every romance needs to contain certain important events, whether internal or external. Internal story beats deal with emotions, while external plot points are what is happening in the world outside of them.

There are three basic kinds of key plot milestones:

>> **Key setup points:** The couple's first meeting and the seeds of their emotional tension need to come out quickly.

>> **General romance-novel developments:** These include the basic progression of any romance: the back-and-forth progress of their growing physical and emotional intimacy, including the realization (and eventual admission) of love.

>> **Book-specific points:** These are the key events only you can decide, because they relate only to your book and your characters, not to anyone else's.

You can use all of these points to pace your story. What they share lies in the reader's attitude toward them — anticipation. She wants to see each milestone reached and handled.

REMEMBER

In the order they normally occur, the milestones that all romances share are

1. **The first meeting:** Whether they knew each other before the book begins or are literally meeting for the first time, the scene in the book where your hero and heroine initially see each other is the first milestone you reach — and the first one the reader is eager to reach with you, even before she's read page one. It's also the one time you shouldn't delay in giving the reader what she wants. (For more information on choosing a starting point for your novel and creating that all-important first meeting, see Chapter 12.)

2. **Confrontation:** At least once, and often several times throughout your book, your hero and heroine need to talk or, more likely, argue about the external issues keeping them apart, the external tension that creates a structure for working out their internal and emotional issues. They may also discuss their emotional conflict at some point, but be careful: Discussing it can conceivably lead to solving it, which can't happen until the end of the book.

3. **Physical attraction:** Whether these scenes contain only a meaningful touch of the hand or a chaste kiss (the most you're likely to find in an inspirational or sweet romance), fully consummated lovemaking, or anything in between, the reader is expecting to find love scenes in your book. That expectation keeps her turning pages.

4. **The realization of love:** This realization actually happens twice, once when the heroine realizes she loves the hero and once when he realizes he loves her. She's usually the first to figure it out, but the order is up to you. Go with what works for your characters and their story.

5. **The mutual confession of love, The End:** Although the confession may not literally be the end of your book — you may need an epilogue to tie up loose ends, for example — you should keep it as close to the actual end as possible. The moment when the hero and heroine admit their feelings, talk out the last of their issues, and assure each other (and the reader) that happily ever after is in the offing presents everything that your reader has come for — and everything you've paced the story to reach.

In many cases, your book follows one of the well-known romance plot tropes, which I describe in Chapter 19, and each of those tropes comes with one or more milestones of its own. A *trope* is simply a well-loved plot device you see often, like enemies to lovers or a marriage of convenience. Table 10-1 contains some major milestones associated with (but not limited to) specific tropes.

TABLE 10-1   ## Common Setups and Related Milestones

Trope	Milestone	Comments
Pregnant heroine	Baby's birth	If your heroine's pregnant, your reader's going to be waiting eagerly for this moment.
Marriage of convenience	The wedding	If you set up a marriage-of-convenience story, you want to show the wedding — and the wedding night. Whether everything happens between them or nothing does, the tension — both sexual and emotional — is bound to be high, so use it to your advantage.
Amnesia	Memory regained	Ninety-nine percent of the time, an amnesiac character regains their memory, or at least they discover their past, even if their actual memory never returns. Your reader is as eager to know the whole story as the characters are, giving them an additional reason to turn the pages.
Woman in jeopardy	Danger and escape	A successful suspense plot involves putting your heroine in genuine jeopardy and then getting her out of it. Unless you're writing a series of books built around the pursuit of the same bad guy, you want to either kill off your villain or bring him to justice, too.
Secret baby	Parentage revealed	The fun of a secret-baby plot lies in knowing that the secret of "Who's the daddy?" doesn't stay secret forever. At some point, the hero finds out, and the reader knows all sorts of hell will break loose then and looks forward to seeing it.
Mystery	Key clues revealed	If you're building your plot around a mystery, you need to dole out clues as the book progresses and effectively time the solution for the greatest effect.

In the course of your own story, though, you set your reader up to expect all sorts of individual milestones. I can't pretend to know all the milestones you may want to put in your story, but here are some examples, which I've made reasonably specific, just so you have an idea of what I'm talking about:

>> **Who wins?** If your hero and heroine are rival Thoroughbred trainers, both hoping to win the Kentucky Derby, your reader needs to know how the race turns out. The same principle applies to any kind of contest: Let your reader know who wins.

>> **The outcome of a legal case.** If you write about a custody case and your hero and heroine are opposing counsel, you need to tell the reader how the case turns out.

>> **A holiday or family gathering.** The simplest things can create the most stress, and your reader wants to know how your characters fare when they meet each other's families or celebrate the holidays — always an emotional time. You can add that stress to the emotional tension they're already dealing with.

>> **Can the ranch be saved?** Can the business stay solvent? Will the restaurant go under? If you ask the question as part of your plot, your reader expects you to answer it.

Plot-related milestones are only part of the picture. Your characters' emotions and the slow dance of the developing relationship provide the other piece.

Reaching key emotional moments

Every step in the development of the romance is like something out of a dance — two steps forward and one step back — until finally the music stops and your hero and heroine end up in each other's arms. (For more on this two steps forward, one step back approach to plotting, check out Chapter 5.)

The biggest steps — the characters recognizing their own feelings, love scenes, the final declaration of love — are so big that they operate as plot points. Throughout your book, there are also smaller developments that don't act as turning points for the plot, but are still important.

REMEMBER

Every encounter between the hero and heroine should have the development of the romance as its subtext. The reader is looking for that development in their scenes together. If they had a fight, how does it affect them the next time they see each other? What happens the next time they have an opportunity to make love? After they've made love or just shared their first kiss, how do they react to each other the next time they meet?

Every action has a consequence, and nothing matters more to the reader than emotional consequences. Just as she looks forward to seeing each plot point settled, she anticipates even more *how* each new development in the romance will be settled. Keep each of these emotional steps in mind. Those steps, combined with the milestones of your plot, are the building blocks of your pacing.

It's not only what happens, it's when and where

After you can recognize the key elements of your plot, you're ready to start thinking about pacing. Everything's in how you present your key elements, both when and where.

REMEMBER

Pace yourself and you pace your book. Don't be in a hurry to tell the reader everything you know or everything that's going on. Be stingy. Keep your reader wanting more, and she'll love you for it. By introducing elements as you need them, when and where they can do you the most good, you give the reader reason to keep going. There will always be something happening and she will always be compelled to know what's next. *Key exception:* You definitely shouldn't make your reader wait for the first meeting between the hero and heroine. But from that point on, you, as the author, should be doing the same two steps forward, one step back dance that the hero and heroine do.

Even though your reader assumes the book's going to end happily, she doesn't know every step of the journey she, along with the heroine, must take to get there, so don't spoil the surprise. Imagine picking up a book and reading this first paragraph:

> *Melanie woke up and stretched, and then looked down at her sleeping husband. Her brand-new, gorgeous, sleeping husband. To think she'd once thought he was a killer in an angel's body. Instead, he was one of the good guys, the DEA's top agent. He'd saved her life, and now, as she lay back down beside him and cuddled up against his muscular chest, she realized that he'd saved her heart, as well. She sighed contentedly and thought back to how it all began.*

Okay, I'm exaggerating, but don't take away the reader's fun. Don't rush through things in the mistaken impression that hurrying equals pacing. Take all the key elements of your plot and your romantic development, and introduce them one at a time in ways that make logical sense. Let each element act as a question, a case of "What happens next?" or "How can this problem be fixed?" Then delay answering that question.

I'm not advocating that you diagram every chapter (unless that works for you, in which case . . . go for it), but I can lay out the beginning of Melanie's story the way it should be told in the following list so that you can see what I mean:

>> **The meeting:** Melanie, who's just been downsized, is at the bank depositing her final paycheck, when masked and armed robbers burst in. The cops come and round up two of the robbers; the third gets away, taking Melanie hostage. He forces her, at gunpoint, to drive him away in her car. When he takes off his mask, she realizes he's gorgeous — but he's also tough, and the situation's terrifying. The day has just gone from bad to impossibly awful.

>> **Confrontation:** Melanie wants out, offers him the car, and promises not to say which way he was heading. But he's not buying it. They retreat into silence. She's terrified, but at the same time, she doesn't feel in any physical danger, because something about the man tells her he won't harm her. He's too gentle with her. Rafe (the robber) wishes he could tell her the truth, which isn't specified, but he knows she'd be in even more danger if he did.

>> **Physical attraction:** They're forced to spend the night in the car. Rafe ties her to him with some rope he finds in her trunk. Sometime in the chilly night, they

end up snuggled together for warmth. When they wake up in each other's arms, they're both embarrassed and feeling awkward — and strangely attracted. The next day, as they drive, the conversation is far-ranging and fascinating. She finds herself wishing he were a normal man, not a criminal. And she keeps remembering how good it felt to wake up in his arms.

>> **Suspense:** Melanie tries to escape when Rafe stops for gas and a phone call. He drags her back into the car, but not before she overhears him talking to someone about "what he should do with her." Suddenly really scared, she withdraws as they continue to drive. He feels terrible because earlier, when they were talking, he'd found her the most interesting — and attractive — woman he'd ever met.

>> **The kiss:** That night, he finds a cheap motel, barricades the door with his bed so she can't escape, and they warily get ready for bed. She asks him again to let her go and tries a little flirting to sweeten the discussion. They kiss, and both get carried away by the passion, but then she remembers it's all an act, that he's a criminal, and he reminds himself that she has ulterior motives. They break off the kiss, both breathless, both wishing things could be different. The inner conflict grows here, because they both want to find love, but neither thinks it's possible.

That's probably two or three chapters, at least. This is how I parcel out information and introduce complications (plot-related and emotional) to keep the reader interested throughout:

>> **Start the action with a bang.** Begin at a point that intrigues the reader, that involves her emotionally or makes her want to see what happens next. I start with the heroine having a lousy day, something every reader can identify with, and then getting caught in a life-and-death situation, making the reader want to see what happens next.

>> **Withhold information.** Instead of revealing right away that the hero's with the DEA (Drug Enforcement Administration), I hid that fact, not only from the heroine but from the reader. I made it clear that there's more to him than meets the eye, but I didn't say what he's hiding, so the reader keeps reading because they want to figure it out. Many authors would explain right away, to the reader and possibly even the heroine, that the hero was with the DEA, but revealing his real position gives away a useful tool for pulling the reader along through the book.

>> **Create sexual tension.** I made Melanie and Rafe clearly attracted to each other, but I didn't pay off on the sexual tension right away. When I did let them get close, I cut it off at a kiss and left them both wanting more — and thinking more is impossible.

>> **Take two steps forward and one step back.** I let Melanie and Rafe talk and feel more comfortable with one another, developing a level of intimacy between them, and then introduced additional suspense, which made her reassess the situation and back off, just as I let them kiss and forced them to stop.

You could try and cram all those things and more into the first chapter, but it would be too fast-paced and wouldn't hold the reader's interest. First, you can't keep up that level of pacing, and second, you must give your reader time to care about your characters. If you go too fast, your reader won't care enough about your characters to keep reading.

Knowing what to tell and what to leave out

Understanding the structural side of pacing your book involves not only knowing how and when to introduce information, but also knowing what information to include and, just as important, what to leave out.

You're telling a story, and your job is to take away everything that doesn't contribute to that story. Everything that's left is what belongs in your book. If you make sure that everything you include has a purpose, and structure the book according to the key elements I discuss in the previous section, your pacing can work for you, not against you.

A good storyteller picks and chooses what to tell because it serves the story and because it moves the story forward. Including any one of the following items is a problem. Many novice writers indulge in two or even all three, which makes the story drag:

>> **Factual digressions:** Whether a piece of information you want to include is really interesting or not, if the story doesn't need it, cut it. Be ruthless. Yes, the farming practices of 16th-century France and the state of 21st-century genetics are fascinating (well, to some people), but if information you turn up in your research doesn't move the story forward, leave it out. (See Chapter 13 for the complete scoop on avoiding information overload.)

>> **Every thought and feeling:** Unedited, stream-of-consciousness writing doesn't belong in a romance novel. Real people's thoughts go all over the map. They're momentarily distracted by sounds or smells, and they go off on long mental digressions about childhood and favorite meals. To make their characters seem real, many novice authors include all those digressions in their books, stopping the action dead and causing the reader to lose interest.

>> **Too much description:** You absolutely need some description. Description sets the scene and helps the reader enter the world of the story. On the other end of the spectrum, too much description — passages that go on too long or descriptions of every single outfit, room, city, or minor character — slows the book down. The reader stops wondering what's going to happen next because, from her point of view, nothing is happening at all.

TIP

Never fall in love with your own prose. That's a sure way to forget what matters and slow your story down to the point that it gets lost in a welter of pretty but ultimately useless words. After you write a chapter, take a pragmatic look at it and ask yourself, "What happened in this chapter?" If nothing much actually happened, go back and look for what you can cut, or where you can add some action to move the story forward.

Avoiding the Dreaded Sagging Middle

One of the most common problems aspiring writers run up against is the sagging middle, when a strong beginning and a compelling ending bracket a central section that can be slow at best, and boring at worst. This problem is one of the biggest that you can have in terms of pacing, because it can go on for a hundred pages or more. Some readers may be willing to forgive a paragraph or two that go off on a tangent, but no one's willing to skim the entire middle of a book in hopes that things eventually pick up at the end.

Recognizing a sagging middle

Seeing your book's sagging middle can be tough, because you like your characters and your story, so everything that happens interests you. You need to make yourself look at your novel objectively and see if your story has any of these tell-tale signs:

>> **A lot of time with the hero and heroine apart:** When your hero and heroine are apart, the romance can't move forward. The reader sees them leading separate lives rather than working through their issues so they can lead a life together. Like every rule, this has exceptions, where your characters might be able to grow fonder of each other while they are apart, but in most cases this backfires and the romance stagnates. My advice is to keep them together on the page as much as possible.

>> **Lack of tension:** The reverse of having the heroine and hero apart is to keep them together and essentially perpetually dating. They spend a lot of time in

each other's company and getting along just fine; any tension is dealt with or, worse, forgotten.

» **Much ado about nothing:** Everyone seems busy, but nothing's really happening. People are shopping, eating, rounding up cattle, negotiating contracts, renovating houses, hosting parties . . . all kinds of busy work, but nothing's moving the story forward, and the romance is static. Maybe the hero and heroine are never alone together in the middle of all the pointless action, or maybe they're just too busy with the mundane details at hand to deal with anything important. Either way, it's like sleight of hand, with all the fuss trying, whether consciously or subconsciously, to divert the reader's attention from the fact that the middle of the story tells her nothing important.

» **A lot of recapping and repetition:** Characters either spend a lot of time talking about things the reader has already seen earlier in the book or the same kinds of scenes and conversations recur, so that the story and, more importantly, the romance, never move forward.

» **Sudden focus on secondary characters:** The secondary characters move abruptly or inexplicably into the foreground, shifting the focus away from the central romance and on to the secondary characters' lives and relationships.

Basically, if your book suddenly seems to lose momentum, if you lose your focus, the middle is sagging.

Stopping the sag before it starts

If you find fixing a sagging middle difficult, the best thing you can do is keep your book lean, mean, and moving from the get-go. There are some techniques you can use during your writing process to avoid a sagging middle. This advice is especially applicable early on in your writing career, when you use the process less intuitively than you may after you have a few manuscripts under your belt. By keeping these strategies at the top of your mind, you increase your chances of avoiding Sagging Middle Syndrome (hereafter SMS):

» **It all starts with plotting.** The single biggest cause of SMS is poor plotting. You simply don't have enough story happening to support the length of the book. You haven't added enough complexity to the emotional issues. This problem is as common in shorter books as it is in longer books. If you're an outliner, go back to your outline and add in complexity. If you're a discovery writer, add more complexity into the plot as you write. (See Chapter 7 for more on both writing methods.)

» **Keep the action incremental.** After the first few chapters, it's easy to feel as if you need to tell the reader what's going on and make your characters hurry up and deal with things, both emotionally and plot-wise. Don't do it. Keep things moving piecemeal and remember all the lessons of pacing that this chapter offers. Those lessons apply throughout the entire book, not just long enough to get the reader hooked. Effective pacing not only engages her in the beginning, but also keeps her reading until she's reached the final page.

» **Make sure everything that happens matters.** Knowing that the middle of your book is a potential danger zone, keep an especially tight rein on yourself during the crucial central section of your book. Consciously focus on the key elements of the romance and the plot. Don't let yourself get sidetracked by your research, your secondary characters, or anything else.

» **Stay flexible about your goals.** Some romances can't possibly be satisfactorily told in 75,000 words (in which case, SMS is never going to be the problem), while others can't be made to fill 100,000–150,000 words, no matter how talented a writer you are. In some cases, you may set out to write a 125,000-word mainstream book and then realize that the story you're telling, and already emotionally involved with, just isn't big and complex enough. In that case, you have to decide whether to abandon it or rethink your goals and aim for a shorter length and, often, a different market. Your idea may be perfect for series romance, and a well-told series romance trumps a sagging mainstream any day.

Dealing with it

Sometimes, despite your best efforts, you end up with SMS anyway. You may not even know it until a critique partner or an editor tells you that your book's sick and you need to get it to the ER (Editing Room), stat. The situation may be critical at that point, but it's not necessarily fatal.

You have a couple of options to consider. Truthfully, they don't always work. Some books, despite the author's best intentions, will never be publishable. If that happens with your manuscript, you need to look at it as a learning experience and move on to other story ideas. (Several well-known authors suggest writing five or six books before trying to publish, and with good reason. Practice is very beneficial.) Before you reach the point of no return, here are a couple of operations — er, options — you can consider:

» **Major surgery:** Despite being the most dramatic-sounding option, this procedure is actually the simplest. You may find that you can simply delete whole chunks of your book, sometimes whole chapters at a time, write transitions to stitch together the remaining important pieces, and end up with a shorter, tighter romance that works.

>> **Grafting:** If the problem is with a lack of complexity in the emotional tension or the plot, you may have to start rethinking from the beginning and create believable complications that let you replace the sagging section with components that are more effective.

You may have more challenges with grafting than with the surgical option, because it's much more complicated and requires a lot more rewriting. You will need to go to the beginning of the book and thread in new information little by little in a lot of different places — conversations, thoughts, and events. You can't just drop it into the story in big chunks, or it feels clunky and artificial, and the book still won't come together. If you do it well, though, you can effectively save a book that wasn't working otherwise.

TIP

If neither major surgery nor grafting can save your manuscript, don't consign it to the garbage or use it to light your next fire. Put the manuscript at the bottom of a drawer, in a file on your hard drive, or wherever else it will be out of sight and mind. Get it out again in a year or two, and you may be surprised to find that you've learned so much during that time away that now you can fix it. At the least, you'll see how much your writing skills have improved.

Show It, Don't (Always) Tell It

There is more than just structural considerations related to plot and conflict that controls pacing. Storytelling choices also have a strong effect. I discuss two key aspects of your writing — your voice and your characters' voices — in chapters 8 and 9, respectively, but I talk about them here specifically in terms of pacing.

Keep the writers' adage of "Show, don't tell" in mind when you're thinking about pacing, but be aware that it's an oversimplification. Both showing (through dialogue) and telling (through narrative) have a role to play.

Harnessing the power of dialogue

Generally speaking, *dialogue* (which, for the purposes of this chapter, means only the characters' true spoken words, and does not include point of view and internal monologue) moves more quickly than narrative. Spoken sentences, generally shorter than the more "writerly" ones you create for the narrative sections, have a momentum of their own. One character's dialogue leads naturally into the next, so the reader doesn't stop to think or get distracted. At the same time, you also have to avoid the trap of using too much dialogue.

Speeding up the pace

The more well-written dialogue you include, the more quickly your book moves. Some readers even flip through a book before they buy it to see whether it has a lot of dialogue because, whether consciously or subconsciously, they're looking for a fast read, and they know a dialogue-filled book gives it to them. Written dialogue, if it sounds natural, makes for quicker pacing for a number of reasons:

>> **It feels like a real conversation.** Like a real conversation, the reader doesn't want to turn away, to stop paying attention even for a moment, because she may miss something. The dialogue isn't going to disappear if she looks away, but the illusion works. You're in much less danger of your reader putting the book down while she's reading dialogue than when she hits an extended narrative passage.

>> **It provides a direct link with the characters.** Dialogue creates an immediate "you are there" feeling. Instead of observing a scene, the reader feels as if she's right in the middle of it. Her identification with the heroine increases, making the reader feel as if everything that's happening to the heroine is really happening to her. That sense of identification allows her to read more quickly — she has something personal on the line.

>> **It's easy to read.** Dialogue also works to power your pacing in a purely visual way. As I discuss in Chapter 9, good dialogue sounds real. Most of the time, people speak briefly — short sentences, short paragraphs. Then the next person speaks, and then back to the first, and so on. Because of that natural back-and-forth pattern, formatted dialogue results in a lot of white space on the page, which looks a lot less daunting than long, dense paragraphs of narration. In a way, this pacing tool is purely psychological, because words are just words. However words are arranged on the page, readers process each individual word at a consistent rate. Dialogue-heavy pages read faster than pages filled with prose simply because they contain fewer words. The quicker the page reads, the more quickly the reader can turn it. The act of turning pages quickly is exciting for a reader, making her speed up even more to keep turning them.

Avoiding the pitfalls

Over-using dialogue as a pacing tool has its pitfalls:

>> **Dialogue has its limits.** Using dialogue as a way to describe a scene, relate action, or convey a character's thoughts is often a mistake. Having two characters sit down and deliver a bunch of explanation disguised as dialogue is awkward. You can have one character explain to another what's going on at times, but those times are few and far between, and you need to keep the

explanation relatively brief. Otherwise, the speaker stops sounding like a real person. The minute that happens, the reader's pulled right out of the book and back to reality.

For the same reason, having your characters talk about their feelings endlessly, or describe what they're physically doing at every moment, doesn't feel believable. It's stiff, fake, and turns readers off.

>> **Too much of anything gets boring.** Readers love dialogue for a lot of good reasons, but a steady diet of it bores them. Hundreds of pages that look and, essentially, sound the same are a turn-off.

>> **All your eggs are in one basket.** Excessive dialogue means your dialogue-writing skills have to be perfect. With a book full of dialogue, the reader has no other elements to fall back on if she's turned off by a particular character's voice or can only take so much of "listening" to a particular person. You run the same risk if you tell a story purely from the first person point of view, which is something to be aware of especially if you're writing in first person. If the reader likes the character's voice, you win, but if not . . . you lose.

A book that relies too heavily on dialogue ends up one of two ways:

>> **Too little:** The telling of the story may sound shallow and incomplete, because you have to leave out so many things that the reader wants to know. In this case, the story is weak and not captivating.

>> **Too much:** The characters explain every detail, making your story sound false and uninvolving. In this case, the story is annoying and tedious.

Telling it like it is: Using narrative effectively

Narrative is just as much a part of good pacing as dialogue, even though writers frequently don't think of it that way. In fact, it seems to me that many writers think that narrative gets in the way of good pacing. I think too many writers tend to view pacing as something speedy and nothing else. Plus, authors misuse narrative more often than dialogue. Overall, readers are more likely to complain when they think a book is boring, which often means slow, rather than too exciting or too fast-moving. (It's also much more common to see books that move too slowly than books that move too quickly.)

Narrative allows you to compensate for what dialogue can't do. Narrative and internal monologue let you do everything from laying out the basics of what's happening to letting the reader know your characters' most secret thoughts.

All those things are crucial to creating a great romance novel, but in order not to trip up your pacing, you need to know how to use narrative effectively.

REMEMBER

Here's the key: As much as possible, break your narrative sections into bits. Tactics include:

>> **Avoid long paragraphs.** Pages filled with long paragraphs of densely packed prose look off-putting, even intimidating. Just from a visual standpoint, shorter paragraphs are more approachable, more manageable, and read more quickly. If you have paragraphs that fill almost an entire page, break that paragraph into three or four. If you do have a lengthy paragraph, follow it with one that's only a few lines long, almost as a reward for the reader. The opposite is also true: Too many short paragraphs can make your work look choppy, so be aware of this as well.

>> **Cut off a scene before it's actually over.** This tip goes along with what I say in the "It's not only what happens, it's when and where" section earlier in this chapter. Don't end every scene with things resolved. Sometimes you can leave the reader hanging without telling her how things turned out. She wants to know what happened, so you're urging her to keep reading — pacing at its most effective.

>> **Move between points of view.** Whether you're using full-blown internal monologue or just dropping into different characters' points of view for a line or two, if you move between different characters' minds, you're creating the kind of variety that keeps a reader interested. Just don't do this so much that it becomes confusing.

>> **Punctuate narrative with dialogue.** Instead of paragraph after paragraph of description, action, or internal monologue, break up narrative with dialogue. You may be able to add just a line, or you may have room for an exchange of several speeches. No matter how long your dialogue, it makes the page look more readable and keeps the reader directly connected to the characters and their world.

If true dialogue isn't possible — if only one character's on scene, for example — you can always have them talk to themselves. Be careful that you don't overdo it, though. It can start to seem self-conscious and awkward, even silly.

>> **Work narrative into dialogue tags.** As much as you can, break the narrative bits down into small, discrete pieces that you can attach to a line of dialogue. Rather than just using *she said,* go for *she said, picking up her suitcase and heading out the door.* This small change camouflages the narrative bit, slipping it under the radar, and gets the information across without calling any attention to itself.

Working together, the last two points in the preceding list can really keep your book moving without giving short shrift to getting across the necessary information. You also want to use narrative for the important task of slowing things down when you want to give the audience a breather or time to think, or to vary the pacing to keep the reader fresh.

As with dialogue, you may encounter some dangers in overusing narrative. You're probably already aware of the first — and biggest — danger: Too much narrative, no matter how interesting the subject, can bring your book to a screeching halt. A second danger, one that you may easily overlook, comes with the temptation to put things into narrative that you can put into dialogue simply because it's so easy to just keep going and explain things in what's essentially your own voice.

As a general rule, if you can put something in dialogue, you probably should.

Finding the balance between showing and telling

To create successful pacing, you need to reach the most effective balance between showing and telling. That balance is different for every book you write, so you need to make conscious decisions as you go. It's not just a matter of deciding on a ratio of x percent this to y percent that, or of creating some kind of diagram that you can apply to every manuscript.

First, you need to think about the ideal pacing for the story you're telling. Here are a few examples:

>> A suspense or adventure plotline probably moves more quickly than a more intimate, family-oriented novel.

>> The pace of life in the era you've chosen influences a historical romance. If it was a time of high tea and leisurely social calls, that needs to be reflected in your storytelling.

>> A steamy book feels driven by the characters' passion for each other, which adds intensity and a push to the pacing.

>> An inspirational romance probably makes room for slower-paced, thoughtful scenes as the characters consider faith and its place in their lives.

After you've decided on the ideal tempo of the pacing, you need to keep that in mind as you write, making sure that your pacing fits with the kind of story you've chosen. As you write each individual scene, think about its role in the overall story. Does it galvanize things? Or does it slow them down to provide a breather? Does it give the reader key information? Does it lull the reader into a false sense of security? Does it make her think? Does it shock her? After you answer the question of each scene's purpose, you will know how to pace that scene and how it fits into the whole.

Once you know the pacing you want to achieve with a scene, you can look at the practicalities of that scene — whether it consists mainly of conversation, action, description, or whatever — and figure out the most effective way to execute it. You can figure out where you can — and where it makes sense to — use dialogue, point of view, or internal monologue to tell your story, which all have a more personal feel. Don't forget that you need narrative, too, and you can use that narrative thoughtfully, for the fullest effect. Ask yourself which style works better in every scene and at every moment.

Vary the proportions of one style to another, always being conscious of how each comes across to a reader. Not only should you make every word in your book the result of a conscious decision on your part, but you should also plan out your bigger choices, too. Your awareness of everything you do pays off in the end. To the reader, everything feels smooth, natural, and seamless; the reader never sees the work you put in and the way you're pulling strings all the way through. She only knows that the book works — and moves.

During your final read-through of your manuscript, pay special attention to your book's pacing to see whether you've achieved the overall effect you set out to capture.

Prose That Goes and Prose That Slows

The most important parts of getting your pacing right involve the big decisions: structuring your story properly (not to mention making sure that you have enough story there to structure) and determining what to tell the reader through dialogue and what to tell through narrative. If you get those decisions right, you've already done 90 percent or more of your work.

You can tweak your prose to support your goal, whether that's making things move faster or slowing them down. Here are some tips to keep in mind:

>> **Choose prose that moves.** Instead of saying *He didn't take time to think. He just ran to the car and jumped inside, then took off in pursuit of the kidnappers,* use gerunds. Make the reader participate in the action, and say *Without taking time to think, he found himself running to the car, jumping inside, and taking off in pursuit of the kidnappers.*

>> **Avoid the passive voice.** Passive-voice constructions, by their very nature, distance the reader (and the characters) from what's going on. In an active-voice construction, the character feels or does something: *Rachel felt unhappy with her new job. The attacker hit Jake over the head.* Passive voice involves something being done to the character: *Rachel was made unhappy by her new job. Jake was hit over the head by the attacker.* It puts everything at a distance and makes for a much less effective way of telling a story.

>> **Use short sentences, which move faster than long, complex ones.** This tip especially relates to dialogue, where short sentences in sequence reflect a quicker, more clipped way of speaking. They create a faster rhythm, whether a single character is saying several brief things in quick succession or two characters are exchanging just a few words. In narrative, however, too many short sentences in sequence can end up sounding choppy and off-putting.

By the same token, longer, more complicated sentences — spoken or in narrative — slow the pace, in part because the reader has to put more thought into reading and interpreting those sentences. Their rhythms are different, more flowing, so they pull things back. You can let your reader know that she can breathe again after any kind of an intense scene by shifting the rhythm of your prose from quick and short to medium-length sentences, and then to slower and more thoughtful long ones.

>> **Go for short words that pack a punch.** If you want to make a scene move or create intensity, use short, sharp words, which have a different impact from longer, smoother ones. This distinction is like the one between short sentences and longer ones, only on a mini-level.

>> **Use punctuation to affect pacing.** Ellipses create pauses, and dashes indicate sharp breaks. Commas, which authors frequently don't think much about and often misuse, represent pauses that are shorter than those pauses indicated by ellipses. Because of that, I'm a big fan of using commas inconsistently, leaving them out when you want your prose to move more quickly, putting them in when you want the reader to slow down. Exclamation points reflect excitement and intensity, which speeds up the pacing, too.

>> **Be sparing with your adjectives.** The more adjectives, the slower the pace. Description slows your story down, so don't interrupt a scene that you want to move quickly by interjecting a long description of something. In almost every case, no matter what's going on in your story, you only need one adjective, maybe two. In breakneck scenes, even one adjective may be too many. Describe only what's absolutely necessary, especially in fast-moving scenes.

REMEMBER

As you write, your mind is multitasking to the max: focusing on characterization, logic, narrative versus dialogue, and every single word choice. Don't worry if you don't get it right every time, because that's what you use revisions and multiple drafts for. If you need to dedicate a draft to each part of the process, do it. It's time-consuming, but well worth it.

IN THIS CHAPTER

» **Creating characters through love scenes**

» **Using love scenes to support tension, not diffuse it**

» **Writing love scenes that fit your book's style**

Chapter **11**

Taking It All Off: Writing Love Scenes

A man and a woman who enjoy each other's conversation and company are friends. Add sexual attraction, tension, and, ultimately, lovemaking or the promise of it, and you have a romance. In this chapter, I talk about the key component of any romance, written or real: love scenes. I give you tips on where to place the love scenes in your novel, how to let those scenes help you create your hero and heroine's characters, and how to write the steamy moments so that they contribute emotionally to your book, instead of reading like purely physical asides.

Comparing Sex and Romance

Though sex and romance have a strong and crucial bond in romance novels, they're not the same thing. At its most basic, sex is a purely *physical* act. Romance, by definition, involves *emotion*. Although not every romantic act (flowers on a special occasion, breakfast in bed) is physically sexual, every sexual act in a romance needs emotional underpinnings. In a romance novel, a love scene involves just that: *love,* even if the characters don't realize it yet.

Emotion mixes with the physicality of sex, and the proportions of each vary based on the specifics of your intended market, your characters, and your plot. Ultimately, no lovemaking scene is ever purely sexual, even though it can be highly sensual, physical, and erotic. Even the most erotic romances (which aren't the same as pure erotica) are still romances, and the sexual encounters between the sheets lead to a romantic conclusion.

REMEMBER

The focus of a traditional male/female romance novel is on the developing relationship — both emotional and, in most cases, sexual — between one woman and one man. (Sweet romances are the exception in that they don't include steamy love scenes.) Whatever their romantic pasts, your hero and heroine should be monogamous in the course of your book, because the idea that they're meant to be together and just aren't interested in anyone else is part of the fantasy the reader brings to the book. (Of course, there are exceptions, reverse harem being one, but for the most part I recommend that you don't set out to break this rule.)

Knowing Where and When

You have to know where to place the love scenes in your book to make them really effective. Even a beautifully written love scene jars the reader when you put it in the wrong place, making her question the characters — and stopping the book in its tracks. Place the love scenes properly — after the proper buildup — and half your job is done, because the reader will want your characters to get together just as much as the characters themselves do.

Creating sexual tension

A well-written, well-placed, and effective love scene is the result of the sexual tension between your hero and heroine, which slowly builds over the course of your novel. Sexual attraction and tension should begin the minute your characters meet and should be components of every subsequent scene between them, building alongside their emotional tension, so that by the time you finally write that first full love scene, your characters and your reader are ready.

Simply put, *sexual tension* is the inevitable result of making your hero and heroine physically attracted to each other but unable to act on that attraction. The reasons why they can't act are limited only by your imagination — you can place physical, circumstantial, or (best of all) emotional barriers between them. An emotional barrier might be, for example, a past hurt that has scarred the character, making it difficult to overcome those feelings. Every time they get close, those feelings of betrayal and mistrust come up. They want to act, but they can't. Sometimes they get a taste of what they're missing (a touch, a kiss, or even the beginnings of love-making) before they pull back. And that tease only makes the tension stronger.

Think of a kid in the days leading up to Christmas, looking at those presents under the tree, shaking them, trying to read through the wrapping, but unable to open them until Christmas comes. Your hero and heroine should feel that way about each other — only they're not sure that Christmas will ever come. For all they know, they may never be together fully and physically. Every time they see each other, every time they talk, you need to make sure an undercurrent of unresolved sexual tension hums between them.

TIP

Here are some helpful ways to ramp up the tension on the way to a love scene and throughout your book:

>> **Make it obvious.** They may fight it, but your hero and heroine need to be undeniably attracted to each other. A sidelong glance, a casual touch that leaves heat in its wake — subtle signals like these are effective precisely because the characters are fighting their attraction. These signals demonstrate the strength of that attraction because they override common sense and the characters' own intentions. And don't just let the reader know; let the characters know, too, adding an extra edge to their encounters. Even when they're at odds, keep the physical awareness humming in the background.

>> **Keep them on each other's minds.** They may not be happy about the fact that they can't stop thinking about and being attracted to each other, but they can't do anything about it. The longer the book goes on, the more they want each other — and the more the reader wants them to get together, too. Right in the middle of a contract negotiation, the hero is assaulted by thoughts of the heroine. And she's thinking of him right then, too, as she tries to call a fractious class of third graders to order. It doesn't always have to be in a positive "wish he were here" kind of way, but they need a gut-level awareness that just doesn't go away.

>> **Make them wait.** Don't let the hero and heroine act on their attraction right away, even — or especially — if the circumstances seem perfect: a moonlit night on the beach, or a hot summer day and a pond just right for skinny-dipping. Frustration feeds tension, so let them feel frustrated and drawn to what they can't have because of those emotional barriers you have set up in previous chapters.

>> **Let them start and then make them stop.** Whether you end a kiss abruptly or allow it to go on for long, slow, wonderful minutes but never let it go any further, give your characters a taste of how good they are together but don't let them go all the way until they just can't stand to be apart (and the reader can't stand for them to be apart, either) anymore.

>> **Leave them wanting more.** No matter how much time they've spent together, whether they shared a single kiss or have spent all night and half the morning tangled up in the sheets — and each other — never let them feel satisfied. The more they have of each other, the more they want of each other.

Deciding when the time's right

Everything in a romance should be character-driven. Your love scenes especially need to follow this rule; those scenes should feel like the characters' decision, not yours. The reader should never see your hand because, to be blunt, no one should be forced into having sex. If the timing doesn't feel natural, you lose the larger sense of romance, of two people being perfect for each other.

As I discuss in the preceding section, sexual attraction and tension should build from the start. Despite that, every time the characters have the chance to act on that tension, they don't (or not all the way). So why now? I can sum up the answer in just one word: motivation. Your characters' motivations should be the true drivers of every aspect of your plot (see Chapter 5), and motivation plays an especially crucial part when it comes to love scenes.

HITTING THE SHEETS BEFORE SHARING THEIR HEARTS

Good love scenes are the natural conclusion to increasing sexual tension. But sometimes physical sex comes before the sexual tension. Or rather, sometimes sex follows immediately after sexual tension becomes evident. For example, the common romance plot of sex with a stranger doesn't work with a long buildup of sexual tension. In a case like that, the sexual tension often follows, when the strangers discover they need to spend time with each other and can't stay strangers. In some of today's most sensuous romances, the hero and heroine are looking for no-strings sex, which they think they've found with each other, so it's only after they get sexually involved that their emotions come into play, too, and sexual tension grows. In both these cases — and quite possibly in others that you can think of — the sexual and emotional development of the relationship turns the usual pattern on its head, following the hero and heroine's sexual involvement rather than preceding it.

When your characters finally get sexually involved, you (and they) need a reason. That reason can't be simply that *you've* decided it's time for a love scene; it has to be *their* reason. That reason is rarely as cut and dried as "(S)he's cute, let's get it on," because most of your readers don't think that way about getting sexually involved, so they don't want the characters to think that way, either. The reader wants to know that the hero and heroine's feelings for each other are involved in their decision, not just their hormones.

REMEMBER

Because you're writing a romance, and because nothing's more intrinsically tied to romance than *love*making, your characters need an emotional basis for their decision to make love. In fact, they may each have their own reason, or even multiple reasons (because people are complex and your characters can be, too). Bringing out these reasons helps develop their characters.

>> **Hero:** Usually the hero is much less conflicted about making love than the heroine. He may hold back because he doesn't want to hurt her or feels he can't offer her a future. Guys connect the physical act with emotion much less than women, and that holds true in romance novels, just as it does in real life. Generally speaking, he doesn't realize that his heart's on the line until later — often much later — in the book.

>> **Heroine:** Your heroine is most likely the one with the most doubts about making love, usually stemming from the fear that a relationship can't possibly work out with the hero, so she's afraid of being hurt beyond repair when (she feels) the inevitable collapse comes. For that reason, she needs to have a definite reason for thinking *now* is the right time.

As the book progresses, sexual tension grows, and emotional conflict (which I discuss in Chapter 5) slowly moves toward resolution. Her decision to make love should come at a point when the tension feels irresistible and the conflict has progressed to a stage where she recognizes this man's importance to her. She must be willing to risk the inevitable pain of a breakup for the sake of storing up memories to live on later. As she reaches this point, she's willing to take the emotional risk of making love to him, leaving herself totally vulnerable. As long as you explain her decision to the reader, who's already feeling the sexual tension and longing to resolve it, the timing of the love scene will be just right.

Using love scenes to increase the tension

Love scenes, properly placed, help build the tension in your book, and create character development as well. They add an extra edge to the emotional tension that's a key component of the relationship and, contradictory as it sounds, love scenes can also help build the sexual tension. Just as a number of factors meet to lead *into* your love scene, you can take real benefits *out* of the scene as you move forward with your story.

Upping the emotional ante

Your characters should move into the love scene thinking, on some level, that making love can resolve things between them. Having made the decision to take their sexual relationship to the next level, they expect exactly that conclusion: a leveling out of the situation, including the emotional roller coaster they've been riding with each other. Instead, they need to discover that nothing's been settled at all. Instead of bringing relief from emotional turmoil, lovemaking leaves things more stormy and confused than ever.

In fact, just as the heroine has to do the most soul-searching going into the love scene, the hero often feels the most confused coming out of it. Heroes, as I discuss in Chapter 4, usually consider themselves impervious emotionally. Your hero most likely thinks that making love with the heroine can be a wonderful, sensual experience that will leave him untouched on any other level. Imagine his surprise to find that his heart's become involved in ways he can't deny. Usually, the last thing he wants to do is to own up to that — to the reality that love makes a person vulnerable, and he's not about to let himself be vulnerable — he has to find ways to hide what he's feeling. He can be angry, curt, condescending, reduce their meaningful interaction to the level of a joke, or anything that fits with his character and doesn't let the heroine know what he's really feeling: that life without her feels emptier than he wants to admit.

Whether in reaction to his behavior or because she's afraid of being hurt and decides to make a pre-emptive strike, the heroine doesn't let on about her feelings, either. So the characters end up feeling more for each other than ever, yet they keep pulling even further apart. The result? The act of lovemaking, which should bring two people even closer together, instead ups the ante on emotional tension and creates more problems for them to spend the rest of the book overcoming. These are all critical aspects to use in your character development arc.

TIP

You can use the couple's emotions to your advantage both during the love scenes and afterward. By shifting into one or both characters' points of view, you let your readers see how much lovemaking means to them. They feel how deeply the characters' emotions are engaged, and how much not being able to confess their true feelings hurts them. Love scenes build a sense of what's at stake for the hero and heroine and, through them, the reader.

Sexual tension feeds . . . on sex?

Sounds contradictory, doesn't it? If you build sexual tension chapter after chapter, until the hero and heroine finally make love, then their lovemaking should release that tension. And it does — for as long as it takes them to exhaust themselves making love. After that, the tension starts building all over again — and it can become even stronger, because now they know how great their lovemaking can be.

Suddenly every accidental touch is filled not only with imagined potential, but also the memory of how wonderful lovemaking was — and increased longing and sexual tension. Their relationship is still a mess, so they can't be like any normal couple and make love whenever they want to, but want to they do. After all, one chocolate chip cookie can't satisfy, and making love with the perfect partner is a whole lot better than cookies. The problem is that cookies are pretty easy to come by, and their feelings don't get hurt. Your characters need to be painfully aware that making things work with the perfect partner is a little tougher.

Using love scenes to support your pacing

After they make love, your characters are still emotionally messed up and filled with sexual tension, the very things that drew your reader eagerly into your love scene in the first place. Because your reader still wants resolution, you haven't lost any steam by letting your hero and heroine — and your reader — have a little fun.

Your reader, like your characters, lands back on square one, still hoping everything can work out, still turning pages waiting to see how things end — and hoping for some more lovemaking along the way.

REMEMBER

That's the beauty of love scenes. Because they don't resolve anything, you can ratchet up the tension, diffuse it temporarily with another love scene that brings your characters closer for a moment and shows them how wonderful things could be between them. Then ratchet it up some more and take the whole roller-coaster ride all over again. Your book keeps moving, and your reader keeps turning the pages.

TIP

All of the advice for effectively timing love scenes, and using them to keep your tension high and your book moving, also applies to any scene involving sexual contact: kissing scenes, unconsummated love scenes — even dreams of lovemaking.

Writing the Scene

After you figure out where to place your love scenes for best effect, you still need to write the scenes themselves. Remember to keep your market and the readers' expectations in mind when you progress to the writing itself.

Knowing your market

As I discuss in Chapter 2, the romance market is a varied one, and just as you don't want to mix Regency mores with a contemporary mystery, you don't want to put a sexy love scene in an inspirational romance or have your medieval characters using birth control. In other words, even readers who read a wide variety of romances — from contemporary romances to western historical romances to romantic comedies to inspirational romances — have varying expectations regarding the frequency, content, and sensuality level of love scenes based on the subgenre they're reading.

Readers who specialize are even stricter in their expectations, so you need to know what's appropriate for the sort of book you're writing. Readers of inspirational romances want a very low level of overt sensuality and no premarital sex. Highly sensual series draw readers who expect a lot of love scenes, a high level of sexual tension, and characters who are inventive when they make love. Mainstream contemporary romances and historical romances have room for varying levels of sensuality, based on the particular characters and plot, so you have a whole continuum along which you can find a spot that feels comfortable for you and your characters. (Check out the "Suiting your language to the market" section later in the chapter for more on market considerations and choosing appropriate love-scene language.)

REMEMBER

What are the best ways to gauge the readers' expectations for love scenes?

>> **Read.** I can't say it often enough: You need to read. Even if you, like many successful authors, don't like to read within your field while you're actively writing, it's important to do your homework before you start. You should read enough that you have a good sense of what your readers are looking for. If you're planning to indie publish (see Chapter 16), read as many successful indie books as you can.

>> **Get the guidelines.** Not every publisher has guidelines for aspiring writers, and some guidelines talk only about what romantic subgenres the publisher is interested in or what length manuscripts they want to see, without addressing levels of sensuality. Other guidelines, however, are more specific. Series

TIP

publishing, because of its nature, often has very specific sensuality requirements, and series publishers do provide guidelines outlining what's appropriate.

If a publisher has guidelines, visit their website to find them and make every effort to follow them. I list other types of writers' resources in Chapter 3, and many of those resources can tell you good sources for guidelines.

It's not what they do, it's how you describe it

Here's where everything I talk about previously in this chapter comes together: in actually writing an intriguing love scene. Most writers think of love scenes as the difficult part. I think that writers who struggle with love scenes often have trouble because they're thinking of the scene in isolation, basing it solely on the mechanics of lovemaking.

REMEMBER

Instead, think of a love scene as an outgrowth of the characters' emotional needs. Love scenes are a key step in the development of the overall relationship, and in the pacing of the book. With emotions in mind, the actual writing becomes easier. You'll have the motivational basis for your scene already figured out, and you don't have to count on the physical act of lovemaking alone to carry the weight of the scene.

Because you can feel fairly sure that everyone in your audience has a pretty good idea of the mechanics of sex, that frees you up from having to describe the whole "Tab A into Slot B" thing. You need to indicate what's happening, but not in clinical terms — in emotional ones.

Focusing on feelings

Don't just explain what the characters are doing, but focus on how they feel about what they're doing. What goes through the heroine's mind as the hero strokes the soft skin of whatever body part you choose? She's aroused, of course, but use her point of view to give emotional weight to the act, as well.

>> Is she a virgin? Perhaps she's surprised that a man — especially this man — can make her feel a pleasure she never dreamed possible.

>> Is she a total tomboy? Feeling so feminine, so much a woman, may amaze her. And she also can be amazed by finding a man who appreciates her strength yet sees into her vulnerable heart.

>> Is she divorced from a man who made her feel inadequate in every way, especially in bed? How delightfully shocking to find out he was wrong, because *this* man clearly finds her a total turn-on, and yet how sad to think it can never last.

The same idea holds true for your hero, who finds your heroine both physically exciting and unexpectedly emotionally affecting. Be sure to include his point of view and feelings, as well.

As I discuss earlier in this chapter in the "Deciding when the time's right" section, everything grows from your characters, so think about what each of them needs and how you can fulfill that need via their lovemaking. So long as neither confesses it to the other, you can even use lovemaking as a catalyst for one or both of them to realize that they're in love and that they want this — both the lovemaking and the relationship — to go on forever, in and out of the bedroom.

Matching language with the moment

You're writing about a sensual moment in the relationship, so use words that go beyond the basics and have sensual implications. The hero can just touch her, but even better, he can stroke her or slide his palm along her flesh. She can kiss him back, or she can nibble his earlobe and tease her lips along his jawline to his mouth. Although I'm a big proponent of "less is more" when using adjectives and adverbs, a love scene is a good place to loosen up on that rule a bit. Kissing, caressing, and lovemaking are a lot more interesting to the reader than any other landscape. Your reader won't mind spending some extra time on both what's going on and how the characters feel about it. In addition, love scenes are all about building up feelings and connections in an atmosphere that's conducive to both. Extra descriptors can be a big help on that score.

Feel free to use words with emotional implications. Your characters can't say that they love each other, but they can love what they're doing to each other. Their hearts, not just their bodies, can respond to each other. They can exalt, celebrate, triumph, and more. The feelings they can't admit to themselves, much less to each other, out of bed can surface during lovemaking. Even though they can't be expressed openly, those feelings color everything that follows.

TIP

You don't want to use an adjective or an adverb to modify everything, but carefully used, they can bring an extra dimension to the scene. No "wham, bam, thank you, ma'am" here. Even if your hero and heroine are so excited that they practically race to the finish line, they do so because they feel an insatiable hunger for each other, so sounds (like the quick rasp of a zipper) shiver along the heroine's aroused nerve endings. Or maybe seduction happens slowly. Sensations are soft, textures are silky, and heat rises in waves along the hero's skin.

Suiting your language to the market

Here's where all that reading comes in handy. If you know your market, you know how far you can go not only in terms of what the characters do (see the "Knowing your market" section earlier in this chapter), but in terms of how explicit you can be in describing it. Sometimes you need to stick entirely to euphemisms and vague descriptions, but in other cases, you can be as explicit as you want in naming body parts. Most of the time, you find yourself falling somewhere between those two extremes (sort of the way movies show breasts and butts but not full frontal nudity, even though they make it clear what's going on). But don't try so hard not to call a spade a spade (or a penis a penis) that you resort to euphemisms that sound more silly than sexy.

Using all five senses

Lovemaking is a sensuous experience, so use the characters' senses to add effect. Naturally you want to rely on touch, because the scene is all about how your characters are touching each other. Don't forget to include the arousing powers of the other four senses:

>> How does her hair smell when he wakes up and leans over to kiss her?

>> How does the light fall across his face, highlighting his cheekbones and deepening the shadows around his eyes?

>> Is he further aroused to hear her moan in abandon as he parts her thighs?

>> Is his skin salty as she runs her tongue across his chest to his nipple?

TIP

Don't just stick to what's going on when they're together, either; use sense memory to bring them closer by recalling feelings later on. The scent of gardenias reminds him of her signature scent. The feel of a denim jacket as she throws it over her shoulders makes her fingers itch to unzip the jeans he always wears. Let them infiltrate each other's lives on such a basic level that it seems they can never be free of each other.

Letting your setting work for you

Setting can do more than just identify locale; it can work for you in bigger and better ways. (See Chapter 6 to find out how to set the scene.) The setting you choose can also work for you in smaller, more intimate ways, and setting is especially important in a love scene. Your setting can heighten the experience by working in tandem with the hero and heroine's responses or by providing a striking contrast:

- **Work with the moment.** Start with a big, airy bedroom; a king-size four-poster bed with a sheer canopy; satin sheets; candles burning and adding light to the moonlight streaming through the windows; and the scent of roses from a vase on the dresser. Add a hero and heroine slowly exploring each other's bodies and learning each other's responses, reveling in each sensation. Fill the room with sensual cues to enhance your characters' feelings and make the moment sensual on every level.

- **Create a contrast.** Contrast the sensuous magic of lovemaking with an anti-romantic setting, like a cheap motel room with bad lighting, a squashed double bed, threadbare covers, and the sound of a TV from the room next door coming through the thin wall. The heat of passion and the private paradise two people can create can override the handicap of such an unlikely setting, even transform it into something romantic and wonderful, proving the power of the hero and heroine's feelings for each other.

BIRTH CONTROL: NECESSARY OR NOT?

You don't have a problem integrating the birth control question if you're writing historical romances, but you need to think about contraception of some kind if you're writing contemporary romances. Some people feel very strongly that you have to mention condoms, but I think that you need to stay true to your characters and yourself — and also the realities of the situation. If your characters are on the run in the jungle, neither one probably has any condoms on them. But if your hero plans a romantic evening, he can logically stash a few in the drawer of the bedside table. Decide what you and your characters feel comfortable with and let that be your guide.

4

Putting It All Together: Mechanics Count, Too

Chapter **12**

Starting and Stopping

The single most important section of your romance novel that you'll ever sit down to write is the beginning. You want to write a beginning strong enough to compel a reader to spend her money. But even after the first hook, the pressure's not off of you as a writer just yet. Even after you get the opening right, you need to keep your reader's rapt attention on every page. One of the best ways to do that is to start and stop every chapter with enough punch to hold your reader's interest and keep her eager to see what happens next. Then, even within each chapter, you need to structure scenes to create mini-cliffhangers and maintain your hold on the reader's attention.

In this chapter, I talk about the aspects of starting and stopping throughout your book, paying particular attention to the all-important opening, as well as chapter endings and beginnings.

Mastering the Winning Beginning

Any form of entertainment needs a great beginning, and that beginning is even more important when you're talking about a novel. A movie viewer has already paid for their ticket before they sit down in the theater, so they're not likely to walk out unless the movie's really, *really* bad. TV comes right into the viewer's living room, so they can just stay on the couch and keep watching easily enough.

But a novel has to sell itself *before* a reader pays for it. A compelling beginning is your best tool for making them reach for their wallet.

The opening of your romance novel gives you an opportunity to introduce your characters in the most intriguing way. It's where you highlight your plot's most fascinating twists and immediately demonstrate your abilities as a storyteller, all of which combine to convince your reader that she can trust you to hold her interest all the way to the last page.

REMEMBER

If you blow the beginning, you may lose your only chance to win a fan. Ace it — and follow through — and you have a fan not only for that book, but quite possibly for every book you publish.

When you first sit down to write, page one may look very intimidating to you. But for your reader, page one should seem like the exciting beginning of a great adventure. You want to involve your reader from the very first line so that your book stands out in her mind, even if she's not quite sure why your book seems so much more interesting than every other book she's seeing.

TIP

You know your story better than anyone, so you're the best judge of its strengths and which hooks can most likely get — and keep — a reader interested.

You need to begin with a bang, not with a slow buildup. Start with something that grabs your reader and refuses to let go. You need to engage your reader's attention right from the get-go, both intellectually (in terms of what's happening with your plot) and, more importantly, emotionally, because romances are all about feeling — your characters' feelings and what those characters can make your reader feel.

How to hook your reader

A lot of elements need to come into play right at the beginning of your book. Your reader is looking for an immediate introduction to as many of the key components of your novel as possible — character, plot, sexual and emotional tension, and writing style.

REMEMBER

Here are two techniques to hook a reader right off the bat (I explain the actual mechanics of these techniques at length in the "Putting Theory into Practice" section later in the chapter):

>> **Choose an exciting place to begin your story.** If you start your novel in the middle of the action, when something interesting is already happening, your reader wants to keep going to see how it turns out. If the book begins with the

hero and heroine in the middle of an argument, for example, the reader wants to know who wins. Emotional excitement and plot-based excitement are both effective, and a combination of the two is more than the sum of its parts.

>> **Involve the reader right away.** If you make her care about what's happening, she has a vested interest in your story. If you start with your hero and heroine on a sinking ship, you engage your reader on a gut level because you've put her in the middle of a life-or-death situation. She tries to stay afloat right along with your characters — and she keeps reading to be sure everyone's safe. You can't make every situation literally life or death, of course, but you can make every situation *feel* like it is. If you start inside a character's point of view as they deal with something that matters to them, you can make that thing matter to the reader, too.

You're writing a romance, so the hero and heroine — and sparks — should figure prominently from the very beginning. Not every book can or will begin with both the hero and the heroine in the scene together, but whether one or both are present, you have to provide compelling characters from the start. The advice I provide in Chapter 4 on developing strong characters is particularly applicable to your hero and heroine in the beginning — if you don't grab the reader's attention now, she won't give your characters the chance to win her over later, because she'll stop reading. Here are a few points to keep in mind:

>> **Make the reader empathize with your heroine.** Get your reader to identify with your heroine from the start and you increase the likelihood that she'll keep turning pages (and plunk down her money for your book).

>> **Make the reader fall for your hero.** Romances are all about falling in love. When you give your reader a reason to care about your hero from the start (beyond his undeniable good looks), she'll be his 'til the end — and will keep reading to get there.

>> **Make sure your hero and heroine are attracted to each other.** Even though your hero and heroine should be at odds — often quite dramatically — from the beginning, the minute they're together, there should still be an unmistakable spark between them that tells the reader these two people belong together — and assures the reader that she's going to enjoy watching them fall in love.

REMEMBER

From beginning to end, make your reader ask questions. Design your opening so that the reader wants to know the answers to questions like *What's going on? Why is she mad at him? What's he rescuing her from?* Questions and curiosity get your reader involved and keep her reading.

How to bore your reader

Right along with beginnings that guarantee you can hook a reader, there are beginnings guaranteed to turn her off immediately. You want to avoid these open-ing don'ts, because if you turn a reader off at the start, you've probably turned her off forever.

>> **Don't recap the background.** Your reader doesn't care about the details of the Battle of Hastings or the trials of modern-day ranching when she's reading a romance. She'll just move on to another book that gives her the emotional excitement she's craving. Don't start with long descriptions of scenery, the political situation, or what in the heroine's life made her end up in this place at this time. All that information can come later. At the beginning, it just gets in the way of the good stuff.

>> **Don't create a laundry list of character descriptions.** Finding out who your characters are, not what they look like, makes your reader care about them. Instead of providing boring descriptions, use dialogue, character thoughts, and piecemeal details to tell your reader the basics of what a character looks like while also explaining who the character is. Writing *Sabrina's green eyes snapped with anger as she strode into Drake's office* engages the reader much more effectively than writing *Sabrina had bright green eyes.* The first sentence makes the reader ask why Sabrina is angry at Drake. The second sentence is a narrative dead-end that doesn't encourage the reader to find out more.

>> **Don't spend time on unimportant info when you have a story to tell.** Nonessential information only delays your reader from getting to the elements that keep her reading. If you start out with a heroine who's a police hostage negotiator in the middle of a life-or-death situation, no one cares that she has a sister and two brothers, all younger, along with a dog named Murphy — unless one of them is a hostage she's negotiating for. The reader

just wants to know whether the hostages can be saved — and where she will find the hero. Get in the reader's way and she'll put down your book and pick up (and pay for) someone else's.

The cute meet: Necessary or not?

Writers often ask me at conferences whether starting with the cute meet is necessary. This question is usually followed by someone else asking what a cute meet is. A *cute meet* means that you begin your book by introducing your hero and heroine in some unique, memorable, and often humorous way. The possibilities are endless, but here are some examples:

>> Your heroine accidentally backs her car into a handsome stranger's luxury SUV in the company parking lot, and then goes up to her office and discovers that he's her new boss.

>> The hero and heroine are both in law enforcement, and they're investigating the same case, but neither one of them knows it. Approaching from opposite sides of a building, they round the corner and end up aiming their guns at each other.

>> Your hero's furious because his son has been suspended from school and storms into the principal's office to complain — only to find out that the principal's the woman he was flirting with at a party the night before.

>> Strangers Julie Denton and Blake Denton are assigned to share a cabin on a sold-out cruise because someone mistakenly assumed that they're husband and wife.

>> Heroine Jaimie Dickson reports for her first day of work on an oil rig, where her good-looking new boss is shocked to discover that he's hired a woman, not the man her name had led him to expect.

REMEMBER

Should you start your romance novel with your characters' own cute meet (which I hope you can make more original than the examples I just gave)? Ultimately, only you can answer that question. A cute meet has both pros and cons, so you need to weigh both sides of the equation.

First, here are the pros of using a cute meet:

>> **It starts with action.** Action involves the reader immediately, which is one of the two things that a good opening scene does (see the "How to hook your reader" section earlier in this chapter).

- **It helps define the characters.** By showing how they react in an interesting, unexpected, and even stressful situation, your characters stand out as individuals right away. That gives your reader an immediate chance to identify with the heroine and fall for the hero.

- **It can immediately introduce the source of tension.** Even if additional complicating factors show up as the book goes along, the cute meet gives you an opportunity to immediately set up at least part of the conflict the hero and heroine need to overcome, which lets the reader get right to the heart of the story.

- **It's memorable.** Because a good cute meet is unique, the characters and their situation stand out in the reader's mind. A reader wants to follow a story line that's memorable and more than just the same old, same old.

Here are some potential pitfalls to using a cute meet:

- **It can be a cliché.** The first and last examples I give earlier in this section really *are* clichés. These days, you really can't use those examples in a book and make your characters seem unique and their story worth reading. To use a cute meet, you have to work hard to make sure that it's something readers haven't seen before.

- **It can feel contrived.** Cute meets often feel contrived, like something the writer's forcing the characters into, not something real people would ever do or a situation they'd ever find themselves in. If the meeting feels contrived, the reader never believes in the characters. If she doesn't believe in the characters, she won't care about them or their story.

- **It undercuts your characters.** Instead of showing your characters as well-rounded, admirable, interesting people, the cute meet can make them come off as shrill, selfish, sexist, petty, just generally unpleasant, or even stupid. In short, a cute meet can show them as exactly the kinds of characters no reader wants to get to know any further.

- **It sets the wrong tone.** As a word, *cute* implies a certain lightness, and many cute meets *are* light and humorous in tone. That tone works perfectly if you're writing a romantic comedy, but your opening may mislead the reader if the rest of your book is suspenseful or dramatic. She'll either expect a different kind of story than she's going to get and be disappointed in the book, or she won't realize it's actually going to turn into a book she'd like.

- **It misrepresents your conflict.** Sometimes a cute meet tries so hard to be as cute as the name implies that it makes the conflict seem as if it has no depth, because the characters end up arguing over something minor and silly. Instead of introducing the real — and compelling — source of conflict that occupies the rest of the book, the cute meet puts something silly front and center, which can turn off a reader looking for substance.

TIP

After you've weighed the pros and cons in relation to the characters and story you have in mind, ask yourself one all-important question: *If I had never met these characters before and had no idea what their story was going to be, would a cute meet make me more or less likely to continue reading?* If the answer is "more likely," then you definitely want to go for the cute meet.

Putting Theory into Practice

After you realize that you need a sense of excitement to capture a reader's interest, you can decide what point in your story makes for the most effective beginning and how to handle that beginning. You can also create the necessary sense of connection in the reader, making your story matter even more to her.

In the hands of a capable writer, reading about watching paint dry can be exciting. Although I don't recommend that scene for the opening of your romance novel, it does make the point that an exciting scene doesn't have to involve running, driving fast, gunfire, or karate. The excitement comes from watching your character go after what they want, trying to overcome the obstacles you've put in their way. This almost always involves some action on the part of your character, like a conversation with a boss, but it doesn't need to be a car chase to be exciting.

Finding your starting point

The best way to make something — anything — exciting is to start in what writers call, thanks to the ancient Romans, *in medias res* ("in the middle of things"). Don't start your story at the beginning, because beginnings often move slowly and don't seem very interesting until events reach critical mass. You can always go back later and fill your reader in on the details (see the next section, "Backtracking to the background"). Start your romance novel in the middle, when something interesting is already going on.

The *real* beginning of a story — not the place where a novel *should* begin — is often slow, a buildup of details that may seem unimportant and unrelated, even just plain boring, at first. If your romance novel begins at this beginning, you're probably looking too far back in time. Even when you communicate relevant and necessary background info, the reader is likely to find it uninvolving and way too time-consuming, so where *should* you start?

TIP

You need to choose an exciting moment, a moment when something is happening that lets you show off your characters and their situation to best effect. Think of it as the beginning of the story the characters share together, rather than the beginning of the entire story.

Suppose your heroine is sure that her brother has been framed and sent to prison for a crime he didn't commit, and she thinks that the hero is the one who framed him. She decides to confront the hero with her suspicions. That scene's bound to be exciting and full of fireworks, along with the first hints of sexual tension. So why not start with the moment when she walks into his office, ready to bombard him with her suspicions?

Be sure you have a handle on your heroine and hero so that they seem real to you — and therefore to the reader — as soon as they're introduced (see Chapter 4 for more on building characters). Then let your story rip. Get the reader involved — emotionally, intellectually, any way you can — from the first line. Drop her into the action, get her adrenalin flowing, make her care about your characters, and she'll turn pages as fast as she can.

Here are a couple of alternate takes on the scene I just described, where the heroine walks in on the hero, gunning for metaphorical bear. These examples demonstrate not only why this is an effective place to begin a book, but also two techniques for writing that beginning: narrative and dialogue.

You can start with a line or two of narrative:

> *Melody Smith knew she was treading on thin ice when she marched into Derek LaMott's office unannounced, but she was past caring. This man had ruined her brother's life and, by extension, her own, and there was no way on earth she was going to let him get away with it. Derek LaMott was about to pay for what he had done.*

I make a point of staying inside the heroine's point of view to add immediacy to the scene and to create a connection between her and the reader.

You can also start with dialogue and mix in some narration to give your reader a bit of context:

> *"Did you really think you could get away with it?"*
>
> *Derek LaMott looked up from behind his impressive walnut desk. Against her will, Melody Smith found herself momentarily mesmerized by the deep blue gaze he turned her way. Then she caught herself and remembered why she was there: for justice.*
>
> *"Get away with what?" LaMott asked, his deep voice shivering its way up Melody's spine.*

Both approaches work, though I prefer the one that uses dialogue, because I think dialogue adds immediacy to the scene. I also think that you can best get to know someone through the way they speak, and that fact is as true of fictional characters as it is of real people.

Both approaches immediately draw the reader into the story, which is why they both work. They start in the middle of "the thing" and put the reader in the heroine's head so that she cares what happens next. Both approaches also get the reader asking questions: How did Derek ruin Melody's brother's life — and hers? What does she think he got away with? What kind of justice is she looking for, and how does she plan to get it? If the reader is asking questions, she's going to want to keep reading to find out the answers.

The second example also introduces a few salient points about each character and establishes the beginnings of sexual attraction. Every romance needs that element of attraction. The sooner you demonstrate that your hero and heroine feel it for each other, the better.

Both openings avoided the time-wasting — and interest-killing — traps I point out in the "How to bore your reader" section earlier in this chapter. Instead of force-feeding details to the reader (whatever Melody's brother supposedly did, full descriptions of Melody and Derek) before they care about the characters and their situation, these openings hit a few key points and save the specifics for later, when the reader has the time and interest to deal with them.

Backtracking to the background

After you choose the best place to open your story, you're almost certainly left with information your reader needs to know. That information would be out of place in the beginning. Your job as the author is to figure out where and how to share the relevant info with your reader.

Suppose your heroine just quit her job in the wake of her boss's unwanted advances, and then went home, hoping for a good cry, and found her fiancé in bed with another woman. Luckily for her, the heroine recently inherited a ranch from an uncle she hardly knew, so she heads out West and makes a new life for herself, far away from the bad memories. The smart place to open the book is with her arrival at the ranch, where she immediately meets the hero. The reader will wonder why she's there. What was bad enough to make her leave everything she knew behind and start a whole new life?

Those questions eventually need to be answered or your book won't make sense. Your next challenge is filling in the blanks in the background, without stalling the story's forward momentum. You can use three tried-and-true techniques to do that. The first method involves taking a moment relatively early in the story to *briefly* review necessary background. Or you can dole out information piecemeal throughout the book, so the reader's never stopped in her tracks for a history lesson. The third technique involves the use of a flashback, which takes the reader back in time for (usually) a few paragraphs or pages, or (sometimes) even a chapter or more.

Picking a quiet moment

After you start your novel at an exciting and involving point, you can fill in the background later, where doing so doesn't take much time or get in the way of your story. Many novice writers think that they need to actually show everything — including all the relevant background — or, at least, provide the reader with all the details. Not true. Most of the time, an overview works just fine. Often a paragraph or two, or even just a couple of key sentences, can do it. In the preceding section, I fit most of what a reader needs to know about the heroine's background into a few sentences (the boss's advances, the fiancé's philandering, the uncle's ranch). Fleshed out with a few details to give it weight and lend interest, that background can still fit into a paragraph, and you can frequently fit a paragraph like that into a quiet moment shortly after the book gets going. For example:

>> The heroine arrives at the ranch and runs smack into the hero, the foreman who's been running the place since her uncle's death (and, truth be told, for the last few years before he died). They immediately have a run-in, based on a combination of her not belonging on a ranch she hasn't ever visited — which he sees as an insult to her uncle, a man who was like a father to him — and her attraction to him, which makes her distant, even rude, because she's in no mood to think well of *any* man at the moment.

   After their set-to, she wanders around the ranch, feeling at loose ends, maybe meeting some of the secondary characters, seeing the hero again from a distance and again tamping down her interest, or having another run-in of some sort, before finally collapsing on her bed (a bed in a room and a place that feel totally foreign to her), reflecting briefly on what led her to make the trip to a new life.

>> You can also use the alternate approach of making one of the secondary characters someone friendly and welcoming who gets her to talk, and the whole story of the sleazy boss and even sleazier ex-fiancé comes spilling out.

Either approach lets you present the basics of the background briefly and in one go. Later, if the reader needs more information, you can write in a line or a paragraph containing the necessary bits and include it in a similar way, where it doesn't call attention to itself or interrupt the flow of the narrative.

Doling out details as you go

You can also take your time and dole the facts out slowly, one at a time. The heroine may reflect on quitting her job but not reveal why she left until several pages or more later. You can even leave the whole story of the ex-fiancé as a mystery, using her point of view to indicate that something major happened but never specifying what, until it all comes out in an emotional scene with the hero.

TIP

Saving key facts and hinting at their existence without revealing them is especially effective when you're dealing with a romantic mystery or suspense plot. By withholding information and making the reader try to figure out what's going on, you're essentially presenting additional clues — whether those clues deal with the plot or the characters' emotional state — to the reader, who's already in mystery-solving mode and primed to enjoy the additional challenge.

Making use of flashbacks

Flashbacks get a bad rap, I think, because too many writers tend to overuse and just plain misuse them. When they're handled properly, though, they can be extremely effective. The key lies in knowing when and how to use them.

Sometimes you really need to include a crucial scene in its entirety for full emotional effect, but it happens before the true action of the book begins or just doesn't have the right characteristics to be an opening scene. That scene can become an effective flashback.

TIP

How do you know whether a scene is worthy of a flashback? Most of the time, you need to base your decision on whether or not it features the hero or the heroine (usually both) and strongly impacts the relationship. Occasionally the flashback isn't relationship related but features one or the other of your main characters and is necessary for the plot. In either case ask yourself whether the book would be weaker without it. If you answer "yes," you have a flashback on your hands.

Authors most commonly use a flashback to fill in the past relationship between a hero and heroine who knew each other before the book began. Don't use a flashback if they only knew each other as passing strangers or business acquaintances, though. You should use a flashback if they were lovers, spouses, or otherwise romantically involved. Their past relationship colors everything that happens in the present and forms the basis of your book, so just saying that they used to be involved doesn't get across the emotional impact you want.

You can, and should, have the two characters talk out their issues at some point in the course of the book. Keep in mind, when they're talking about a shared past, it feels awkward if they go so far as to recount every detail of what happened. They don't need to remind each other of events they lived through together. (I talk more about this issue in Chapter 9, when I discuss natural and believable dialogue.) This situation just begs to be dealt with in flashback.

Choose an appropriate point — usually following an encounter between the two of them, often an emotionally intense one, maybe even right after the first scene — and have one of the characters think back to how things used to be, how everything fell apart . . . or whatever makes sense for the story. You need a sentence or two of transition, and then you can present the flashback in the same tense as the rest of the book.

Depending on your story and how much of the past you need to show, you can use a series of flashbacks or even one long one that's composed of multiple scenes and can go on for a chapter or more. The bottom line lies in something I say all the time to writers: It's all in the execution. I've seen successful romances where nearly half the book was a flashback. I also see books with one brief flashback that doesn't work for one reason or another — the scene itself is unnecessary or the placement is jarring, for example — and it's off-putting. This just demonstrates that it really isn't *what* you write, it's *how* you write it that really counts.

TIP

How should you format a flashback? If you're lucky enough to get feedback from an editor, they may have a specific format they'd like you to follow, but if you're working independently, you have several possibilities. You can italicize the entire thing (much like a dream), but that font is awkward and hard to read (especially for multiple flashbacks or flashbacks longer than one page). You can also present it as part of your regular text, without any special spacing or other formatting. The clearest approach is to set it off with time/space breaks (see Chapter 14 for a description) before and after the flashback.

Opening lines that work

The first page, the first paragraph, and especially the first line of your book are so important that you should put some extra time into thinking about what makes your opening work. There are several practical techniques you can use to make sure yours is a winner. Have fun experimenting with them until you find the one with the biggest impact.

Going solo

Visually speaking, a single, relatively brief line really catches the eye. If you can craft a strong opening line, one that intrigues the reader, you can increase its impact by letting it stand alone. Here are a few examples:

The man in the corner wouldn't stop looking at her.

It wasn't until the arrows stopped flying that she realized she'd been hit.

When I sent a text to my late husband, the last thing I expected was a reply.

Each of those sentences puts the reader right in the middle of a situation where the stakes are high, whether in terms of curiosity (the first: Why is the man looking at her? Is he the hero?), suspense (the second: Will she live?), or emotionally (the third: Is it his baby? Why didn't she tell him before he left?). Each opening line makes the reader ask at least one question that's interesting and important enough to make her keep reading.

Keeping it short

Even if you can't come up with a single line as an opener, or if your story doesn't lend itself to such an abrupt beginning, try to avoid starting with a long, dense paragraph, especially one that takes up all or most of the page. A big chunk of text, whether it's description, internal monologue, or anything else, looks intimidating. Try to make your first paragraph relatively brief, and follow it with several manageable-looking ones, not one that takes up the rest of the page. That makes your book look more inviting to the reader.

Talking the talk

Don't start with just any dialogue — start with something exciting that puts the reader right into the scene and a key character's head. Use a brief, punchy line — one that makes the reader wonder what's happening and where things are going. Here are some dialogue examples:

"What the hell are you doing here?"

"What do you mean, it's my baby?"

"I'm going to get out of here, and when I do, Mr. Kirkland Martin the Third is toast!"

Any one of those lines can stand alone, but you can also add a dialogue tag or an ensuing line of description. Here are the expanded versions:

"What the hell are you doing here?" She knew she was shouting, but she couldn't stop herself. She'd traveled 2,000 miles to get away from him, and now here he was, standing on her doorstep, as large as life and even more handsome than she remembered.

"What do you mean, it's my baby?" he growled, moving to stand threateningly over her and the tiny blue-clad bundle she was cradling in her arms.

"I'm going to get out of here, and when I do, Mr. Kirkland Martin the Third is toast!" She felt stupid talking to herself, but after three days locked in a bank vault — damn long weekends, anyway — she was desperate for the sound of a voice, any voice, even her own. Besides, threats always sounded better aloud.

Asking questions

Two of the previous examples ask a question. You want to make the reader curious, to get her asking mental questions about what happens next. If you can find a natural way to ask a question for her, which makes her try to think of the answer herself, so much the better. Just be sure that the question sounds natural; you don't want the reader to hear your voice talking to her, only your character's.

Setting deadlines

This technique doesn't work for every storyline, but time pressure in your book can work on your reader the same way that time pressure works in real life — increasing a sense of urgency — which makes the reader even more eager to keep reading. You can work in a built-in deadline easily if you're dealing with suspense, but you can make it work just as well in nonsuspense stories. For example:

> *Five minutes. Five minutes, and then, if the stick turned blue, her life was going to take a dramatic turn straight into booties, babies, and boy, would she be in trouble.*

> *Lisa tapped her foot impatiently and checked her watch. Again. She would give him another 30 seconds, and then she was going hunting for another husband.*

Bucking conventional wisdom

How you approach this option is up to you. Sometimes you have an idea so good that you just have to toss the rules out the window and go with it. If you think that's happening to you, commit it to paper, let it sit for a day, and then go back and read it, asking yourself one question: If you went into a store, picked up this book and, knowing nothing about it, read this opener, would you want to know more? If you can honestly answer yes, go ahead and give it a shot.

Constructing Can't-Miss Chapters

Just as the opening of your book is crucial to catching a reader's interest, every chapter — the ending of one and the beginning of the next — needs to keep her interest high and get her to keep turning pages instead of putting the book down and going off to do something else.

WARNING

A reader is most likely to put down a book at the end of a chapter, a natural and logical break. Any time a reader puts a book down, they're in danger of never picking it up again. If that happens, the reader ends up looking at that author as a waste of time and money and avoiding them in the future. For that reason, the end of every chapter you write needs to leave your reader at a point where she's dying to know more.

You can't guarantee that a reader will *never* put your book down — some things, like the call of a crying baby or the need to finish lunch and get back to work, have to take precedence. But you *can* do your best to ensure that your reader picks it back up again the minute she has a chance.

Treat your chapter openings with as much care as you put into your chapter endings. For one thing, before putting the book down at the end of a chapter, your reader may sneak a peek at the opening of the next chapter. If the story is captivating, she will feel compelled to see whether the action that ended the previous chapter will continue into the next. She will be eager to know how it will turn out. In addition, when a reader picks the book back up, you have to lock her back into your story as quickly as possible and draw her away from her real life. This is why chapter openings and closing are so critical.

TIP

Aim to keep each chapter at about 20–25 manuscript pages. This length keeps the book from feeling choppy, as if it's been broken into too many sections, and minimizes the number of chapter endings, each of which poses the risk of your reader putting down the book for good. At this length, each chapter also stays short enough not to be daunting, so if your reader's tired or only has a little bit of time to read, she feels capable of managing "just one more."

Viewing every chapter as a new beginning

Think of every chapter opening in the same terms you think about the opening of your romance novel itself. You don't introduce your characters every time, of course, and the physical attraction between them should be clear even by Chapter Two, but you can always reveal something new about them or emphasize and deepen the attraction.

REMEMBER

The beginning of every chapter needs to grab the reader's attention right away. Whether you pick up where the action of the previous chapter left off or switch to another scene (or another character's point of view), make sure that what you're doing is exciting and interesting.

As with the opening of your book (see the "How to hook your reader" section earlier in this chapter for tips on how to start), you may again want to start subsequent chapters right in the middle of something. But because you have the weight of your book's initial hook behind you, giving the reader the impetus to go on, you could also start at the beginning of a scene as well. This technique can work throughout the book, as long as you make the opening sequences interesting.

Avoid opening a chapter with a long period of setting the scene or of an introspection that doesn't also raise questions in the reader's mind that she wants to see answered. You've worked hard to keep your book moving up to this point, don't slow it down — or bring it to a halt — now. Give the reader a good reason to go on, and go on she will.

Leave 'em wanting more: Effective chapter endings

Many novice writers succumb to the temptation to finish every chapter as if they're ending a mini-book. They sum up what happened, wrap up the action, and leave the reader with a sigh of relief. Big mistake.

If the reader's feeling good, as if she's gotten a payoff, she has no incentive to keep reading. She's more likely to put the book down and bask in her happiness (and the characters' happiness) for a while. That may be great for your reader, but it's lousy for you. That kind of feeling may even make her put the book down when she doesn't have to — when real life isn't beckoning, when she's wide awake and not struggling to read "just one more page" — and that's a dangerous situation. If your chapter ending doesn't give your reader a reason to read on, you've failed. As you can see in the following sections, you have more than one option for making chapter endings work for (not against) you.

Hanging by a thread: Cliffhangers made simple

The easiest way to compel a reader to keep going (so that she'll be so caught up in the story that she won't even realize it) is to end your chapter with a cliffhanger. Whether you use a literally life-or-death scenario (the heroine hanging off the side of a cliff and hoping that the hero arrives in time to rescue her) or you only make it feel like a cliffhanger (the hero has just stormed out of the bedroom, accusing the heroine of betraying him by not telling him he has a son), you can get the reader's heart racing, her brain whirling, and her fingers turning pages by breaking away from the action at a crucial point.

Some plots lend themselves to cliffhangers more readily than others. Any kind of suspense, mystery, or adventure plot is a natural fit. Historical romances, because they often take place at a time when day-to-day life was more exciting and demanding, also often lend themselves to cliffhanger endings. Any action-oriented scene creates an easy opportunity, but you can make anything in your story feel important enough to build a cliffhanger around.

Is your heroine waiting for word on the outcome of her child's operation? Does the fate of the ranch hang on how well the cattle sell at market? Has the power gone out in the lab just as the hero was about to complete the last crucial equation? Have the horses left the starting gate but not yet reached the home stretch?

Even without an earth-shattering plot twist, every romance has the perfect ingredients to create a cliffhanger: a man, a woman, and romantic tension. Every romance reader wants to see the ultimate happiness of the hero and heroine. Get the characters to an emotionally fraught point and then cut the scene short. Leave them without resolution (even send one of them storming away), and you have a cliffhanger no reader can resist. (For tips on when to resolve cliffhangers, see the "Keeping transitions fresh" section later in the chapter.)

Romances have an advantage over every other form of fiction when it comes to cliffhangers — the extreme importance that the romantic relationship holds for the reader. No other form of fiction can promise that kind of emotional involvement on the part of the reader. Romance novels have access to every kind of cliffhanger in fiction in general — plus guaranteed access to one more.

Sending mixed messages

You can also keep your reader reading by giving her satisfaction on one level at the end of the chapter but withholding the total happiness she's looking for. To do that, get to a point in the plot or even emotionally that seems to offer satisfaction, and then use your hero or heroine's point of view to show that things aren't really as simple or on as even a keel as they look. Another option is to get to what seems to be a resolution, and then throw a monkey wrench into the works by introducing another complication, such as an ex-fiancé suddenly appearing on the scene.

REMEMBER

Be sure that whatever you introduce feels believable — an emotional issue that's been simmering under the surface or an unexpected but still logical plot twist, for example. Out-of-the-blue contrivance — the hero's teenage daughter *who's never even been mentioned before*, for example — is a surefire way to irritate a reader.

By creating a partial sense of satisfaction, and then adding doubt and tension, you give the reader reason to hope that she may eventually get everything she wants. You also give her a specific reason to keep reading: to see what effect the newly introduced or otherwise unresolved issue has on things. You can use this approach with a purely emotional scene or by using action.

>> **Playing on emotion:** Throughout the entire course of every romance, the reader is hoping for one thing — to see the hero and heroine get together. In most cases, that means physically, through lovemaking (or, at least, kissing and other physical intimacies), or another form of commitment. In every case, the reader's hoping for emotional intimacy and for the characters to settle their differences.

You can give the reader a great partial payoff at the end of a chapter by letting the couple get closer physically, whether it's a first kiss or actual lovemaking (see Chapter 11 for more on writing love scenes). But then withhold the full emotional payoff by using one character's point of view to show trouble in paradise, a secret that can break them up, an emotional complication that they think can't possibly be overcome . . . anything that lets the reader know that these characters still have plenty to resolve in the relationship.

>> **Wrapping up the action:** You can wrap up something active or suspenseful (the opposite of creating a cliffhanger), letting the reader breathe a sigh of relief. Nonstop action can be tough. You have to give her a break sometime. Then you can undercut the reader's relief by getting inside a character's head to reveal more trouble — whether plot-related or emotional — to come.

Maybe the hero's just rescued the heroine from a group of South American revolutionaries, and she's fallen into his arms in gratitude. But then the hero hears the sound of approaching footsteps and the click of the safety being released on a gun. Or maybe the hero and heroine have just finished a tough negotiation with a rival company. Their side won, so they're laughing and happy, and he's giving her a preview of just how much happier he plans to make her in bed that night. The reader's happy, too — until the heroine thinks to herself that soon she'll have to start making excuses not to go to bed with the hero or he'll notice that she's pregnant and starting to show.

As a variation on this approach (less effective because it's less immediate, but still viable), you can leave an important issue unresolved earlier in the chapter and then provide a payoff for something else at the end of the chapter. The reader enjoys the resolution you do provide, but she'll keep reading in search of a resolution for the earlier issue, too. Just be sure that the unresolved issue is important enough to stay in the front of the reader's mind, so she's still thinking about it even at the end of the chapter when you're wrapping up something else.

Packing a punch

The hardest type of effective chapter ending to talk about is what I call *ending with a punch*. I'd be rich if I had a nickel for every time I've told an author they need a punchier line for the end of the chapter — and I'm not talking about the punch line of a joke.

Sometimes the punch comes not in what happens but in how you say it. That concept can be difficult to explain: It's both vague and frequently subjective. Essentially, it means ending the chapter at a moment of high emotion or excitement, so your prose is still moving, and not tacking on a final line that slows things down and wraps them up. Keep the reader's adrenaline flowing; don't give her a chance to relax and pull away from the book.

>> **An ending with punch:** Picture a playful scene where your hero and heroine finally let go of their reservations and fill their conversation with flirty subtext. Finally, at the end of the scene, your hero comes dangerously close to your heroine and you say something like: *He pulled her tighter, stared deep into her eyes, and after several agonizing moments, he brushed his lips across hers.*

>> **An ending that falls flat:** Often an author has the right end line, but they've tacked on something extraneous that ruins the pacing and deflects the punch: *He pulled her tighter, stared deep into her eyes, and after several agonizing moments, he brushed his lips across hers. He had never felt so right, so complete, so at peace.* That one extra line slows the pace and makes the scene feel finished in a way the first version didn't, and that makes it less likely to draw the reader forward.

TIP

You can use this technique with any kind of scene. If you end a chapter without a cliffhanger or mixed message (the other techniques I cover earlier in this section), take a look at what you've written and think about each of the last few lines, or maybe the last few paragraphs. Experiment by cutting the last line or paragraph, especially if it seems like you've wrapped things up, and see if you can make the chapter end with a bigger bang.

Keeping transitions fresh

As you move between chapters, you need to vary the way you do it. If you end every chapter with a cliffhanger, your reader starts to find things predictable, and eventually your cliffhangers become increasingly less effective — especially if you immediately solve each one at the start of the next chapter. By working variety and unpredictability into how you handle your chapter openings and endings, you keep the reader interested and on her toes — and eagerly turning pages to see what happens next.

A good technique for moving from chapter to chapter while keeping the reader involved is to end one chapter on a cliffhanger and then start the next chapter with something completely different but also interesting. This strategy keeps the reader's interest on two fronts. She wants to know how the cliffhanger turns out, so she keeps reading for that reason alone. But because you've also started the next chapter with something interesting in its own right, she also wants to know more about what's going on right in front of her.

You can also end with a cliffhanger and then dial things down at the beginning of the next chapter. Don't dial them so far down that the reader gets bored or skips the boring bits in a search to see how the cliffhanger turns out. To keep the writing interesting, you *can* vary the pace, maybe get inside a character's head for some explanation or move into a flashback. You don't always need to move from action to action, and in fact, you shouldn't. The best pacing involves varying the tempo.

Moving from Scene to Scene

Moving from scene to scene is very much like moving from chapter to chapter, just on a smaller scale. Every word you write should be geared toward drawing your reader forward from page to page, so beginnings and endings — whether on the macro or micro level — are key components of your writing and one of the elements of pacing.

Stringing scenes together

Look at scenes as tiny chapters and then use the same techniques to move between them that you use for moving between chapters:

>> **Start with something interesting.** Your book has no room for anything that doesn't earn its keep. Don't think a reader doesn't notice it if you sandwich a filler scene — however interesting you may find the info or however poetic the description — in between two interesting scenes. Unless she's dealing with a fire, an earthquake, or a crying baby, you can't find a surer way to get a reader to put your book down in the middle of a chapter.

Just like the beginning of your book or the start of every chapter, the beginning of every scene has to interest your reader, even if it's not deeply emotional or actively exciting. An individual scene is a smaller increment than a full chapter, so you can paint it on a smaller, less dramatic canvas. In fact, it makes sense to save most of the big-bang stuff for transitions between chapters, where the risk of losing the reader is greatest.

>> **End with something intriguing.** You have more flexibility here than with chapter endings, but overall, you should employ the same techniques as you do when ending a chapter — cliffhangers, mixed messages, and punch. With scene endings, though, you can also end with a genuine wrap-up of that small piece of the action, whether plot-oriented or emotional.

>> **Vary your methods.** As with chapter transitions, don't rely on the same technique every time. You don't want your reader to be able to predict your every move, so mix them up.

TIP

Although you generally don't want an entire action chapter to move into a chapter made up solely of introspection, single scenes can sustain a single tone because they're shorter. If you end one scene on a calm note, try starting the next scene on a different note — exciting, suspenseful, humorous — and see how it impacts the flow.

Seeing scene endings as mini-chapter endings

The way you end each scene is particularly crucial. In addition to employing the same techniques that you use to end any chapter, watch out for one pitfall that I rarely see with chapter endings but frequently see with scene endings: trailing off.

Sometimes, a writer is so focused on making every chapter ending dramatic that they lose sight of their individual scene endings. Each scene may be important, but instead of ending effectively, some or all of them just sputter away. Here are a few examples:

>> **Characters finish the relevant part of a conversation but keep talking, moving on to other subjects, saying extended goodbyes.** Real-life conversations do move in that way, but in a romance novel, that kind of conversation is counterproductive. It bores the reader and takes the focus off what she's supposed to take away from the scene.

>> **The action goes on for too long.** The reader rarely needs to see the follow-up to the important parts. If the heroine's been trying — and failing — to saddle her own horse every day for a week, end at the moment when she finally succeeds. Readers don't need to see her mounting up and riding away.

>> **There's no point to the scene.** Characters often reach key conclusions and revelations about themselves or what's going on during action scenes, sometimes even during scenes of mundane everyday action. The point of a scene like that almost always lies in the character's progress, not the action itself. After you've hit that high point, wrap up the scene and move on to the next.

Intercutting scenes

If you end a scene with a mini-cliffhanger or with the reader in doubt as to how things will work out, don't always be in a hurry to relieve the suspense or answer the questions.

You can follow what's essentially the chapter pattern: Break off the scene at a key point, cut to something else entirely (the equivalent of opening the next chapter without picking up where you left off), and then resolve the cliffhanger a scene or two later. Because scenes are so much shorter than full chapters, you can alternate between two scenes in a way that you'd have a lot more trouble doing successfully if you were working with chapters.

TIP

Experiment with the film technique of *intercutting* two scenes (moving back and forth between them) so that you break each down into three, four, or more bits. This technique works most effectively when each scene is compelling in its own right, so that the reader is equally interested in how both of them turn out.

Each time you cut away, pick an exciting moment, even a mini-cliffhanger, and each time you cut back, re-enter the action *in medias res* ("in the middle of things"). Don't recap, just keep things moving, going back and forth until you resolve each scene.

WARNING

If you have the raw material, in the form of two compelling scenes happening simultaneously, don't be afraid to maximize the excitement by intercutting them. Be careful not to overuse the technique, or you dilute its effectiveness.

Chapter **13**

Getting Your Story Straight: Doing Research

The only time that you can get away with doing absolutely no research is if you're writing a contemporary romance that's set in your own area and deals with jobs, settings, and character types that you already know. You might also be able to get away without doing any research if you're an historian and writing about a period that you know inside out. However, most books require research to make them accurate. Your book *needs* to be accurate, which makes research crucial.

Few people would question the need to research historical romances, and most contemporary romances include at least one or two aspects outside the author's personal experiences or knowledge. Even futuristic and fantasy-based romances require some research, depending on the world you create, because those worlds still need to feel believable and logical to the reader. This is especially true of any story based on current scientific developments.

In this chapter, I talk about everything research related, starting with how to recognize what you need to know more about. I also give you some ideas on where to find the facts you need, how to organize those facts, how to use information to make your book stronger, and how to get legal permission when you need it.

Getting It Right: Priority Number One

Everything — selling an editor on your work and then selling readers on your talents — depends on one thing: getting your readers so wrapped up in the story that the characters' lives, emotions, and the world you've created for them feel real. To make that happen, you have to make the illusion perfect. You can't let anything break the spell — and nothing breaks the spell like running smack into some sort of mistake, whether it's a trunk in the back of your vintage Volkswagen Beetle or a medieval heroine zipping up her wedding dress.

Factual missteps can turn off readers, but if you're trying to traditionally publish and an editor catches a lot of mistakes, your manuscript likely will never even see a bookshelf. Your editor will need to count on you to get things right, because they don't have time to check and fix all the details, though they will keep an eye out for everything they can.

Sometimes, though, despite everyone's best efforts, factual mistakes make it through to publication, and most of the time, readers *will* catch those mistakes, even if it's only one reader in 10 or 100. And every reader who catches you in a mistake may never pick up another one of your books. What she *will* do is tell her friends (not to mention everyone who reads the who-knows-how-many romance-related online message boards). Your reader could even be a reviewer who tells thousands of people what you did wrong.

WARNING

In both traditional and indie publishing, sales are the lifeblood of every author. If your sales suffer because you aren't careful with your research, your career can disappear before it even gets off the ground. Wherever and however you do your research, check and double-check everything you can. Make absolutely sure that your book is accurate.

Making Research Work for You

Research is important, but diving headfirst into the process without thinking it through can be counterproductive. Having a plan before you actually start looking around for information can help you focus on finding what you need, rather than wandering off on tangents that, however interesting, probably just waste your time.

REMEMBER

Efficiency is the name of the research game. As a writer, you want to spend most of your time writing. Being prolific can help you become successful, so you don't want to sabotage your own chances by getting distracted down a research rabbit hole. Too much time researching takes away from the time you could be writing.

Figuring out what you need to know

Most editors focus on the big-picture aspects of editing (characterization, story structure, and so on), leaving the details in the hands of the author and, secondarily, the copy editor. That's why it's your job, as the writer, to do your research and stay one step ahead of any possible questions an editor might — or, more problematically, might not — ask.

It's a good idea to get into the habit of asking yourself questions as you write. Some types of mistakes (in police procedure or in historical fact, for example) can sink an entire book. So if you're one step ahead of an editor and ask yourself questions as you write — and then answer them accurately — you've gone a long way toward writing a factually correct book.

Starting with the basics

In doing research, you first need to figure out what questions to ask and what answers can make your book stronger. These research basics are a starting point for almost any romance novel:

>> **History:** Obviously, this research topic comes into play with any historical romance, but sometimes history even affects a contemporary romance (if a character needs to know information for a plot-related reason, for example) or a paranormal novel (if the modern-day lovers are reincarnations of past lovers, for example).

>> **Professions:** Most of your characters do something other than what you do at your day job — and they probably aren't romance writers, either. Get your facts straight about whatever jobs they hold, whether their profession is ranching, medicine, the military, or anything else.

>> **Geography and locale:** Whether your characters travel to the Grand Canyon, New Orleans, Paris, or the Amazon rainforest, you need to accurately portray the locations you choose for your book. That not only means getting the landscape (or the cityscape) right, it means getting the local flora and fauna right, too. And don't forget the weather, either.

Finding the devil in the details

Within any of the larger categories listed in the preceding section, you can find a whole world of information, some of which will clearly be necessary for your purposes. But realizing which smaller facts matter isn't always second nature.

REMEMBER

Sensitize yourself so that you're aware of every fact, however small, that you use. Question every detail you put on the page (Do I know this for sure or not?). Commit an item to print only when you're 100 percent certain of its accuracy. This can be pretty time-consuming, especially when you're writing a long book or one that has a lot of hard or precise facts in it. The good news is that as you hone your research skills, knowing what to ask becomes second nature, which will help streamline the process.

For example, you may want to know whether a piece of slang that sounds too contemporary was really spoken during whatever era the book is set in, whether DNA tests can really come back within a particular period of time, or whether cowboys really brand their livestock in the spring. These are the sorts of questions you need to ask yourself. Whether you ask them before you write, during the writing process, or after you complete your first draft, you will need to be confident in the answers.

REMEMBER

Watch out for mistakes as seemingly simple as having your heroine take a New York City taxi uptown on Fifth Avenue — which actually runs downtown — or sending your hero north on Interstate 82 — which actually runs east/west (north/south interstates have odd numbers). Streets and highways may not seem like research-worthy subjects, but assumptions like that lead to mistakes. Take nothing for granted and, when in doubt, check. The smallest facts can trip you up:

>> Is 100 acres large enough for a cattle ranch? If you live in a city, 100 acres sounds like a lot of land, but the answer is no, it's not nearly enough.

>> Do you want an English saddle, a Western saddle, or a cavalry, racing, side-, or some other kind of saddle on your hero's horse? Be sure that you have the right one for the right use.

>> When were zippers invented? If you're writing an historical romance, you need to know, so you don't put one in the back of your Regency heroine's dress.

>> Does the Canadian postal service deliver mail on Saturday? Not the last time I talked about it with a Canadian.

>> Are sparkling wine and champagne the same thing? Laypeople call a lot of sparkling wines champagne, but a vintner hero knows which ones really are and which aren't.

>> What time does the evening news come on? Viewers in the Eastern and Pacific time zones get the news at a different time than those in the Central or Mountain time zone.

>> When did CDs start replacing cassettes?

>> When did streaming movies replace renting DVDs?

>> When did England do away with primogeniture?

>> Does mincemeat really contain meat?

Avoiding information overload

Not only do you have to decide what you need to know, you also need to recognize what you *don't* need to know. Too much information creates problems of its own.

Weighing down the reader

Too much information can stop your story in its tracks. You end up boring your readers. Even if they find it interesting, it will create the tone of an informative book, which breaks the spell of your romance. Your tasks as a writer are to provide just enough information to make the world of your story feel complete and to accurately portray every locale and profession — but no more.

REMEMBER

Just because something interests you doesn't make it interesting and/or useful to a reader. An interesting tidbit belongs in your book only when it contributes something necessary in terms of characterization, plot, or setting. It's up to you to scrutinize every detail and decide whether including it serves a purpose — if it's necessary for the reader to really enjoy the book or if, like Mount Everest, it's just *there*. During your research you're going to find out all kinds of things that your reader doesn't need to know. Be ruthless as you pick and choose what to put in the book. Save the rest for writers' get-togethers and cocktail-party trivia. Check out these examples on what to include/exclude:

>> If you're writing an historical romance, you probably need to describe a typical meal at some point, but you don't need to describe every detail of what the kitchens are like, how many cooks and servants are needed to prepare the food, or how long the meat hangs to cure before it's cooked. If any of these things play into your story, though, you should include them — but *only* if that information is relevant to your plot.

>> If your hero and heroine are doctors, you need to use — and use correctly — enough medical terminology to make them seem real. You may also need to accurately identify an operation or procedure, along with a few general facts about how it's performed. You don't need to describe the operation in detail, though; remember, you're writing a romance, not a medical thriller. (And, unless you want a large portion of your readership to get queasy, you also shouldn't describe it too graphically.)

>> When describing a landmark building, the reader doesn't need to know who the architect was, how they designed the building, and how a particular construction company built it.

>> Does the hero drive an SUV? You may want to mention the color, the make, and the fact that it has 4-wheel drive (if that's going to be important later on). But the size of the engine, every detail of the interior, and how much it cost . . . not so noteworthy.

TIP

You can easily avoid giving too much information — especially of the "how things work" variety — by cutting away from describing the specifics of the action and entering into another scene, and then coming back when the characters have finished that action, whatever it is. Or you can cut away from description to how your hero or heroine is feeling and what he or she is thinking, which the reader is much more interested in knowing, anyway.

Delaying your writing progress

The more you can decide ahead of time what you need to know and what you don't, the more time you can save yourself as you research — time that can be better spent actually writing your romance. Discipline yourself as you research so that you're capturing only the information you need. You're bound to be tempted at some point by all kinds of fascinating stuff, no matter how much you try to narrow your focus only to what you need. Sometimes you'll succumb, so don't beat yourself up. Just resist as much as you can. You'll thank yourself later (and me, for telling you to be tough on yourself) when your book is done and on its way to an editor, while your writer friends are still having fun researching and stumbling across all kinds of interesting but ultimately useless trivia, their books still unwritten.

TIP

You may come across information that falls into the "maybe" category: info you may end up needing later in the book, depending on how things develop, or that spurs an idea for another story. I don't want you wasting time later retracing your research steps or losing an idea for the next bestseller. So save it, either as a note for your current book (in the following section in this chapter, I talk more about organizing your research) or in your idea file (see Chapter 5). You can always go back later and incorporate it.

Getting Down to Business

Before you crack open a research book or open a browser, it's worth taking a few minutes to get yourself organized. Choose the best time in the writing process for doing research, or at least the bulk of it. Determine how you plan to keep track of the information you will find — what organizational system you will use — so you can pull the necessary facts out of your hat (or filing cabinet) when you need them.

Timing is everything

When should you do your research? Try to do your big picture research ahead of time — after you've outlined the book, or brainstormed (if you're a discovery writer), but before you start actually writing. You can work more efficiently that way because, if you research before you write, you can have most of the information that you need already in front of you. That way, you never (or rarely, anyway) have to leave your creative zone.

Inevitably, though, you'll realize as you write that you need to know something else. If you only need a small detail that doesn't have any repercussions for your characters or your plot, you can probably just make a note and check it out later. As I'm writing I like to type XXX in the manuscript to indicate I need to go back and research something. (Just be sure to search for the XXXs when you do your final edit to make sure you addressed them all and removed them!) If, however, the answer to your question is going to affect how the rest of the book plays out, you need to check it out right away. As frustrating as pulling yourself away from a manuscript might be when you're really into the writing, it's a lot better than having to go back later and redo everything because you made an assumption that turned out to be wrong.

Doing your research and, as much as possible, getting it all organized ahead of time may sound like a lot of work, but the investment pays off as you write and it saves you time in the long run. That investment can also make the difference between becoming successful or not, and that's the best investment of all.

Organizing like a pro

Organize your research in whatever way works for you. The key lies in literally *organizing* it, so that you don't find yourself muttering, "I *know* it's here somewhere," as you turn over every inch of your office and comb your hard drive, wasting time looking for something you know is there. Somewhere.

REMEMBER

Organizing your research as you go makes it easy to access as you write, and that streamlines the process. In case you haven't noticed, I'm all about efficiency. I want you to get your book written and out into the world. As long as your book is still at your house being researched, it can't sell!

TIP

File everything the minute you get it. I know firsthand the perils of the "I'll put it in this pile and deal with it later" approach to filing. It either never gets done at all (I usually end up having to go find the information all over again), or it gets done in a big rush at the least convenient time, because that's when I simply *have* to have some particular thing I just *know* is in there.

Backing things up

I recommend saving hard copies of your research because, as much as I love computers, I'm very aware of their fallibility. Saved documents and URLs are vulnerable in a crash, not to mention that URLs seem to change with the wind. At the very least, download and save your research on a thumb drive or on the cloud as well as your hard drive.

TIP

When you save hard copies of information that you get off the Internet, you're making things easier on yourself, because you probably don't do all your research online. And, as you can see in the next section, having all your research organized and in one location makes life easier.

Keeping info handy

In the course of your research, you may end up with articles saved from magazines and newspapers, photocopies of relevant bits from books, stories and information printed from the Web, and even pictures you pulled from catalogues or took on vacation (for advice on finding resources, see the "Finding the Facts" section later in this chapter). To save your research, subdivide it into related groupings, for example:

>> Geographical/locale-based information

>> Job-related information

>> Historical facts

>> Miscellaneous

The "Miscellaneous" group can be broken down into as many smaller specific categories as you want. Include things specific to your book, such as fashion, news stories that relate in some way to your plot, and so on.

Store your loose research materials in a filing cabinet, a multi-pocket expanding file, individual folders, manila envelopes, or whatever works for you. One exception: If you use entire books in your research, keep them together on a designated shelf.

If you organize everything together, you can find a particular piece of information more easily when you need it. You will only have to look in one place, not two dozen. Whatever storage method you use, develop a system that's logical for you, and keep things clearly labeled and accessible. (Make files on your computer for any information you save there, too, and name them something that will make sense to you later.)

As you're working, you may find keeping some of your research around you especially useful if you know you'll be needing it frequently. (A historical time-line, a list of military ranks, or specific technical terminology may fall into this category.) This list of necessary facts can also include pictures — your hero's estate house, for example, or just landscape photos that help you stay in the right mindset for the book. In Chapter 3, I talk about setting up your home office, which involves giving yourself space to tack up papers and pictures or paste sticky notes.

Completing the project

After you're done writing a book, save your research. To make room so that you can start on the next book, you may need to box up the research or rubber band it into a stack and put it under the bed. But don't get rid of it. For one thing, if an editor asks you to revise, that research may come in handy for rewrites — or for answering their questions when they want to know if such and such is really true. For another, it may be useful for another book someday — perhaps a sequel — so why go through the effort of gathering it all again?

Finding the Facts

You can do your research in all kinds of places, and many writers use several different methods for each book. In fact, one method can lead you to another. An article cites a book, a book leads you to another book, an online site leads you to another site or yet another book, and any one of those sources can give you the name of someone you want to talk to personally, if you can. Even family and friends can be sources.

Surfing the Net: Great information (and misinformation)

The Internet is wonderful, and you can find pretty much everything in the world there — if you know how to look for it, and you're skeptical enough not to believe everything you read. To use the Net for research (something you almost certainly will do, at some point) keep the following in mind:

>> **Narrow your search parameters.** Whether you choose a search engine that works with key words or lets you pose an actual question, experiment with different words and combinations of words, or with asking your question in different ways, so that you get a list of results that can actually help you. If at first you don't get what you need, rephrase and try again. Over time, the process will become more intuitive, and you'll go through fewer trials, make fewer errors, and waste less time before finding what you want.

>> **Consider the source.** Not all opinions are created equal. One of the things that gives the Net its richness and makes it so interesting is that anyone who has something to say can have a voice. But the complete lack of censorship, the fact that no one has to offer proof of what they say, and the ability of "facts" — unproven though they may actually be — to spread in literally moments if they catch the interest of enough people, means that all opinions can *look* equal, even though they aren't.

Before you accept something as the truth and use it in your romance novel (or anywhere else), take a look at the credentials of the person who said it and the site where you found it. Make sure you're not looking at the result of axe grinding but at unbiased, accurate reporting. Check and double-check — and be sure that your backup sources aren't just quoting the original and each other in an endless round robin.

Basically, look at the Internet as if it had "Researcher Beware" stamped on its metaphorical forehead. If you do, you can find it a fabulous resource in every way.

>> **Check the date.** Errors can live forever online. Books tend to go out of print as they —and the information they hold — become dated. Magazines and newspapers carry obvious dates. Online, you often have to look harder to find out how old a piece of information is. Look around the site to see if you can find the date when the site's creator entered the information. If you can't find one, getting independent confirmation, with a date attached, becomes even more important.

If you're writing a Regency historical romance, a site that hasn't been updated in years can be just as accurate as one updated yesterday. Because the Regency period ended in 1820, nothing about it has changed in a while. But even when dealing with historical periods, it pays to keep track of any new theories and discoveries. The older the period and the less well-documented it is, the more likely this is to be true. Scholars of ancient Egypt, for example, seem to rewrite history with the discovery of each new tomb. And if you're checking into cutting-edge medical treatments, artificial intelligence, the political situation in the Middle East, or anything else where timeliness counts, be sure that the information you use is both accurate and as up-to-date as possible.

The Internet is also a great source for hard-copy research materials that you can't find anywhere else: out-of-print books or old magazines and newspapers. I strongly recommend buying new copies of texts whenever you can. Other writers need their royalties just as much as you hope to one day receive yours, and newspapers and magazines need to make money or they go out of business. Sometimes you can't find something new, only a used copy. When you can't find a source anywhere else, the Internet turns the world into your marketplace.

Supporting your local library and bookstore

With the Internet available from the comfort of your own home and offering everything you can possibly want, you can easily forget that you have all kinds of other research options available to you. For in-depth information, the Net can't compare to a good book (though it can often steer you toward one). Look to a book for an in-depth exploration that lets you get the full experience.

When you're writing an historical romance, don't worry so much about immersing yourself in the grand history of the time but rather in the rhythms and events of the day-to-day life of the period you've chosen. Doing so allows you to write from the same position of comfortable knowledge that an author writing a contemporary book can (as long as you know that you can resist the siren call to include every fact you've discovered). Frequently, you can find books — sometimes even firsthand accounts — that let you enter the past. You can rarely find that kind of extended sojourn online, where you're more likely to see summaries of what life was like in other times or other general information.

TIP

Basic textbooks (not the complicated grad-school kind, but textbooks geared for high school or even junior high students) are a great research resource. They contain as much information as you usually want or need, and they present that information clearly, concisely, and in easily understood language: You won't need to do research to understand your research. Be sure that you have a current edition, though.

Which books should you borrow and which should you buy? Glad you asked!

>> **Head to the bookstore.** You should probably buy any book that you think you'll need for a while — whether for an extended length of time as you write this book or later, for another book. Bookstores are useful when the book is relatively easy to find.

>> **Check out the library.** Research often involves a lot of books that you read once and don't need again or books you'd love to own but that just aren't

available anymore. To get hold of these books, start at your local library. What your library doesn't have, it may be able to get on inter-library loan. If you're lucky enough to live near a public university, its library (or, often, libraries, because individual departments often have in-depth research collections) is another resource to look into.

THE UNLUCKY SEVEN: PLACES *NOT* TO DO YOUR RESEARCH

Plenty of pitfalls are waiting to trap you if you don't do your research carefully and thoroughly. Plenty of unreliable sources exist, and even reliable sources can sometimes fail you. Maintain a healthy skepticism about everything you discover, double-check every fact, and you can't go wrong. Here's a sampling of places and sources to avoid, or at least to treat with extreme caution:

- **A friend of a friend:** Urban legends always supposedly happened to a friend of a friend. Rumors follow the same chain. Distrust anything that comes to you this way. Most of the time, the info is so off base that it would be funny — if so many people didn't believe it. Check, double-check, and triple-check any fact or story you hear second- or thirdhand.

- **Email fun-facts lists:** These lists claim that a duck's quack doesn't echo, a swan is the only bird with a penis, and all sorts of other weird information that *could* be true. But most of it isn't. Email warnings about terrible things that happen to women in mall parking lots, kids in public restrooms, and the like fall into this same general category. The stories are usually exaggerations at best, and fabrications at worst, so don't refer to one as reality in your romance unless you have independent confirmation that it happened.

- **Spoof sites:** Some online sites look incredibly real — but are total nonsense. They may be parodies of official sites (like the FBI) or created to look as if they represent the voice of reason, and they often contain well-faked photos. Don't be taken in. If something looks too funny, freaky, or generally unbelievable to be true, it probably is.

- **Tabloids:** Whether they deal in celebrity gossip or Bigfoot sightings, no tabloid practices what's called mainstream journalism. Take what they offer with a grain of salt. They're designed to entertain more than to report, so be entertained, but check everything twice.

- **TV dramas and the movies:** Some TV shows and films are scrupulous in their own research, others extrapolate from real-world information or fudge a few details, and still others may as well be set on Mars. I can almost always tell when an aspiring author has based their research into police procedures, for example, entirely on Hollywood's version of reality. You can find useful information on TV and in the movies, but consult other sources to sort the wheat from the chaff.

- **Other novels:** Fiction can spread misinformation just as effectively as TV or the Internet. I'm forever reading published books that are filled with major errors — and I can only imagine how many mistakes get published that I don't know enough to catch. Don't be guilty of spreading others' errors.

- **Memory:** The mind is unreliable. Your recollection of something you read, heard, or saw in the past may be 100 percent accurate — or far from the truth. Before you build a book around something you remember, check to be sure your memory isn't playing tricks.

Developing a nose for news

To find the most up-to-date information, magazines and newspapers are a terrific source to use. Whether you subscribe to an online newspaper or magazine or buy what interests you on the newsstand, you can find plenty of ideas to spur twists in your current book or entire plotlines for future romances. If you're looking for information on a specific topic, you can often find the most timely developments written up in newspapers and magazines.

Even when you don't need cutting-edge knowledge, you can find a lot of specialty magazines that can give you information — maybe all the information you need or, at least, information enough to help you formulate additional questions and figure out where you can go to find the answers.

If you can't find the kind of magazine you need even at a big newsstand or your library (and the more specialized or scholarly the magazine, the less likely you are to find it just lying around somewhere), your library has a periodicals directory that can help you track down what you want so you can order it directly.

TIP

Many newspapers (and magazines) archive their stories online. Depending on how old the article you want is, you may be able to find it by checking the paper's website. Libraries are another great source of old newspapers (especially local papers that you can't find anywhere else), usually saved on microfilm or microfiche. Several CD-ROM and online searchable cloud storage sources are also available for newspapers. Depending on how far back the records go, you may even find old newspapers helpful when you're writing an historical romance, especially for a story you've set locally.

Taking time to stop, look, and listen

News magazines, made-for-TV documentaries, documentary films, and even the plain old nightly news . . . all of these sources can give you great information. Record what you think may interest you, if possible, but you can also get a lot of these sources on video or DVD. You can even buy transcripts of many news magazines and interview shows directly. Stay tuned after a show to see if it offers a transcript service.

Entire cable channels are devoted to all kinds of special interests. Check into what's available to you (or to your friends and family, so that you can ask them to record a show for you) and see what's on the schedule. Look for nonfiction videos and DVDs, too.

REMEMBER

Be sure that the broadcast material is of the nonfiction, news variety. TV police dramas, infomercials, and last summer's blockbuster action movie don't count as credible sources. (For more info on avoiding less-than-stellar sources, see the sidebar "The unlucky seven: Places *not* to do your research" in this chapter.)

You can find good sources of information in news radio, talk radio, podcasts, and public radio. Be sure you don't mistake one person's opinion for absolute fact. This problem comes into play most in talk radio and podcasts, which are for the most part open, uncensored (other than a several-second delay so that censors can bleep out profanity) forums, so anyone can talk and say pretty much anything. Double- and triple check anything you hear just to make sure it's accurate.

Traveling for fun and profit

Travel — whether to the museum in the center of town or overseas to an entirely different world — is a great method of researching everything from locale to culture to history to anything else you can think of. Travel can also cost you a pretty penny (but see Chapter 3 for some basic information on writing off your costs), so don't go broke running around the world.

When you *can* travel, though, take full advantage of the opportunities it presents. Take all the pictures that you can (wherever you have permission for picture taking), talk to anyone who can help you (locals, experts at historical sites, tour guides), and buy research material (postcards, books, newspapers, whatever looks helpful) that you don't have access to at home.

Most people are happy to talk to a writer, so ask questions wherever you go — as long as the person, the locale, and the situation seem safe. Do be careful in any situation that looks dicey. Trust your own instincts and don't take chances.

If you can't get up and go, become an armchair traveler. Read articles and books by people who've been there, especially firsthand accounts that give you that "you are there" feeling. Check out coffee-table books, which usually have great pictures. Read travel guides and look at maps — including street maps of major cities you plan to include in your book. Get to know everything you can about a place or time, just as if you were really planning to go. Just be careful not to sound like a tour guide when you start writing.

Talking to experts

Nothing beats talking to someone who actually walks the walk and talks the talk, especially when you're trying to uncover the ins and outs of a particular profession — not just how to do the job but what life is like when that's how you make your living. An expert in any field (history, science, or whatever) is always a helpful resource, especially when you need in-depth information or a real-world sense of things.

Here's a quick step-by-step guide to landing and conducting an interview:

1. **Find an expert.** In the course of your online, print, and broadcast media research, you may come across names of people — or the people themselves — who can help you. Talk to your family and friends, too, because they may know just the person you should talk to.

2. **Ask the expert for their help.** After you've identified a possible contact, introduce yourself, whether in person, or through a call, letter, or email. Explain what you're looking for and ask for help. Not everyone has the time or inclination to oblige, but a lot of people do.

TIP

   When in doubt, pick up the phone and make a cold call; you'd be amazed how many people are happy to talk to you about their specialties. Pity the poor expert who often has no one to talk to in detail about their specialty, family and friends having long ago tired of hearing the details of how to run a candy company or research the space-time continuum. Imagine how happy they'd be to talk to someone who really wants to know what it's like.

3. **Conduct the interview.** When you're interviewing someone, be polite and respectful, friendly but not in an imposing way, and don't take up any more of the expert's time than you need to. Take careful notes or, if your expert's willing, record your conversations. In the end, you probably have a lot more detail than you need, but you also get an irreplaceable sense of reality to bring to your writing.

4. **Follow up after the interview.** After you're done, don't just write a thank-you note. Let your expert know that you'll send a copy of the book if it's published,

and then be sure that you do. You should also publicly say thanks for the help in your book's acknowledgments section.

TIP

You can also, in some circumstances, actually live your research, at least to a degree. If you're writing a police procedural, call your local police department and ask to go on a "ride-along." Talk to your local firehouse about hanging around and watching life at the station. You may be able to spend time on a working ranch, go out on a commercial fishing boat, or spend a day watching your local veterinarian in action. Sometimes insurance regulations and legal concerns make things impossible, but you never know until you ask, so it can't hurt to give it a shot.

Getting Permissions

When you're writing a romance novel, you're much less likely than a nonfiction writer to need legal permission for anything you want to put in your book. Still, from time to time, permissions may be an issue — whether you want permission to use a quote from a song, a script, a poem, or another book, or because you're using proprietary information from any source, or you want to reference a particular person or business by name in your book.

Determining when permission is necessary

When you sign a contract with a publisher, something I talk more about in Chapter 17, one of the clauses almost certainly deals with *warranties and indemnification*. Basically, that clause says that you, not your publisher, are legally — and financially — liable if someone sues because you quote a source without permission, use information without permission, base a character on a real person without that person's consent, *libel* a person or business (meaning you defame them in writing), or leave yourself open to legal action in any other way through something you say in your book.

REMEMBER

Bear in mind as you read this section that I'm not a lawyer. I'm giving you a layperson's legal advice, albeit a layperson who's been in the publishing business for a long time. My basic recommendation always comes down to being cautious, not taking chances you don't have to. Whenever possible, avoid writing anything that may require getting legal permission. If you're not sure how much of a chance you're taking, or if you don't want to do something that you think may cause trouble, get legal advice. It may cost you, but undoubtedly less than losing a lawsuit would.

Here's a list of things to avoid if you can — and how to avoid them:

>> **Don't name real people.** Other than historical figures (Abe Lincoln, Geronimo, and so on), you're better off avoiding the issue of real people altogether. For example, if you're writing a contemporary romance with a political setting, make up the name of the president and other officials.

>> **Don't stray from the facts.** If you must use a real person, contemporary or historical, stick to the known facts about that person. Don't speculate on people's personal lives, sexual kinks, or anything else you can't support with research.

>> **Don't base characters on real people.** You want your characters to feel real, but base them on traits and qualities you compile from various sources. Don't write about your ex-boyfriend, your neighbor, or your best friend from college, making them fictional just by giving them a new name. By the same token, don't base a business, whether a giant corporation or a local restaurant, entirely on a real business.

>> **Avoid direct quotes.** Refer to *a popular love song* instead of quoting one directly, for example.

TECHNICAL STUFF

Stick to sources that are in the public domain: Shakespeare rather than Neil Simon, for example. *Public domain* refers to works that are no longer covered by copyright, but the laws governing when a works falls into the public domain are complex and are based on the type of work — song, book, and so on — and when it was created. Something hundreds of years old, like Shakespeare's plays, won't be a problem, but a specific translation of an ancient work may be, as may more recent works, so you'll have to research the work you'd like to use. You should also look into the laws governing *fair use,* which allows excerpts of a certain length and of certain types of work to be used in certain circumstances. Again, the laws are complex, but you can use the same skills that help you research facts for your book to research these legalities.

>> **Don't say anything negative about a real person or business.** This mistake is the biggest taboo of all. If your characters eat fast food and get food poisoning, don't name — or in any way describe so that the reader can identify — a particular restaurant or franchise.

There are books everywhere that undoubtedly do everything I've just told you *not* to do. That fact doesn't matter. Whether you end up in legal trouble or not, it's not worth taking the chance. Let someone else make headlines — and take legal chances — for writing a scandalously tasty page-turner; you're writing a romance, and that's something else entirely.

Even if you do everything you can to avoid needing to get legal permission, sometimes you may find it unavoidable. You may not see any way around using a quote or mentioning a real person in a way that's completely neutral or even complimentary. If you talk to an expert, get written permission to use the information they give you. Depending on the specific circumstances, you may or may not need it, but when in doubt, play it safe and get permission. You can't go wrong covering your assets.

TIP

After you're under contract, feel free to ask your editor if you're unsure whether you need to get permission for something or not. Your editor has access to their company's legal department and can get you a specific answer, one no general book (like this one) can provide.

Filling out the paperwork

Every publisher probably requires something different, even if only slightly, in terms of an acceptable permission, so when you're unpublished and need to come up with something for your source to sign, you're really flying blind.

I recommend that you come up with a basic letter for your source (or whoever) to sign. The specifics of what you're asking (to use a direct quote, to use information, and so on) vary, but you're asking to be allowed to use whatever it is in your book at no cost and to be released from any future legal action. You may find a cost is involved in using a quote or other material that requires permission, and you need to decide whether the quote is worth it or if you're better off doing without it. That letter may or may not be good enough to satisfy your publisher if you sell the book, but it gives you a starting point. Your editor can tell you what else they need if and when the time comes.

Chapter **14**

Neatness Counts — and So Does Grammar

To be a successful romance writer, you need to be a storyteller, but you can't be *only* a storyteller. You need to get all the writing mechanics right: grammar, punctuation, spelling, formatting, word count . . . every detail plays a crucial part in getting your story past an editor to the reader. If your manuscript has mistakes that are obvious as soon an editor or reader picks it up, they won't even read your work; mistakes can stop a reader dead in their tracks before they've even read a few pages.

Making a manuscript as clean as possible before it goes out should be a writer's top priority. An editor's job isn't to teach you to write or to fix all the "boring" details you don't want to be bothered with. Their job is to take a good book and make it better. The mechanics are easy enough for every author to get right, so the editor can spend their time offering you their expertise where it counts, such as with content flow and story arch.

In this chapter, you learn what you need to know about grammar and punctuation, and where to go to get your grammar questions answered. You also get pointers on how to format your manuscript so it looks professional and is easy to read.

Knowing the Importance of Good Writing

Good writing helps tell the story instead of getting in the way of it. A big part of good writing is good grammar. Knowing the fundamentals of good grammar will help you go far in your writing journey. Even though you will have an editor, you still want to learn the basics so your editor can make your writing shine.

Good writing shouldn't call attention to itself. Instead, it should allow you to see through the words to the story you're telling, much like a window: You don't notice the glass; you notice the beautiful views beyond. Learning the craft of writing allows you to write in a way that keeps the reader engaged in the story and not distracted by the words or grammar. Good writing doesn't only sell your book, it sells your next book, and the one after that.

Poor writing calls attention to itself, like smudges on the window. It takes away from the story you're trying to tell. If you can't see the story through the writing, you'll lose readers. The good news is that writing well is a skill that can be learned. Don't lose heart if your first attempts aren't where you'd like to be. If you can tell your writing needs work, you're in a good place. You have a discerning eye, and you'll be able to improve as you practice.

Before you can play fast and loose with the rules of grammar, you need to know what they are. Don't just count on your ear to tell you what's right or wrong. You may have grown up hearing regionalisms or particular quirks in the way people speak that aren't technically correct, even though they sound fine to you. Your parents' speech patterns may have influenced you more than anyone else's. Those peculiarities of language can be useful to you in dialogue, but they can really trip you up in narrative.

Finding good references

The first thing you need to do is get a good grammar book (or two) and keep it where you can refer to it whenever you need to. There are hundreds of good ones out there, some serious, some classic, and some that take a lighter, quirkier approach. Any grammar guide is fine, as long as you have one. Here are a few that I like:

» *The Deluxe Transitive Vampire: The Ultimate Handbook of Grammar for the Innocent, the Eager, and the Doomed* by Karen Elizabeth Gordon (Pantheon)

» *The Elements of Style* by William Strunk, Jr, & E. B. White (independently published)

» *Grammar Essentials For Dummies* by Geraldine Wood (Wiley)

» *Eats, Shoots & Leaves* by Lynn Truss (Avery)

» *English Grammar in Use* by Raymond Murphy (Cambridge University Press)

You can find more suggested grammar books at becomeawritertoday.com/best-grammar-books.

The biggest grammar problem most writers face isn't digging up an answer when they have a question. It's knowing when they should be asking a question in the first place. The best way to learn what you don't know is to hire a freelance editor and pay attention to the mistakes you're making on a regular basis. Ask yourself why your editor corrected your grammar in a particular place. The more you study your mistakes and learn why they needed correcting, the more likely it is you won't make those same mistakes in the future. You can be on the lookout for them as you write and correct them before they ever catch an editor's eye.

Using grammar and spell-check programs

A lot of word-processing programs have a built-in grammar-checking capacity. There are also separate programs that check grammar, such as Grammarly (grammarly.com), which offers a free plan and a Premium version. Before you write an entire book and find out you've made the same mistake(s) over and over, grammar-check a chapter and see what your program points out to you, and then consult your grammar book to see how you can fix your mistakes.

Grammar checkers are strict taskmasters, and sometimes they point out grammar mistakes that don't really cause a problem, at least when and where they appear in your manuscript. The rules of language sometimes lag behind common usage. Don't blindly follow where they lead you, or you can end up with a book so stiff and formal it can never cut it as popular fiction.

For example, proper English usage has a whole prohibition against dangling prepositions, but sometimes you can't avoid them without sounding ridiculous. Technically, it's wrong to say "That's something I won't put up with." But wrong or not, it's preferable to "That's something with which I won't put up." Most of the time, you're not going to run into anything quite so extreme (or silly), but it still pays to think about every example and not just accept what an impersonal program tells you.

TIP

You should also be using a spell-check program as you write. This can help you avoid a manuscript riddled with typos and spelling errors. But be aware a spell-checker can't catch if you've used the wrong word, as long as it's spelled correctly. In the end, no program can totally replace a human proofreader.

Taking a course

Take a grammar course or, if one's not available locally, a writing course that focuses not just on storytelling but on mechanics. You can even ask your instructor to focus on grammar when they review your work. In-person courses aren't your only option, though. Look online for a course available from a college or writers' resource site, or get a grammar workbook so you can focus specifically on understanding the rules and then applying them to your romance-novel-in-progress.

Asking a friend

If you have a willing friend with the right expertise, ask them to look over some of your work and mark it up specifically for grammar. This is a great thing to do before you submit your manuscript to an editor. The more eyes on a project before you try for traditional publishing, the better. If you don't have any friends who can proofread, it's a good idea to hire a freelance proofreader.

Making a Point with Punctuation

Grammar involves not just word order and sentence structure, but also the use of punctuation. For an in-depth look at all the rules of punctuation, refer to a dedicated guide, but a few things make such a difference that bringing them up here is important.

Comma placement

Comma placement can literally change the meaning of a sentence. Take a look at these examples:

>> *Let's bake, kids.*

>> *Let's bake kids.*

>> *I love cooking, my grandmother, and my children.*

>> *I love cooking my grandmother and my children.*

As you can see, the placement of the comma makes a *big* difference . . . and in some cases, can save lives!

REMEMBER

Most of the time, your comma usage isn't going to save your grandmother, but commas can still help or hinder your prose. I'm a big believer that it's better to use commas inconsistently but for effect rather than use them strictly by the book. Punctuation really is a tool, which means you control it, not vice versa. Think carefully about your commas, because if you get them right, they can really enhance the way your prose flows. If you get them wrong, though, they can make it stutter along like a leaky balloon, or completely change your meaning.

Here are some examples of the correct and incorrect way to use a comma:

>> **Correct:** *I would love to learn to fly a plane, ride a horse, and skydive.*

>> **Incorrect:** *I would love, to learn to fly, a plane ride a horse and, skydive.*

>> **Correct:** *I will, unfortunately, miss your graduation ceremony.*

>> **Incorrect:** *I, will unfortunately miss, your graduation ceremony.*

These examples are extreme, but it's easy to see how incorrectly placed commas can mess up the flow of a sentence. A quick brush-up on where commas are supposed to be placed will take you far.

TIP

`prowritingaid.com/punctuation-checker` is one of many online tools that offers a free punctuation checker.

Using ellipses and em dashes

Many writers confuse when to use an ellipsis versus an em dash. An ellipsis (. . .) represents a pause if it comes in the middle of a sentence, or a trailing off if it comes at the end. An em dash or long dash (—) in the middle of a sentence marks an abrupt change or denotes emphasis; at the end of a sentence, it shows that the dialogue has been cut off, often mid-sentence or even mid-word. Use an ellipsis as part of slow, thoughtful moments; em dashes usually come when a character is angry or upset. Em dashes can set off a phrase the same way commas can (though they imply greater emphasis); ellipses can't.

Here are some examples of the correct use of ellipses:

>> *She thought she could like him, but maybe . . . maybe that was just too much wine talking.*

>> *"I can't even think how you could . . ." She let her words trail off, unsure what to say next.*

>> *"Would you . . . I mean, could you . . . could you ever love me?" she asked slowly.*

Here are some examples of the correct use of em dashes:

>> *She immediately thought — though she had no idea why — he was the man she was destined to marry.*

>> *"I can't — I won't — I refuse to — to —" She stopped speaking abruptly, unable to put her thoughts into words.*

>> *"I'm so furious I could —" Afraid she would say something unforgivable, she turned away without another word.*

TIP

Set off only one phrase at a time with em dashes:

>> **Correct:** *He was the most irritating — the most infuriating — man she'd ever met.*

>> **Incorrect:** *He was the most irritating — the most infuriating — the most incomprehensible — man she'd ever met.*

This rule holds true even if what you're setting off comes at the end of a sentence:

>> **Correct:** *She was ready to spring into action the minute she got the word — and he was going to get what was coming to him.*

>> **Incorrect:** *She was ready to spring into action the minute she got the word — and he was going to get what was coming to him — and she was about to become his worst nightmare.*

Used in a sentence, em dashes often come in pairs. I often see writers using them in threes, which makes it impossible to see which phrase is actually being set off and emphasized. For example:

>> **Incorrect:** *He was making her crazy — infuriating man that he was — crazy enough to scream — and she had to get away.*

>> **Correct:** Rephrasing is almost always the only way to correct this sort of error: *He was making her crazy enough to scream — infuriating man that he was — and she had to get away.* Or you can break one sentence into two: *He was making her crazy — infuriating man that he was — crazy enough to scream. She had to get away.*

Talking about Dialogue and Narrative

Handling grammar in fiction, especially popular fiction, can be tricky. You need to look at grammar in different ways depending on what part of the book you're talking about.

>> **Dialogue:** You can use the language a lot more freely in dialogue than you can in narrative. Even university professors (and editors) have been known to misplace the occasional modifier or split an infinitive when speaking, and most people are a lot less formal — and a lot less accurate — when they talk.

>> **Narrative:** Even in narrative, editors apply the grammar rules much more loosely for popular fiction than for literary fiction or most nonfiction, especially of the scholarly sort.

REMEMBER

Even though you know the rules of grammar and punctuation, you may sometimes find yourself choosing to break them. In fact, you may find, on occasion, that you not only *can* break the rules, you *should.* The key is in knowing the rules first and respecting them where they're helpful. Only break them when you know why you're doing it.

Dialogue generally offers the most compelling reason to break the rules in order for your characters to sound both natural and like the individuals they are. (I talk in more detail about this license to break the rules in Chapter 9, when I discuss giving your characters voices.) Very few people speak as if they've walked straight out of the pages of a grammar book. You don't want to make your characters speak so ungrammatically that the reader gets a headache trying to decipher what they're saying, nor do you want to ladle on the colloquialisms, regionalisms, and everyday sloppiness so your characters sound like constructs, not real people.

TIP

You want your characters to sound informal and conversational. Because of that, when you're writing dialogue, your ear for speech (not the analytical part of your mind that handles the rules and regulations of grammar) should take charge. It's helpful to immerse yourself in dialogue, studying how other writers walk this line. Watch a few movies with the dialogue in mind, studying how the different characters talk. Your own characters will develop their dialogue as you figure out what sounds right for them.

Narrative, or the parts of the story being narrated, should be told to the reader in your author voice. In narrative, you may find it helpful to think of yourself as *telling* a story as much as *writing* one. A romance novel needs to move, to carry the reader along, so your language needs to have a casual quality to it because that keeps the book moving. Don't stop your reader dead in the middle of a paragraph too ponderous and stilted to stand up to its own weight.

Unless you're writing in the first person, your narrative should be less conversational than your dialogue. While most of the time your narrative should follow the rules of grammar, feel free to bend the rules occasionally when they make your novel read too stiff. (See Chapter 10 for more about using narrative effectively.)

Making Thoughtful and Relevant Word Choices

The wrong word choice can ruin even the most grammatical (in an appropriately informal sense, of course) prose. Part of the reason to play just a bit fast and loose with the rules of grammar involves creating a tone that sounds comfortable and natural to the reader, because that familiarity pulls them in. If you punctuate that natural prose with strange word choices — even if that word accurately describes what you're after — you break the mood you've worked hard to create on every level with both the creative and the mechanical aspects of your book.

Don't choose a fancy word when a simple one will do

Sometimes writers try so hard to vary their vocabulary that they end up replacing common words that don't — and shouldn't — call attention to themselves with outlandish choices that yell, "Look at me!" The reader may even laugh at them because of their silly, awkward, or inappropriate appearance.

A car is a *car*. Maybe it's a *sedan*, an *SUV*, or a *pickup truck*. It rarely needs to be called a *vehicle*, even though, technically speaking, it is one. If an author starts talking about a character's *mode of transport* (or just *transport*), the editor is likely to pull out their pencil in frustration and write in *car*. And that example isn't even particularly extreme!

WARNING

Particularly in descriptions, fewer adjectives are usually better than too many adjectives, and normal, comprehensible ones are almost always better than the incomprehensible exotic variety. As a general rule, make a cliff *steep*, not *declivitous*; your room *well-lit* rather than *refulgent*; and your hero's background *secret*, not *recondite*.

In popular fiction, you never want your reader to have to consult the dictionary. Make the meaning of any unusual word, including technical terms, clear from context, or explain it unobtrusively in the text.

Don't use incorrect synonyms

I find another kind of trouble writers get into even more irritating to read than the high-falutin' word syndrome, because it's not only intrusive, it's incorrect. The writer chooses what they think is a synonym, but the word they choose really isn't a synonym — at least, not for the word as they use it.

The English language not only features inconsistent rules of grammar and pronunciation, but many words — even common ones — have multiple meanings. Too often, an author tires of a common term or just decides to have a little fun with language, but because they don't really think about multiple meanings when they grab their thesaurus, they don't come up with a synonym at all. Moving with *easy* grace isn't the same as moving with *elementary* grace, much less *commodious* grace, but both of those ten-dollar words turn up in a thesaurus as synonyms for *easy*.

TIP

If you absolutely have to consult a thesaurus and you choose an unfamiliar word, double-check it in a dictionary to make sure that it means what you want it to mean.

Watch for repeated words

Sometimes repeated words may creep into your writing without you realizing it. Reading your work out loud will help you find those instances where you repeat words. It also helps to know the common words that creep in often. Here are a few I search for when I'm editing: *just, that, so, really, seems, actually,* and *quite*. Be sure to read your manuscript with an eye for the words you repeat so you can edit them. It's a quick way to elevate your writing.

AVOIDING COMMON MISTAKES

Many people get a number of expressions and words wrong. Here are some of the most common mistakes:

- **A hair's breadth:** The width of a hair is very thin, and that's what you're talking about: the smallest possible distance. For example: *She missed the target by a hair's breadth*. It's not *a hare's breath,* though I'm sure a bunny's breaths are pretty small, too. And *a hair's breath* doesn't even make sense, not that lack of sense has stopped many people from writing it.

- **Soft-pedal:** As a hyphenated verb, this means to play something down. It comes from the music world and refers to using the soft pedal on a piano. For example: *The defense attorney tried to soft-pedal the facts in the case.*

- **Flaunt versus flout:** *Flaunting* something means to show it off, and *flouting* means to ignore or go against. For example: *He flaunted his ignorance as he flouted the law.*

- **Heart-rending versus heart-rendering:** If something's *heart-rending,* it's heart-breaking. *Rendering* is a butcher's term for getting fat from flesh, so . . . ewwww. For example: *It was a heart-rending story about the victim of a heart-rendering serial killer.*

- **Incarnation versus incantation:** An *incarnation* is a life (hence reincarnation), or a version of something that personifies an ideal. An *incantation* is a ritualized formula or statement. For example: *In his incarnation as a wizard, he was given to reciting mysterious incantations.*

Formatting for Success

Even if your book's insides — the story and the mechanics of how you've told it — are perfect, you still need to put the manuscript into an acceptable format before you present it to an editor or before you indie publish it. Looks do count, and for very good reasons.

No matter how you're going to publish, you want to look professional. If you're traditionally publishing, follow the submission guidelines for formatting your manuscript so it's easy for the editor to read. If there are no formatting guidelines, here are some general rules to follow. (See the "Formatting with indie publishing in mind" section later in this chapter.)

Setting your margins

In your finished manuscript, you need to make your *margins*, the blank spaces around the printed area of your pages, consistent throughout. Here are a few general guidelines:

>> Margins should be set to 1 inch wide on all sides. Word defaults to this setting when starting a new document, but you will want to double check this before you submit your manuscript to an editor.

>> Set up your margins so you have the same number of lines on every page, counting the extra spacing between scenes, called *space breaks,* as lines. The exceptions to this rule are the first and last pages of every chapter: You should establish layout rules to make all your first pages the same, but your last pages vary and can't be predicted.

WARNING

Don't make your margins too large. Every editor is on to that trick and knows it's just a way to make a book look longer than it really is.

Using the right fonts and spacing

Double-space your book. It really is that simple. You may have places where you need to single-space a particular section — if you're quoting a letter a character has written, for example — but you almost certainly want to double-space 99.9 percent of your book. The last thing you want to do is have an editor send it back unread and tell you to format it correctly before resubmitting.

TIP

Choosing a fun font is not the way to stand out. Times New Roman is the standard and by far the best, because it's easy to read. Avoid anything fancy, too thin, heavy, scripty, or compressed. A whole manuscript in these types of fonts will makes your editor's eyes spin and their head pound. Size matters, too. Go for 12 point because it's big enough to be clear and easy to read, but not so big that it looks like large print.

TIP

Send all manuscripts as a Word document, in either a .doc or .docx file format. Even if you draft your manuscript in another program, it's standard to send a Word document to an agent or editor.

Breaking your story into paragraphs

Paragraph a romance manuscript just like a published romance novel. Don't put an extra space break between paragraphs (unless you're indicating a time or place break, which I get to in just a second), and make sure you indent the first line of each paragraph. Don't follow the format of this book, because nonfiction is a different animal altogether.

You can indicate a time or place break in one of two ways:

» **Double-space:** You can just include an extra blank line to alert the reader to this shift.

» **Double-space, type — # — and double-space again:** Because simply double-spacing can look like a mistake to an editor, I recommend using this method.

Don't simply add four or five (or more) spaces, leaving a large gap, to indicate a break. That technique looks unprofessional and wastes space unnecessarily.

When you start a new chapter, be consistent. For chapter openings, I recommend spacing about a third of the way down the page, and then centering and typing *Chapter [Whatever]*. Space down from there to the page's midpoint and start the text of your chapter there.

TIP

Use the header and footer feature to add your name and number your pages. If your editor decides to print your manuscript it will be helpful for them to have your name on each page, and numbering the pages helps them keep them in order.

Avoiding common formatting mistakes

Here are a few general formatting tips to keep in mind as you write:

» **Don't use a tab to indent your paragraphs.** I've seen many manuscripts messed up by this simple practice. Or worse, the author has used the spacebar to space-space-space an indent. Don't do that. Word has triangles in the ruler above your work that you can use to indent text. Select all your text and move those indent markers.

» **Use headings to indicate new chapters.** As you're drafting your manuscript, if you're using Word, don't forget that styles will help you format. When you start a new chapter, use the Heading 1 style for the chapter name. (Just click on Heading 1 in the Styles Pane to apply that style to your text.) When you go to format, this will help separate your chapters. This also helps you skip around your manuscript if you're utilizing the Review Pane to the left of your work.

» **Use a single space after periods.** If you were taught to double-space after each period, it's time to give up that old habit. Two spaces are no longer needed, and this can mess up the document's formatting. If you think you have double-spaces stuck in your manuscript, use the Find and Replace feature to weed them out.

Formatting with indie publishing in mind

Most editors I've worked with prefer the manuscript to be submitted in Microsoft Word. While writing is a fairly solitary endeavor, you will need to coordinate edits with other professionals to get your work published, and Word is the industry standard.

I also highly recommend purchasing a formatting program so you can format your own book. While you can hire someone to do this for you, if you later find a typo you need to correct or a sentence you'd like to rework, you will have to pay to have these things changed. It's not only frustrating to you, the author, but it's also frustrating and tedious for the professional you've hired.

Here are two formatting programs I recommend:

>> **Vellum** (`vellum.pub`) has been around longer and is very well-reviewed in the indie space, but it currently is only available for Macs. I use Vellum myself and have been very pleased with the results. It's easy to get professional formatting with a few settings and clicks.

>> **Atticus** (`atticus.io`) is available for both PCs and Macs, and I've heard many good things about it. It, too, is also fairly easy to use and produces a professional product.

If you're well-versed in using Word, you can use Styles to format your entire manuscript and make it look fantastic, but there is a learning curve. You can purchase templates for formatting in Word, which might help you. I've done this before and they weren't too difficult to learn, although I will say that Vellum was easier and faster.

In the end, whatever you choose to do, make your book look professional to the reader. The last thing you want to do is turn away readers with a poorly formatted book. On the other hand, a well-formatted book will make you look like the professional you are.

Checking Your Work One Last Time

There probably won't be a second chance to resubmit your manuscript to an agent or editor, so you want to make certain it's the best it can be before you submit it. Use this handy checklist to make sure your manuscript is ready for submission.

❑ I've checked my grammar and spelling using a grammar-checking program, spell-check program, and a reference book.

❑ I've checked for punctuation errors.

❑ I've made sure the grammar is appropriate for my book's dialogue and narrative.

❑ I've checked for unnecessarily large or complex words.

❑ I've checked for incorrect synonyms.

❑ I've checked for repeated words.

❑ I've asked a friend, colleague, or professional editor to read my manuscript.

❑ My story meets the formatting guidelines for the publishing house.

5

Traditional or Indie Publishing — Which Is Best for You?

IN THIS PART . . .

Choose the publishing path that's right for you.

Find success with indie (self) publishing.

Submit your manuscript with traditional publishing.

Handle rejection letters and revision requests.

Chapter **15**

Choosing Your Publishing Path

So you've finished your manuscript and polished it until it shines. Now you're ready to decide if you're going to indie publish or look for a traditional publisher. This is probably the most daunting point you'll ever reach in your writing career, especially if this is your first time publishing. The good news is that there are more options for authors today than there ever have been before. Indie publishing has opened many doors, and has empowered authors to take their careers into their own hands. Traditional publishing can bring your book into bookstores across the country, and even around the world.

Traditional publishing means you submit your manuscript, or a query letter, to a publisher and they decide if it's something they want to publish. If you choose to traditionally publish, you also need to decide whether you need an agent. If you're going to submit to smaller publishers, you may not need an agent, depending on the publisher. There are benefits to going with a smaller publisher. However, if your dream is to publish with a large house, you'll definitely want to begin querying agents.

Indie publishing, also called self-publishing, means you publish your own work using a website like Amazon's Kindle Direct Publishing. Indie publishing can give you a lot of freedom, but it can be daunting. Some authors thrive in the indie world, while others find themselves wallowing in obscurity. It can be difficult to navigate if you've never published before.

Both are valid paths authors can take. This chapter details the pros and cons for each, so whichever choice you make, you can feel comfortable knowing that path is right for you.

Weighing Your Options

Before you choose traditional or indie, you'll want to look at all your options. You may be surprised to find out the direction you originally decided on might not be the best fit for you. Taking a step back and looking at all the advantages — and disadvantages — for each choice will help you decide what is right for you and your goals.

TECHNICAL STUFF

It's important to know the reason we have options today. The invention of the *ebook* — an electronic version of a printed book — and devices that can read those ebooks, has opened up the world of indie publishing. Indie publishing existed long before the ebook, but not many self-published books ever sold more than a few copies. The problem was distribution. You could publish your book yourself, but you ended up with a garage full of paperback books that you then had to hand-sell. Bookstores, for the most part, purchase traditionally published books they know they can return if the books don't sell. Indie published books hardly ever graced their shelves.

When ebooks began to take off, this suddenly gave authors a way to sell books directly to readers, without having to go through the gatekeeping of traditional publishing.

REMEMBER

Indie authors still don't have great print book distribution. If you choose to indie publish, your focus will most likely be selling ebooks, not printed books. Print sales will come if your ebook sales are robust, but your focus will need to be on marketing your ebooks. If your goal is to get your book in bookstores, you will want to traditionally publish, because that is the way to get wide print distribution.

Knowing the pros and cons of how you publish

There is no one right way to publish. Neither path is better than the other, and don't let anyone tell you otherwise. They are different, and each comes with benefits and difficulties. I often see these two camps — traditional publishing and indie publishing — pitted against each other. This is silly to me. We are all authors, no matter how we publish. We should join together, embrace our differences, and celebrate our love for writing. And the reality is many authors choose to do both, as you'll see later in this chapter.

REMEMBER

Whether you traditionally publish or go the indie route, certain tasks will be your responsibility:

>> **Marketing your book:** Many authors mistakenly think that if they traditionally publish, they won't need to market their books. The reality is that every author needs to market their books, no matter how they publish. While a traditional publishing house might set aside a specific budget for marketing, it's not a guarantee. They will list your book on their website and get your book on Amazon, but they may not be able to spend a lot of dollars marketing your book. Especially if you're a new author, you'll need to bring quite a bit of marketing power to the table.

>> **Managing your social media:** It's true, some of the more successful authors have a personal assistant who can manage their social media. But, for the most part, you'll be in charge of handling this yourself. There are so many social media sites out there, and many more that crop up over time. Find the social media sites you enjoy and stick with doing one or two really well. You might also talk with other authors about what works well for them.

>> **Creating and maintaining a website:** While you can hire this out, when you're first starting out you may want to do it yourself. There are many drag-and-drop options out there for creating a simple website. If you find this daunting, grab a teenager you know and have them help you. All you basically need is one site that points fans to your social media, has a place to sign up for your newsletter (which I discuss in Chapter 16), and offers a simple form people can fill out to contact you.

Changing course

As you make publishing choices, you don't have to continue with the choice you've made. For example, if you decide traditional publishing is the path you'd like, you don't have to go on traditionally publishing if you find it's not working out the way you had hoped. The same goes for indie publishing. Just because you start by indie publishing, it doesn't mean you have to stick with indie publishing forever. This is a misconception I often see.

Yes, it's true that traditional publishers will look at your work more closely if you've had raging success as an indie author, but even if your books haven't sold extremely well, if you're shopping a new book that hasn't been published, traditional publishers will look at it as a new entity. Don't try to traditionally publish a book that you've already indie published, unless it's sold over 100,000 copies within the first year. If you have had this kind of success, you may get a traditional publishing deal if the publisher feels there are still markets they can tap into. If the book had been selling well and sales dropped off, it's possible no one will want to take it on, feeling that the book has already sold to everyone who might want it. When in doubt, if you've already indie published a book, don't then submit the same book to traditional publishers. Submit new work to them.

TIP

Don't close any doors as you're deciding which path to take. Indie publishing can supplement your traditional publishing path, or vice versa. Many traditional publishers only like publishing one or two books a year. If you're prolific, you may find indie publishing is a great way to bring in more fans and more income in between traditionally published books. As you begin down the publishing road, don't turn away from the idea of switching paths along the way, or doing a mixture of the two.

Staying on top of a quickly changing landscape

The publishing world has been shifting and changing almost constantly, and it can be difficult to navigate through these unstable waters. This is why I tell authors they need to be a part of at least one online author group where regular discussions are taking place. Authors in general are helpful people. Being in a group with many authors who are able to share thoughts, ideas, and the latest publishing news will help you make wise publishing decisions.

It's almost impossible to read every article, listen to every podcast, or keep up with every tweet. You'll miss things if you try on your own. But if you're involved in a large enough group, if something is going on in the world of publishing, you'll most likely hear about it.

Here are the makings of a great group:

>> **It's large:** You'll want to join a group with enough authors in it to be sure to generate discussions. If you join a group that is too small, you'll risk missing important news in the publishing world. I recommend looking for an online group with more than 10,000 members.

>> **It has both indie and traditionally published authors:** You will want to keep up with both the indie world and the traditional world. If a group has authors from both publishing paths, you can stay on top of what is going on in both worlds.

>> **They chat about publishing:** The group won't be helpful if there are not regular discussions about publishing. Ideally, the group should have new and more experienced authors so there are questions being asked, and answers given. You will learn a lot as new authors ask their questions.

TIP

Look for writers groups in the social media you frequent. If you're on Facebook, search there. You'll find quite a few groups on Facebook, and hopefully you'll find some that check all the boxes for you. If you're not on Facebook, try looking on the platforms you frequent. Even if you don't care for social media, you might want to join at least one site. It's very important not to be left behind in this business. Don't let the world pass you by because you're still trying to publish like it's 1995.

Here are a few writers groups I recommend for staying on top of the publishing world:

>> **20Booksto50K:** This Facebook group, started by Craig Martelle and Michael Anderle, has made it their mission to help authors be successful. They have an extremely helpful all-star document with many tips on how to make the writing business work for you.

>> **The Writing Gals:** This is my Facebook group that I started with three other sweet-romance authors. We talk about the craft of writing, publishing today, and how to write to market. Our goal is to be helpful to authors no matter where they are in their journey.

>> **SPF Community:** The Self-Publishing Formula Community is a Facebook group where many authors discuss writing and publishing. Founded by Mark Dawson, this group is a free resource he gives to all authors.

Comparing and Contrasting the Paths

The easiest way to figure out which publishing avenue is best for you is to compare and contrast them. In this section I explore the pros and cons of each direction you can take so you can decide for yourself. (See Chapter 17 for more on traditional publishing, and Chapter 16 for more on indie publishing.)

Traditional publishing

Traditional publishing has been around for hundreds of years. Many of the large, well-established publishing houses are based in New York City, and they employ teams of professionals who help get books ready for publication. Traditional publishers pay the author with advances and royalties.

With traditional publishing, you will submit a query letter (which I talk about in Chapter 17), sample pages/chapters, or the full manuscript to a publishing house. An editor will read it and decide if they want to invest in your manuscript. There are different sizes of publishing houses. Some larger publishing houses, or *presses*, will only take agented manuscripts, which means you will need to first acquire a literary agent who will then submit your work. (See Chapter 17 for more on finding an agent.)

Some publishing companies make themselves look like traditional publishing houses, but they do not operate in the same way. These are called *vanity presses*. I talk about vanity presses in detail later in this chapter; for now, just be aware that if the publishing house is asking you to pay for any services, they are not a traditional publishing house. They are a vanity press.

Here are the advantages to traditional publishing:

>> **There are no upfront costs to you.** The publishing house will provide all the editing, cover design, formatting, and so on. You will not be asked to pay any fees. Because the publishing house is investing in you and your work, they will want to make sure your manuscript is well written and has a market. They will control all of the decision making during each of these steps.

>> **A marketing plan is usually included.** While not all contracts provide an extensive marketing budget, your publisher will probably provide some marketing for your book, and it's possible you could get quite a bit of marketing. The amount of marketing will depend on how large the publishing house is, if they are paying an advance, and how large that advance is. The larger the advance, the more they will most likely spend on marketing. (See Chapter 17 for more on advances.)

>> **There may be opportunities to sign your book.** Your publisher may set up some book signings for you. Again, this will depend on the size of the publisher and the size of your advance. Check the contract you're offered to see what the publisher will set up for you.

>> **You get a sense of validation.** Having a publisher who believes in your book enough to invest in its future not only gives you validation, but also a great sense of accomplishment. Someone else who knows the publishing business has read your work and they believe it has a chance to sell well.

>> **A publishing team stands behind you.** If you traditionally publish you'll have a ready-made in-house team of publishing experts behind you to walk you through the process.

Traditional publishing also has its disadvantages:

>> **There's no guarantee.** It can take years of submitting manuscripts before you finally get an acceptance, if you ever get one. It can be a long, tedious process paved with many rejection letters, and this can be disheartening.

>> **The process is slow.** If you do get accepted, it can sometimes take two or more years to see the book actually published and into bookstores. This includes time for revision and content edits, copy editing, formatting, and publishing. Indie authors can publish much faster.

>> **You might get dropped.** If your book doesn't sell as well as your publisher would like, or if market conditions change, they could decide not to publish your next book. Actually, at any point in the two-plus year process, they could pull the plug.

>> **You may find unfavorable contract clauses.** Some contracts might have clauses in them that are not advantageous to the author. Hire an intellectual property attorney to read the contract to make sure you're not signing something unfavorable to you. For example, you wouldn't want the publisher to own your characters and world, giving them the ability to hire another author to continue writing your series if you get dropped. (See Chapter 17 for details on contracts.)

>> **Your royalties are smaller.** You're sharing your royalties with your publishing house, and in some cases, your agent as well. Your take-home pay will be a small percentage. An average range is 15 percent to 25 percent.

>> **You get paid less frequently.** Your publisher will cut you a check once every six months, or maybe once a year, depending on the publisher. Most people have monthly expenses, and budgeting for an annual paycheck can be difficult.

>> **Sales reports come months later.** You will probably get sales reports as you get paid, but they will come months after those sales are recorded. If you're spending money every day to market your book but you can't see if it's making a difference in sales until you get the report months later, it's hard to know how to assess your marketing plan.

>> **You have less control.** If you're traditionally published, you won't have a large say in how the book is presented. The cover, the title, and maybe even the blurb will be decided by the publishing house. This can be a good thing, because publishers often know better than authors what sells well, but the author may feel as if the publisher has made a poor decision and there's not much that can be done about it.

>> **You can't control the price.** This one might not sound like much of a disadvantage, but it can be difficult to promote your book if you can't put

that book on sale. There are many promotional websites that will showcase your book — if it's discounted. Without control over the price, you can't promote your book with them.

Small presses

Small presses are usually independently owned and have a limited staff. Publishing with a small press falls under the traditional publishing umbrella. There are some great benefits to going with a small press:

>> **You don't have to hire an agent.** Most small presses will take unagented manuscripts, meaning you can submit your manuscript directly to the publishing house. This saves you the time and effort of acquiring an agent before you can get published.

>> **You get more personalized attention.** Your book will get the most individualized attention if you publish with a small press. Because they don't publish many authors, they will spend more time working with you to get your book published.

>> **You have a better chance of being published.** If you submit to a small press, your chances for publication increase because they get fewer submissions than the larger publishing houses.

There are some disadvantages as well:

>> **Small presses have a more localized reach.** Most small presses publish *niche* books (that is, books that appeal to a smaller audience, such as LDS romance), and have a small marketing budget. It's possible your book won't make it into the large bookstore chains if you publish with a small press.

>> **The advance is small or non-existent.** It's highly likely if you publish with a small press you won't be offered an advance. If you are, it will be a smaller advance than what the larger publishing houses pay.

>> **You may get an ebook only.** Many small publishers don't publish in print. They will publish your book as an ebook. Some will publish your book as an ebook first to see how well it sells, and only work with print after it is successful. It's possible you won't ever get the book published in print form through a small publisher.

Mid-sized and large publishing houses

While there are some differences between mid-sized and large publishing houses, I'm grouping them together here because there are many similarities. The biggest difference is the more personalized attention you receive with the mid-sized presses, much like attending a smaller school. The other difference is that many mid-sized presses are owned by universities or organizations, whereas most large presses are owned by major conglomerations.

Here are the advantages to working with a larger press:

>> **You get more money.** The larger the publishing house, the more money they have to spend on an advance and a marketing plan for your book. The larger presses have more influence in the book world because they have deeper pockets.

>> **Your book might get into bookstores and libraries.** If you publish with a large press, your book will most likely grace the shelves of many bookstores and libraries across the country. The more your advance is, the more likely you will get prime real estate in bookstores.

>> **Most breakout books are published by large presses.** If your goal is to be the next Danielle Steel or Nora Roberts, you will want to be published by a large press. Don't forget, though, that many large-press authors started out publishing with a smaller press before their work became well known.

Publishing with a large press does have some disadvantages:

>> **You'll be one of many.** The larger the press, the more likely they are working with a lot of authors. The less well-known authors may get less attention because, let's face it, those authors bringing in the high dollars are generally the ones they focus on.

>> **They do not take unagented manuscripts.** You will need to first get a literary agent, who will then submit to the larger publishing houses. It can be difficult to get a literary agent; they get hundreds if not thousands of query letters and only take on a handful of authors each year. (See Chapter 17 for more on finding an agent.)

>> **It's difficult to get published with a large press.** Even if you get a literary agent to take you on, it's still difficult to get a publishing contract with a large publishing house. There's a lot of competition. There are many authors who sign with an agent who never get offered a publishing deal with a large house.

Vanity presses

A *vanity press* (also known as a vanity publisher or subsidy publisher) is a particular type of publishing where the author pays for publishing services. Because the vanity press does not acquire any risk by investing in the author's work, they will publish any book, no matter the quality of the writing.

I'm not going to tell you that all vanity publishing is a scam and all they do is take advantage of authors. I've seen some vanity presses that work very hard to help the author put forth a quality book. But I will warn you that there are some vanity publishers that I would never recommend because they put very little effort into editing and cover design, giving an inferior quality product to the author. There are even some vanity presses that practice predatory behavior, outright lie to authors about what they are going to do for them, and pretend they are traditional publishers when in fact they are not.

The problem with vanity presses is that they don't make money by selling your book; instead, they make money by selling services to authors. They don't lose anything if your book doesn't sell well. They may offer you a marketing package, but look closely at their capabilities before signing up with them. They can't get your book into bookstores, no matter what they claim. (And some are very misleading about this.) They can list your book in the catalog that bookstores order from, making your book available to be purchased, but it's up to individual bookstores to order your book, and most won't if it's published through a vanity press. Vanity presses are also well known for their extremely high prices.

If you do decide to use a vanity press, be sure to vet them by searching for reviews of the company. Try searching online by typing in the company name and "reviews." You can also ask your writers group if anyone has had positive (or not-so-positive) interactions with the company. Also, look into how much it would cost to hire freelancers yourself versus how much you would pay the vanity press. Most indie authors pay much less for the same services by hiring freelance editors, formatters, and cover designers.

Having said all that, there are some benefits to using a vanity press:

>> **It's a one-stop shop.** Most vanity presses offer all services at one place. You won't have to figure out who to hire for editing, cover art, and so on.

>> **They create both an ebook and a paperback for you.** Some small publishers will only publish ebooks. Hiring a vanity press gives you both the ebook and the paperback.

>> **You don't have to be tech-savvy.** Indie publishing is great, but you will need to do a few things for yourself on the Internet, such as creating accounts and uploading files. This can be confusing to some people who aren't comfortable using computers. With a vanity press, all of this is done for you.

While there are a few perks for choosing a vanity publisher, don't go with one before looking at the disadvantages:

>> **You may lose control of your copyright.** Many vanity publishers will take control over the rights to publish your book and not allow you out of the contract without paying high exit fees.

>> **It can be expensive.** Most vanity publishers charge thousands of dollars for their services. You pay upfront, and many times there is no way to get your money back if you are unhappy with their work.

>> **Their work can be shoddy.** Not all vanity publishers hire poor editors and cover designers, but some are well known for their poor quality. Just be sure to check on the reviews and the quality of other books they've published before hiring a vanity publishing company. Printed copies can also arrive with quality-control problems like crooked type or untrimmed pages.

>> **Their practices can be deceptive.** Again, not all vanity presses will lie to you, but some will. Be aware that those companies are out there, and not everything they promise you will be delivered.

>> **There's no distribution and no price control.** You will get several boxes of books, but no way to distribute them. Your ebook will be for sale on Amazon and other retailers, but you can't control the price, and most vanity published books don't sell well because of this.

Hybrid publishing companies

Not to be confused with vanity presses, *hybrid publishing companies* share the cost of production with the author, but they are more similar to traditional publishing houses in that they are selective about who they publish, and they make the majority of their money through selling books. That gives them a stake in your book's success.

Indie publishing

Indie publishing, or self-publishing, has changed quite a bit over the years. There are many indie authors making a living at it, even bringing in six and seven figures a year. Here are the advantages of indie publishing:

>> **You have full control.** You are fully in charge of the end product you put out. There are no gatekeepers to tell you to change something to fit the market better. However, this is also a disadvantage, as you could put out a book that has no market, thus making it hard to sell.

>> **It's faster.** Because you're working directly with freelance editors and cover designers, you can publish your book a lot faster than traditional publishers. You still have to work with their schedules, so if you hire an extremely popular

editor, for example, you could wait six months to get into their queue, but in general you have much more control over how fast you can publish.

>> **You can control the price of your book.** This may be the best advantage you have as an indie author. You can put your book on sale, or even make it free. This is a fantastic tool to use as an author trying to get noticed amongst the thousands of books published each year.

>> **Royalties are higher.** Most ebook publishing websites like Amazon will give you 75 percent royalties, which means you don't have to have a bestseller to earn a decent paycheck as an indie author. More midlist (mid-range-selling) indie authors are able to write full-time than traditionally published midlist authors because their royalties are higher.

>> **Payments come in every month.** If you're selling books, you get paid every month. There is a two-month lag for most retailers, but once you start earning royalties, it's nice to get paid each month.

>> **Sales reports are almost real-time.** You are able to see sales practically as they come in, which is extremely helpful when you're marketing your book. (Sales reports may be delayed up to 48 hours, but for the most part you'll be able to see sales within an hour or so of someone buying your book.)

Now let's look at some of the disadvantages:

>> **You will need to manage everything.** It's your responsibility to hire editors and cover designers, complete the formatting or hire it out, and upload and publish the final product to the websites. As you publish, you'll acquire a team to work with you on your book. You'll be the project manager in charge of making sure everyone is doing their job.

>> **Your book probably won't be in bookstores.** Not physical ones, anyway. Yes, it's true you can take a few copies down to your local indie bookstore and they may put them on the shelf for you, paying you on consignment. But the reality is your book will not be in bookstores across the nation, unless you're a mega-bestseller who then gets a traditional publishing offer from a large press. (It has happened; look at *The Martian* by Andy Weir or *Wool* by Hugh Howey.)

>> **You will cover all upfront costs.** Publishing isn't cheap, even if you indie publish and hire freelancers. Without a publisher, you are in charge of paying all the upfront costs. You can shop around, look into different editors, or buy a pre-made cover to save some money, but the fact remains you have to pay everything yourself if you indie publish.

Becoming a Hybrid Author:
The Best of Both Worlds

In the end, you don't have to choose just one path. You might end up doing both indie publishing and traditional publishing. This is called being a *hybrid author,* where you have some books you've indie published, and others that are traditionally published.

You can become a hybrid author several different ways. If you choose to indie publish first and you become quite successful, you could approach some literary agents and get representation. It's much easier to get a literary agent to take you on if you've had books that have sold well. Or, if your books sell amazingly well, you could be approached by editors or agents. This is what happened to me when my first book hit *The New York Times* bestseller list with my indie published book.

If you indie publish but don't find great success, you still could become a hybrid author if you submit your next book to agents or small presses. (Just don't submit a book you've already published. They're only interested in new books that haven't been published yet.)

I also know a lot of traditionally published authors who have decided to indie publish a book for one reason or another. Maybe they have a few books they've written that don't quite fit with their publishing house, so they decide to publish them on their own. Many authors decide to indie publish the novels that traditional publishers reject. Or, their publisher can't publish more than two books a year, so they publish their other books themselves.

TIP

If you plan on becoming a hybrid author, you'll want to check all your contracts that you sign to make sure the publishing house will allow you to self-publish a book. Some contracts strictly prohibit this, or they prohibit any books set in the same world to be self-published, so make sure to address this when you are negotiating your contract. The publishing house may also want *first right of refusal* for any books you write. This just means they want to see any books you write, giving them the option to publish it if they want.

Being a hybrid author has some advantages. You get to work with professionals on your traditionally published books, but you also get to publish on your own schedule those books you indie publish. Your indie work can help sell your traditionally published books, and vice versa.

WARNING

One disadvantage to being a hybrid author could be pushing yourself too hard. Burnout is real, and if you are publishing both as an indie and traditionally, you could find yourself stretched too thin. Be sure to make adjustments to your publishing schedule if you start to feel overworked.

In the end, however you decide to publish, the choice is yours and don't let anyone make you feel you've made the wrong choice. Everyone is different, and we have different goals when it comes to writing and publishing. Choose the best path for you, knowing that if you find yourself unhappy, you can change your mind down the road.

Chapter **16**

Finding Success in Indie Publishing

ndie publishing, also known as self-publishing, has become very popular, and it's easy to see why when you look at all the benefits, including the fact that you have total control and can publish on your own schedule. Because you have full control you can have a sale whenever you want, which is a great way to attract new readers. You also get higher royalties as an indie author. Elana Johnson, Skye Warren, and Pamela Kelley are just three examples of highly successful indie romance authors.

But success isn't only measured by high sales. All authors should define what success means for them. Many authors simply want to share their stories with the world. Some love to maintain full creative control from start to finish. Others love working with all the different trades and thoroughly enjoy the publishing process. Many indie authors use their book to augment their primary stream of income or use it to pull in customers for something else they do. Determining what your needs are for your book will help you have a positive self-publishing experience.

Indie authors get to wear two different hats: creative and business. Authors who chose the indie path do so because they enjoy juggling those two aspects of writing and publishing. Indie authors learn to intertwine the two dynamics and can look at their creative baby with an equally critical eye. They are able to make business decisions about their book without being emotionally tied to the manuscript. This is important if you're going to create a professional product that will appeal to your audience.

I start this chapter by exploring what success might mean for you. The rest of the chapter is devoted to best practices as an indie author. These are my best tips for becoming a full-time indie author, and being able to support yourself and your family in the writing business.

Defining Your Success

Every writer has their own definition of success. Before you start your indie-publishing journey, take a moment to write down a few of your publishing goals. They can be as detailed or as general as you'd like. These goals are just for you, and no one else has to see them.

REMEMBER

There are many non-sales-related goals you can have as an indie author. Here are a few to spark some ideas for you as you brainstorm what your goals might look like:

>> **Publishing a physical book.** Indie publishing can be highly satisfying in and of itself. Holding a book in your hands that you've written is an incredible thing. It's a wonderful goal to simply publish a book that you've put your heart and soul into writing.

>> **Seeing your book on a store shelf.** While it's true that indie authors rarely get distribution to chain bookstores, many local bookstores are happy to stock indie books on consignment. It's very satisfying to see your book on a store shelf.

>> **Having your book recommended.** Of course, it's everyone's goal to sell their book, but it's even more special to know that your book was loved enough for someone to recommend it on social media.

>> **Receiving a great review.** There's something cool about getting a great review from a stranger who picked up your book and enjoyed it — and they want the world to know.

>> **Getting a fan email.** It takes a special book to motivate someone to contact the author. Receiving a fan email can be one of the most rewarding things about publishing your work.

>> **Collaborating with a favorite author.** Working with an author you admire can be very uplifting, and it's a great way to attract new readers.

While this list is in no way exhaustive, it might give you some ideas for success goals you can adopt.

REMEMBER

Having a sales-related goal is fine; many authors write in order to make money. Just be aware that becoming a runaway success is largely out of your control. Having said that, what *is* within your control is putting in the work. Most authors pulling in six figures have published more than 30 books. If your goal is to make money at this, you should also have the goal to write and publish regularly.

Creating a Professional Product

As you indie publish, it's highly important to create a professional product. All your effort in writing and polishing up your book will be lost if your presentation of it is subpar. I've seen more books sink into obscurity because of poor presentation than I have for any other reason. You've spent all that time writing and crafting a good story, so you should take just as much pride in packaging it well. At the very least, you will need a high-quality cover, a well-written blurb copy, and tight formatting of the text. Formatting the interior text is covered in Chapter 14, so the following sections discuss the exterior of the book. Finally, there are publication details you may want to include in your book, such as an ISBN, a Library of Congress Control Number, and copyright information, which are all discussed later in this chapter.

TIP

You can hire freelancers to help you publish without the high cost of using a vanity press (covered in Chapter 15). Most large author groups have a list of cover designers, formatters, and editors. If you are not a part of a large author group, seek one out to join. I started a group with several other romance authors called The Writing Gals, and we have a Facebook group where anyone can join and ask questions. Groups like mine are the perfect place to find freelancers who can help you create a professional product.

Judging a book by its cover

Besides the story, the cover is the most important part of your book. It's what first catches the eye of potential readers. A cover is not just the front of the book, it's also the back and the spine. Graphic designers know how to use the space effectively as well as how to satisfy the many technical aspects of layout, printing, folding, and shelving that your book requires. They know how to create a cohesive finished product that looks professional and sells your book.

As an indie author, you basically have three options for your cover:

» **Learn graphic design yourself.** Learning the art and science of graphic design involves studying your favorite book covers, knowing how to use the positive and negative space, and familiarizing yourself with graphic design software such as Adobe products or Canva. (Unless you have a graphic design background, though, I highly recommend choosing one of the following two options.)

» **Purchase a premade cover off the Internet.** Finding a premade cover means scrolling through thousands of ready-made covers on the Internet for one that fits your book, and hiring that company to customize it with your title and author name.

» **Hire out the cover design to a freelance graphic designer.** Choosing to hire a professional graphic designer involves researching individual portfolios, emailing candidates, and working with the designer until you get a final product.

No matter which option you choose, your cover should:

» **Be professional.** If your cover isn't up to par, it will be quickly overlooked. Your ebook will be sitting on the virtual shelves with all the traditionally published books in your genre. Premade covers are designed by professionals and there are many created for all the romance genres. They cost less than working with a freelance graphic designer because there's less work for your designer to do. You can find some great, professional-looking covers that won't break your bank.

» **Showcase your genre.** Readers shop by genre, and romance readers are no exception. They won't look twice at your book if the cover doesn't look like a romance novel. It's a good idea before you hire a cover designer to do some research and look at the top selling books in your sub-genre. Do they have couples on the cover? Or do most of them have a single male? Or are they mostly sporting a beach house? All of these, and more, have been trends in the romance genre. If you're writing a rom com, find out specifically what is selling well right now in the rom com space. You want your book to match.

» **Look current.** The last thing you want is a book cover that looks like it was designed twenty years ago. Color, layout, print quality, hairstyles, and clothing can all give a cover a dated feel. Update older book covers to look more like the books published today.

>> **Be easy to read.** Make sure your cover uses fonts that are legible. I can't tell you how many books I've seen where I can't read the title on the cover. Be aware of this as you are designing your cover, and make sure there is enough contrast between the font color and the background colors around it.

>> **Use professional fonts.** Purchase fonts from reputable sources. Design programs like Adobe (adobe.com) have fonts that can be legitimately downloaded to augment their basic fonts.

WARNING

Don't use any fonts that come with your computer. They are not the kind of fonts you should be using to design a book cover. Also, don't download free fonts from the Internet. At best, they are poorly designed; at worst, they are pirated copies that are illegal to use.

>> **Use professional images.** Make sure that the images you select from the internet are legal to use and of a high value print quality. Consider paying for a royalty-free image from one of the many stock photo websites.

Your cover should make a great first impression. It should look like the other covers in your genre, and it should make the reader want to check out the blurb (see the "Writing blurbs" section later in the chapter). If you're having issues selling a book, the cover is usually the culprit. Make sure it's on point, and your job marketing as an indie author will be much easier.

Writing a tagline (it's all in the hook)

Having a snappy tagline is crucial when you go to market your book. A *tagline* is one (but sometimes up to three) brief sentences that introduce your story. Most taglines are fewer than 20 words. Usually the tagline is what you see in advertisements, or you see it before the blurb (see the following section) when you're looking at a book on Amazon.

One of my favorite taglines is from the 1979 movie *Alien:* "In space, no one can hear you scream." That one simple sentence captures the feeling of the entire movie. It's a great example, because it's short, snappy, and showcases the genre so well. It also makes you wonder: Why are they screaming in space? This is what you need to do with your tagline, but of course, yours will showcase the romance in your novel.

When I'm writing a tagline I try to think about the main trope of my story. A *trope* is a plot device that has been used so often it becomes instantly recognizable. Unlike clichés, which you should avoid, tropes often bring people to your story. (See Chapter 19 for the most common tropes in romance writing.) For example, I wrote a modern-day story titled *A Marriage of Anything But Convenience.* The tagline I use is "It was a simple marriage of convenience. Just two years. What could possibly go wrong?" This tagline works well because it puts a spotlight on the trope — marriage of convenience — and implies many things go wrong with this plan, which brings in promised tension. It also gives the reader some questions to ponder: What does go wrong? Why are they getting into a marriage of convenience?

TIP

Your tagline should intrigue your reader and accurately represent your book. Be sure the tone of your tagline matches your book; don't write a cute, funny tagline for a book that has no humor in it. Try writing at least twelve different taglines before you pick the final version. Sometimes stretching yourself to continue to think of options is the best way to come up with something great. If you stop at the first tagline you came up with, you won't know if you could have thought of something better on your tenth try. This is a good rule to follow when writing your blurb as well.

Writing blurbs

Your *blurb* is that two- or three-paragraph synopsis that is on the front flap or back cover of your book, or on your ebook page online. This is the description that potentially sells your book. It needs to pull the reader in and make her want to purchase your book. The importance of your blurb is second only to your cover, so you need to make it shine.

It can be challenging to narrow down a 75,000-word novel to just two or three paragraphs. Where do you even start? One tip I've found helpful is to try writing the blurb before writing the book. Before all the side plots are weaved in it can be easier to sift through your story to find the core conflicts. Blurbs should reveal the main romance plot, and shine a light on the tropes you've used.

As you are writing your blurb, ask yourself these questions:

>> Who is your heroine, what is her goal, and what obstacles stand in her way?

>> Who is your hero, what is his goal, and what obstacles stand in his way?

>> What is the main conflict between your characters?

>> What circumstances shove your characters together?

>> What is going to hook your reader into reading your book?

TECHNICAL
STUFF

Romance blurbs are often different from other genres, so it's helpful to read the blurbs of the best-selling indie romance books in your particular niche so you can learn the way they are written. If your romance is written with the points of view of the two main characters, often the blurb features each character getting a paragraph to describe their situation. If your book is written from the female character's point of view, the blurb often just features her and her conflicts.

Whatever you do, practice, practice, practice. You will not want to write just one blurb and be done. Blurb writing is a skill, and you will get better at it the more you do it. Stretch yourself, just like you did with your tagline. Try out different things. See what works the best. It's also a great idea to ask your friends, beta readers, or critique partners to read over your blurb and get their input. If you'll be working with an editor, be sure to have them check your blurb for mistakes when you hire them to edit your manuscript.

TIP

Test your different blurbs by creating a simple Facebook ad, and duplicating it five or six times, changing the blurb on each one. Everything else should stay the same, just swap out the blurbs. Run these ads for a few days and see which blurb is getting the most clicks. You can test your tagline this way as well.

Building your website

Before launching your first book, it's important to build a simple website where you can link to all your social media, link to your books, and offer visitors a place to sign up for your newsletter. There are many user-friendly website builders out there like Wix (`wix.com`), Squarespace (`squarespace.com`), and Weebly (`weebly.com`).

In addition to being a hub for all of your links, your website should contain a Contact Me page. If your indie published book sells really well you could get contacted by literary agents, foreign rights agents, subsidiary rights agents, movie producers, and more, and they will need to be able to contact you via your website.

Creating Your Launch Team

When you're done with your book, when it's well written, crisply packaged, and ready to launch, you'll want a launch team (also called a review team) to help you get the word out. A *launch team* is a group of people who will read your book and then post a review on retail websites. They will talk about your book on social media. You want your launch team to be made up of people who love your genre.

Your launch team may be small with your first book, and that's okay. Actually, it's preferable. It allows you to work out the kinks in your marketing and test your approach to promoting yourself without the whole world watching. Eventually, your goal might be to grow your team as you continue to publish so more readers will help promote each subsequent book.

I grew my launch team slowly by offering a free copy of my book each time I published. I asked on social media and in my newsletter if anyone would like to join my launch team. If you're new to publishing and you don't have a newsletter (covered later in the chapter), that's fine, you can grow one. That will come over time.

To create a launch team, reach out on social media. It's best if you can get fans of your genre to join your team, rather than friends and family. (Amazon is the largest sales platform, and it's against their Terms of Service to have friends and family review your book.) Try posting on a social media platform like TikTok, or in reader groups on Facebook, to see if you can get interest from readers to join your launch team. Keep a spreadsheet of everyone who agrees to help you, including their email address, so you can contact them to send them your book. Keep this list for the next time you publish, and send out another call for team members so you can grow your list.

REMEMBER

Be sure to coach your team when it's time to launch your book. Remember, they are there to help you spread the word, not only with reviews, but also by posting on social media. One of the best ways to sell books is through word of mouth. If your team understands this, they can help you by talking about your book and recommending it to other readers.

Sending out ARCs

An Advanced Reader Copy, or ARC, is a proof copy of your book that you send out to your launch team and to other reviewers before it's published. It's up to you if you'd rather send out a physical copy of your book or an ebook, although I highly recommend sending out ebook copies instead of print. It's much more expensive to send out physical copies, and there's no real added benefit. Sending ebook copies by email is free, and it's much easier to contact your reviewers when it's time to leave their review.

TIP

I use a self-publishing software program called Vellum (vellum.pub) to create my ARC, but you can use whatever program you have to create an ebook file. An .epub file is the most common for the ebook, but I always send a PDF of the book as well just in case my reader isn't able to open an .epub file.

Finding helpful services

Several different services can help you send out your ARCs, gain readers who are willing to review your book, or help with other tasks:

- **BookFunnel:** This service allows you to upload your ebook in different formats so your readers can pick which one works best for them. They collect emails for you so you know who has grabbed your ARC for review. BookFunnel can also watermark your book to make it more difficult for people to pirate, and it's traceable. You can sync BookFunnel with a number of email services so you can collect those emails and build an email list automatically. Go to bookfunnel.com.

- **StoryOrigin:** Through this website you can list your ARC and readers can download it in order to review it. You can do quite a few other things on StoryOrigin, so I would suggest checking out this website. For more, see storyoriginapp.com.

- **Booksprout:** You can use this website to list your ARC so readers can download your book to review. Go to booksprout.co.

Check with these websites for their fees and decide if this is worth the investment for you. If you're just starting out, you might want to do everything yourself to save money. As you grow, you may want to pay these websites to take care of some of these things. My advice is to start out with a small launch team you've created yourself. Until you start selling your books, you won't be sure what your budget is. Starting off using free resources will save you a lot of money. When you're publishing your second book, you'll know more what to expect in terms of income from your book, and you'll be able to decide if using a service to distribute your ARCs is worth it for you.

Forming Your Launch Plan

Before you launch your book, it's a good idea to formulate a *launch plan*. This simply means you are going to plan how you will launch your book to attract attention and sales. As you prepare your launch plan, think about what you'll do to announce your book, and how you will get readers excited about it.

If you are a new author, your launch plan may simply be publishing the book and creating some social media posts about it. If this isn't your first book, you may already have a newsletter and some followers that you can announce your book to. The more you publish, the more you will establish a launch plan that works for you.

Advertising is an important part of launching a book. Here are some avenues you can use to advertise your new book:

>> **Social media:** Promote your book on all your social media sites. Even if you don't have a large following, keep cultivating your social media so when your next book comes out you can have a larger audience.

>> **Paid ads:** You might want to start rolling out some paid ads as you launch your book. Facebook ads, Amazon ads, and BookBub ads are all good places to start. When you first publish you need to get some visibility, and ads will help with this.

WARNING

Ads from Facebook, Amazon, and BookBub are paid per click, meaning you bid on how much you will pay each time someone clicks on your ad. These can get quite expensive, and it's easy to overspend if you're not careful. Keep a close eye on how much you're spending versus how much you're earning, or you can easily spend a lot more than you're making. If, however, you see your sales increase, you can slowly increase your ad budget until you're happy with the ratio of spending versus earning. I like to earn twice what I'm spending at the very least. If I'm not doing that, I shut off the ad or I lower my bid so I'm paying less per click.

>> **Newsletter swaps:** Your newsletter is one of your most powerful marketing tools, and I talk more about this in "Building a newsletter" later in the chapter. When you launch a book, you can ask other authors to mention your new release in their newsletters, and in exchange, you can mention one of their books in yours. You'll want to swap with authors who write in your genre, because their audience will be the most likely to purchase your book.

>> **Paid newsletter mentions:** A week or two after you publish you might want to discount your book to spur even more sales. It works well to lower the price to 99 cents and purchase some paid newsletter mentions from companies who advertise discounted books. Newsletter companies like these have thousands of readers subscribed to their emails, and they will announce your sale to all of them. This is a great way to introduce your new book to readers looking for a bargain. There are many newsletter companies, some that work better than others, so ask in your author group which ones are working for them. My current favorites are:

- BookBub: bookbub.com/welcome

- Robin Reads: robinreads.com

- Bargain Booksy: bargainbooksy.com

- The Fussy Librarian: thefussylibrarian.com

- The eReader Cafe: theereadercafe.com

- Book Cave: mybookcave.com
- Ereader News Today: ereadernewstoday.com

If you are a new author, I suggest you roll out your advertising slowly, over the first ten days after you publish. The reason for this is because of the way Amazon, and some of the other sellers, look at book sales. A sudden spike in sales doesn't do much for your book, but if you slowly increase your sales rank over a span of ten days, your book will look like it's doing quite well, improving each day. This will trigger some in-house marketing for your book, and you will start to see sales that you can't attribute to your own efforts. This is because the booksellers, like Amazon, are starting to advertise for you. I call this my "slow launch method."

If you are an established indie author with quite a few books already published, you can launch a book with a large marketing push, because your name will continue to sell the book. You may not want to use the slow launch method if you're already an established author and have a well-known name.

TIP

People often ask me if there's a better time of year to publish, or a time to avoid. In general, I've published throughout the year and have not found a bad month to publish. Sales are usually up for me in December and January, so those are great months to publish. I would avoid any holiday as your release day. I would also avoid releasing on Prime Day, which is Amazon's massive sale. Most people are buying big-ticket items on Prime Day, and books get overlooked.

Networking

Networking is getting to know other authors in your genre so you can work together either in marketing or in any number of other projects. Networking is making friends. I know many authors are introverts, so this might seem daunting to you, but it's worth it to get out there and mingle, not only for the opportunities you might come across, but also because making friends helps you feel like you're a part of a community.

Networking happens both online and in person with authors. Online, you can form groups on social networks that allow you to work directly with authors who write in your genre. This is very helpful in finding authors to swap newsletters with, to market together, or to form collaborations. When networking online, it's important to interact with people. Start out by reading conversation threads in author groups. Then, when you can contribute something of value, jump in and start commenting.

In-person networking happens at writing conferences, at local writing groups, critique groups, and at other author events. Try sitting next to someone who is sitting alone and strike up a conversation. Be friendly and willing to ask questions so you can get to know other authors. In-person relationships will also give you opportunities to work together, creating in-person events to sell books, or to chat about where you hire services.

Quite a few opportunities may come your way because of networking:

>> **Author interviews:** Authors are often asked to be interviewed on author websites, YouTube channels, and podcasts. Sometimes the channels are small, but some have wider audiences. Take every opportunity you can to get exposure.

>> **Collaborations:** Authors may be asked to write stories for anthologies, collaborative series, and boxed sets. These opportunities will widen your audience and introduce you to new readers.

>> **Newsletter swaps:** Newsletter swaps (mentioned in the previous section) get the word out about a book on sale, a new release, or any other event that might be coming up.

>> **Group sales:** Joining with other authors to have a group sale can magnify your reach and help you gain new fans.

>> **Backmatter swaps:** Networking with others in your genre can help you find authors willing to put your book information in the back of their book in exchange for you doing the same. This is usually in a section after the end of the book where you recommend other books, often titled, "Other books you might enjoy."

>> **Editorial reviews:** Well-known authors are often recruited to be editorial book reviewers within their genre. Every book you review for someone else is essentially advertising for your own publications. It keeps your name circulating. Just be sure not to agree to swap reviews. It's against Amazon's Terms of Service for authors to review swap, so they must be marked as editorial reviews and be put in that section.

REMEMBER

Networking is essential to keeping yourself on top of what is happening in the indie world, and the publishing world in general. Without being involved in author groups, you can miss out on so much.

Boosting your sales

It's no accident Amazon is the largest online bookstore: They are great at selling books. They use algorithms and sales-tracking features to find the appropriate audience for your book. There are a few best practices you can do to help your sales build over time that work in line with their algorithms:

>> **Sell to fans of your genre first.** You can teach Amazon who would be the most interested in your book by marketing to people who read in your genre before anyone else. Ask other authors who write in your genre if they will announce your book to their fans, and announce in social media groups targeted to your genre so you will teach Amazon who will buy your book. After that, you can tell your friends and family about your book.

>> **Utilize a pen name if you write in a different genre.** Keeping separate pen names for your different genres will help Amazon sell your books to the right audiences. If you write several genres under the same name it can confuse not only readers, but the Amazon algorithms. It's always best to separate them.

>> **Unlink your Facebook account with your Amazon account.** Linking your Amazon account to your Facebook account (or any social media account) can cause issues. If you associate with your readers on social media, Amazon can get the idea that you are friends with them. It's against their Terms of Service for friends to leave reviews, and they regularly ban people from leaving reviews on accounts they believe are connected socially.

Building Momentum

As you publish, there are a few things you can do to keep the momentum going, and help build your author business. Newsletters have been mentioned quite a bit, so we'll start there.

Building a newsletter

As an indie author, your newsletter will be your largest asset. You are the one responsible for marketing your books, and being able to reach out to readers will be invaluable. Your newsletter will not be a paper newsletter, so don't worry about having to print one out. The cost of mailing a physical newsletter would be too high to be profitable for indie authors. You will send your subscribers the newsletter via email.

Here are a few newsletter companies that indie authors are using right now:

>> MailerLite: `mailerlite.com`

>> Mailchimp: `mailchimp.com`

» Flodesk: `flodesk.com`

» EmailOctopus: `emailoctopus.com`

Most of these newsletter companies have a free plan up to a certain number of subscribers. I recommend MailerLite, which gives you up to a thousand subscribers free; they are well established; they integrate with BookFunnel; and the plans are reasonable once you exceed your thousand subscribers. However, compare the companies to see which one is right for you.

Once you choose a company and set up your newsletter, you'll need to get subscribers. There are a few great ways to do this. For starters, you'll want to put a link to subscribe in the back of your book. You can entice readers to subscribe by giving away a free reader magnet. A reader magnet is a free story you give away when someone subscribes to your newsletter. (I talk more about reader magnets in the following section.)

You can also put a link to your newsletter signup on your website. The readers who go to your website are people who have read your work and are looking for more information about you. Adding a newsletter subscriber link to your website entices those readers to subscribe to get to know you better.

TIP

Both StoryOrigin (`storyoriginapp.com`) and BookFunnel (`bookfunnel.com`) have group promos where you can collaborate with other authors to gain subscribers. Each author gives one ebook away free, and together you all market the promotion. Readers have to sign up for your newsletters to get the free books.

Your newsletter can be as simple as you'd like it to be. Many authors start with a short, personal message. You can talk about anything that interests you: your pet, your work in progress, or even your hopes for the future. Next, if you're using author swaps, you can talk about another author's books. Showcase the cover and tell them a little bit about the book, or put in the book blurb. In my newsletter, I like to share books from my genre that are on sale. My newsletter subscribers love a bargain. It gets them excited for my newsletter, and I get more people engaged and opening my email. End your newsletter with a promotion for your own work. You can link to your books, or create a short promotion for one of your upcoming works. Always give them something to buy from you.

TIP

Many authors love to add a poll or ask a question for their readers to answer. You can poll your readers about many different things, like their favorite tropes, or what a character's name should be. Your readers will love to be able to give you input about your next book, or just to share something about themselves with you. If you're sending a November newsletter, ask them about their favorite Thanksgiving pie. Be creative!

If you still need more ideas about what to send in your newsletter, subscribe to a few other author newsletters and see what they send you. They may give you some great ideas. You can also look at their layout and see how they design their newsletters, and what graphics they use. Most newsletter companies have easy-to-use drag-and-drop templates, but sometimes it's hard to come up with what to put where. Getting a few examples is helpful.

How often do you need to send out a newsletter? This is up to you. I send mine once a week, but you can send it out once a month if you're not doing a lot of swaps with other authors, or if you're just starting out and don't have a lot of content to send out. When I first started, I had no one to swap with, and nothing I wanted to say, so I only sent out a newsletter when I had a new book to publish.

Many authors, after they publish quite a few books and grow their newsletters, will hire a personal assistant (PA) to send their newsletter out for them. This is one thing you can look forward to if your goal is to become an established indie author with a large audience.

Giving away a reader magnet

Writing a reader magnet is a great way to boost your newsletter numbers. A *reader magnet* is a book or a story you give away free as a reward for joining your newsletter. It can be a full book, a novella, a short story, a prequel story, or even a deleted scene from your book. Many authors will write a story about a secondary character in their novel, and use this for a reader magnet. The basic premise is to write something that will entice people to join your newsletter. They will get that free story emailed to them if they subscribe.

TIP

As you write more books, you may want to use a book that you're also selling as a reader magnet. This gives readers a choice: They can purchase the book, or they can subscribe to your newsletter to get the book free.

Many companies can help you gain newsletter subscribers with your reader magnet. You can upload your reader magnet to StoryOrigin (storyoriginapp.com), BookFunnel (bookfunnel.com), and Book Cave (mybookcave.com), and use their promotional tools to help get more newsletter subscribers. You can even automate giving your reader magnet by using services like BookFunnel, so that any time someone downloads your reader magnet, they automatically get signed up for your newsletter.

SHOULD YOU SET UP A PRE-ORDER?

When you go to publish your book, Amazon will ask you if you would like to set up a pre-order for the book. This allows you to start selling your book right away, but on a pre-order status. If you set up a pre-order, readers can order the book prior to your publication date. They will get the book automatically downloaded to their Kindle later, on the date you set for it to publish.

Pre-orders can be awesome. You can set up your book to sell before it's even finished. I know many authors who utilize pre-orders to gather up sales before their book publishes. But sometimes setting up a pre-order can hurt your sales.

Amazon is set up to sell books, and the more a book sells, the more it will be shown in search results and on other pages. But the reverse is also true: The fewer books you sell, the less your book is shown. If you're not a well-known author, setting up a pre-order might not be very good for you. If your pre-order sits without sales every day, it can kill your after-launch sales.

It's much harder to get someone to buy a pre-order than it is to buy a book that is already for sale. Readers have to wait for the book. It takes an extra shove to get people to purchase that pre-order. If you're a new author, it's even more difficult because people haven't read your work before. My advice is to not use pre-orders until you have a big enough name to attract steady sales while your book is on pre-order.

Purchasing an ISBN

An ISBN (International Standard Book Number) is a product identifier, or barcode, that goes on the back of your physical book. It includes information about your book such as the title and the author. When indie publishing a novel, you have the choice to purchase your own ISBN from Bowker (myidentifiers.com), or to obtain a free ISBN from Amazon KDP (Kindle Direct Publishing), Barnes and Noble Press, or the other retailers. The only company that does not supply a free ISBN is IngramSpark, so if you want to publish with them you will need to purchase your own ISBN.

There is a lot of debate in the indie world about whether you need to purchase your own ISBN numbers, or if it's okay to use the free ones provided. There are pros and cons for each way of doing it.

Here are some benefits to purchasing your own ISBN numbers:

>> **You get to establish your own publishing company.** When you purchase a set of ISBN numbers, you will need to name your publishing company. You are in essence setting yourself up to be a publisher. Your publishing company name will be listed as the publisher of your book.

>> **You may get your books into libraries and bookstores.** If you publish your book through IngramSpark (`ingramspark.com`), your book will be listed in their catalog. Worldwide bookstores and libraries will have access to purchase your book.

>> **You look more professional.** Having a publishing company with a name and possibly a website will make you appear more professional.

There are also some drawbacks:

>> **ISBN numbers are expensive.** If you live in the United States, you have to purchase your ISBN numbers through Bowker. The current price for one ISBN from Bowker is $125. You can save money by buying in bulk, but even so, it's expensive.

>> **It costs money to publish through IngramSpark.** The current price to publish one book through IngramSpark is $49. It's free to publish both a print and ebook through Amazon KDP and Barnes and Noble Press.

>> **There's no guarantee you'll sell to bookstores or libraries.** Even if you spend the money to get your ISBN number, and spend the money to publish through IngramSpark, you have no guarantee that a bookstore or library will purchase your book.

Before you purchase an ISBN number for your book, look through the pros and cons and decide which way is right for you. Personally, I have never purchased an ISBN number, I've used the free ones. I publish all of my print books through Amazon KDP. My print sales are currently around 4 percent of my income. I sell far more ebooks and audiobooks than I do printed books, so for me, it's not worth it to spend the money on ISBN numbers.

Registering your copyright

If you live in the United States, your book is copyrighted as soon as you write the words on the page. This is a protection that is automatically placed on your work. You do not need to register your copyright in order to have that copyright protection. Having said that, if you have any legal issues, it might be helpful to have your work registered with the U.S. Copyright Office.

Here are the benefits to registering your book with the U.S. Copyright Office:

>> **It creates a record of your copyright ownership.** This may deter others from stealing your work.

>> **It allows you to sue if your work is copied.** If you do not register your copyright, you won't be able to sue.

>> **It allows you to recover statutory damages and attorney's fees if you sue.** You must have previously registered your copyright if you wish to receive damages in a lawsuit.

Registering your copyright gives you advantages in court. If you do not register, you still own the copyright and can still have a copied book taken down from Amazon, or another seller, if someone copies your work. You just can't sue for damages.

It does cost money to register your copyright. It currently costs $45 for an electronic filing. I know many successful indie authors who register their copyright with each book they publish, and I know many successful indie authors who don't. It's totally up to you if you would like to register your copyright with the U.S. Copyright Office.

Obtaining a Library of Congress Control Number

A Library of Congress Control Number (LCCN) is a unique identification number that the Library of Congress assigns to the catalog record created for each book in its cataloged collections. You don't need to obtain a Library of Congress Control Number to publish your book, but there are two reasons why you may wish to:

>> **It helps give your book legitimacy.** You can obtain a Catalog in Publication record before you publish so you can include your LCCN on your copyright page.

>> **It can help your book get into libraries.** While you don't have to have an LCCN to be in libraries, it does help. Libraries use this number for cataloging your book.

You'll need to obtain an LCCN if you want to submit your book to the Library of Congress. Housed in three buildings on Capitol Hill in Washington, D.C., the Library of Congress is the largest library in the world. If you send your book to the Library of Congress, they will decide if they accept your book, or not. Just sending it in does not guarantee it will be added to the Library of Congress. If accepted, it doesn't mean it will stay in the Library of Congress forever. For more information, go to `loc.gov/publish`.

After You Publish

After you launch your book, you may be wondering what to do next. What do you need to do to keep up the interest in your book? Let's take a look at marketing, market research, and some easy and fun things you can do to market your book.

Doing market research

As I've said elsewhere in this book, the secret to selling a lot of books is figuring out what your audience wants and giving it to them. Marketing encompasses your book cover, your blurb, and of course, your book itself. You're not selling a product, you're selling an experience. Marketing is researching the market to know what the reader wants. If that experience doesn't give your reader what they want, they're going to go somewhere else to get it.

Authors ask me all the time what my marketing secret is. The funny thing is, I don't really have a secret. I do a lot of market research before I publish a book so I position myself to sell well even before I write a word. I read widely in my genre, making sure I know what books are selling well and which authors I should pay attention to. I watch what the successful authors are doing. I make sure I know what my readers want.

REMEMBER

Sometimes it's not about marketing. Sometimes it's about continuing to write and publish before you find a book that will hit the market just right. It's much easier to market a book that sells well on its own than it is to market a book that is a slow seller. I have has fast-sellers and slow-sellers. My top-selling book sold more than my 19 slowest sellers combined. This book business is sometimes unpredictable. Don't get discouraged if you do everything you can to sell a book, but nothing seems to move the needle. You may simply have not written your bestseller yet. Keep writing.

Paying for ads

Many six- and seven-figure indie authors have achieved their sales success through purchasing ads. Facebook ads, BookBub ads, and Amazon ads are the most common. If your book is doing well, paying for ads can help it do even better. If your book is not selling well, ads can sometimes help you increase your sales and make your book more visible.

REMEMBER

Ads don't sell books. Your book cover, your blurb, and the premise of your novel are what sell your book. If something about your book is stopping readers from buying it, buying ads will be a waste of money.

There are many courses you can pay for that will teach you how to set up ads and use them successfully to market your book. However, some of these courses are quite expensive. Before you spend money on a course on ads, glean as much as you can from free videos on YouTube. You can learn a lot about how to set up ads with free information that is readily available. Take advantage of this before you decide you need to spend a lot of money on a course. I honestly wouldn't take a course on ads before your book income is enough to cover the expense of that course.

TIP

Spend ad money on your most successful books. You will find spending some ad money on a book that already is selling well will make your ad dollars go much farther than spending money on one of your slow-moving books. I place ads on my fast-moving books and let them sell my other books.

Understanding the power of free

The number one reason a reader buys a fiction book is because they've read that author before and they love their work. As an author, this is valuable information. This means your number one goal should be to get as many readers as you can. Notice I said *readers,* and not sales.

Giving away a book for free is a powerful tool. You can quickly gain hundreds of fans by making one of your books free, and buying some advertising for your free book. Not only does this allow you to gain new readers quickly, it also increases your sales after the book goes back to full price. There are a few reasons for this.

The more books you give away in a short period of time, the more visible your book will become on the sales platforms. Amazon, in particular, has a system that shows your book on other book pages in the form of the "also bought" list, and the more you give away, the more book pages you'll show up on. If you give away enough books, your book can be advertised on hundreds, if not thousands, of other book pages. This is free advertising. Whenever I plan a free book, I will buy up mentions in as many paid newsletters as I can so I can give away a lot of books. (I listed my favorite newsletter advertisers in the "Forming Your Launch Plan" section, earlier in this chapter.) My goal is always to give away at least ten thousand units. Sometimes I don't reach my goal, but my most successful giveaways have been when I have given away more than ten thousand books.

Another reason you'll see sales rise is because some people don't want to read just one book in a series. If you give away one of the books, you'll generally see an uptick in sales for the other books in the series. Even if you're giving away a stand-alone book, you'll see sales rise on your other books because people will either read that book and go looking for more from you, or they will be reminded that they enjoyed your books in the past and they'll pick up some of your books they've missed.

Many authors are resistant to the idea of giving away free books. They feel it's their hard work and they don't want to give it away for nothing. The problem with that logic is you're not giving them away for *nothing.* You're using the giveaway as a marketing tactic. One of your biggest hurdles to jump over is your visibility. Giving away your book for a short time can increase your visibility, which in turn, increases your sales.

REMEMBER

It's been proven time and again: Free works. When the grocery store is giving away samples, they're not doing that because they have extra cheddar cheese chips and don't know what to do with them. They're giving them away because it sells cheddar cheese chips.

As soon as I put all of my audiobooks up on YouTube for people to listen to free, I started selling more ebooks. Why? Because people found out they liked my writing style. Some people read faster than they can listen to an audiobook, so I'm sure I sold some books because of that reason. Or they bought the book because I have ads on my audiobooks on YouTube. Or they bought a paperback because they wanted to give my book to a friend or relative. No matter the reason, remember that number one reason why someone will buy a book, and use it to your advantage.

FREE AND LOW-COST MARKETING IDEAS

It can be overwhelming to look at all the ways you can spend money to market your book. Here are some simple, free or low-cost things you can do to help get the word out:

- **Try TikTok.** Many authors introduce new readers to their work through short TikTok videos. If a TikTok video goes viral, it can help you sell hundreds of copies of your ebook. Try looking up your favorite authors on TikTok to see how they are marketing their books.

- **Post on Instagram.** Quite a few authors love to showcase their book on Instagram. If you love taking pictures and are on Instagram, this might be the perfect platform for you.

(continued)

(continued)

- **Join Facebook groups.** Many Facebook groups are dedicated to readers of a particular genre. You can join these groups and get to know the readers firsthand. Always read the rules in each group to make sure you are following them. Also, make sure the groups you join are not simply full of authors dropping their links, with no readers who want to buy books.

- **Have a launch party.** Consider launching your book with an online (or in-person) launch party. Gather up some friends and invite book-lovers to join you. You can do a special giveaway to generate more interest in your party.

- **Check your local shops.** Many local stores are happy to stock your physical book on consignment. Think outside the box, and don't just focus on bookstores. I know authors who have their books for sale in local coffee shops or small-town grocery stores.

- **Gain author support.** Ask your author friends if they would help you spread the word by posting about your book on their social media accounts. Creating a buzz is a fun way to get noticed, and author friends already have readers who follow them.

- **Hold a book signing.** Many local shops are willing to host a book signing. They will even help advertise the event. Don't be afraid to ask if a local store would be willing to do this. It's a great way to meet new people and gain new fans.

Chapter **17**

Selling Your Manuscript: Traditional Publishing

I f you've decided to traditionally publish, you'll need to start researching the market to know exactly where your book will fit, and which publishers would be most likely to pick you up. It can be challenging to get a book published traditionally, but you can significantly increase your chances of getting published by knowing who's who in the business — publishers and editors — and tailoring your submission so that it's as close to what they're looking for as possible.

When you've decided on the most appropriate publisher, maybe even a specific editor, you've taken the first step, but you have more to think about. Each publishing house has its own submission procedures, so you need to know how to tailor your submission to suit the requirements of each publisher. *Query letter, partial, complete* — you need to understand these terms and know how to meet expectations. In this chapter, I give you tips on negotiating the publishing maze; figuring out the most appropriate publisher to target; answering the question of whether you need an agent; and creating a query letter or partial manuscript that accurately represents your book.

Submitting Made Simple

Submitting your novel is a relatively simple process. Most publishers want submissions through email or through a form on their website. Almost all publishers will have their submission guidelines right on their website, easy to find. The hardest part will be researching who wants what, and tailoring your submissions to each publisher, and if you can, each editor.

Doing your research

Before you can submit your novel, research the market with an eye toward who's publishing what. Don't submit your manuscript to publishers who aren't interested in your kind of book. It does you no good to submit your romance novel to an editor who only works on science fiction and fantasy.

TIP

Start at your local bookstore or library and check other books in your genre. Make a list of all the publishing houses, editors, and agents who have handled that particular genre. Also look online to expand your list. Check with any writers' organizations you belong to, and talk to other romance writers at writing conferences. Pitch to agents and editors at these conferences. All of these things will help you find publishers to whom you can submit your manuscript.

After you figure out which publishers and editors are most likely to be receptive to your manuscript, you need to determine what each house's procedures are, and then target your submission to be exactly what they're looking for. Each publishing house has submission guidelines listed on their website. Read through those guidelines and follow them exactly. They also list the editors who specialize in each genre. After you've submitted your manuscript, all you can do is wait, but waiting will be a lot less daunting if you know you've come as close as you possibly can to giving the publisher what they want.

REMEMBER

Figuring out what a publisher or specific editor is looking for is step one. You're looking for the answers to two key questions:

>> **Are unsolicited submissions accepted?** An *unsolicited submission,* also referred to as a *slush* or *over-the-transom submission,* is any submission that hasn't been specifically requested by an editor and/or isn't represented by an agent. If the house doesn't accept unsolicited material, you can try to get your manuscript in front of an editor via a one-on-one appointment at a writing conference or through a contest. The most reliable option, though, is to look for an agent (which I discuss in the "Deciding Whether You Need an Agent" section later in this chapter).

>> **What form should a submission take?** There are three basic ways of submitting a novel:

- Query letter
- Partial manuscript
- Complete manuscript

Every house makes its own decisions as to which form it wants to see and from whom. Some houses accept unsolicited submissions only in the form of a query letter, while they look at partial or complete manuscripts from an agent or by direct request.

REMEMBER

There are exceptions to every rule. Though most publishers and editors prefer to see either a query letter or a complete manuscript from a new author, some are open to seeing partial manuscripts. The key is to find out exactly what the publisher or editor you've targeted is willing to consider or specifically asks to see.

Writing a successful query letter

A *query letter,* or *query,* is the briefest form of submission, required by some publishers (and also some agents). It's also the most common form of submission for unpublished and/or unagented authors. Your first approach to an agent is likely to be through a query letter as well. The basics are just the same, although you may need to tweak your query letter slightly, since you're asking the agent to consider you as a client, not publish your book. While your wording may change slightly, the query letter includes the same information for a publisher as it would for an agent.

TIP

Search on websites like AgentQuery (agentquery.com) to find out which agents take romance novels before you query them.

A query letter consists of four basic parts, and should be less than one page:

>> Introduction to your work: your genre, word count of the manuscript, and your book's title/subtitle

>> The hook: a brief description of your story, 200–300 words

>> Your bio: 50–100 words

>> Short thank you and closing: one sentence

Your *hook*, or the description of your story, is the most important part of your query letter. Make sure you think about these questions as you're crafting your hook:

>> Who is your main character?

>> What is their problem?

>> What do they want, and why do they want it?

>> What keeps them from getting what they want?

>> What drives the story forward? What is the main conflict?

You can use the same tips from Chapter 16 on writing blurbs to help you write your hook. You want your description to be enticing to the agent or editor who will read it.

The most common question I hear about queries is "How can I get an editor to buy my book if all they have to go on is a short description?" The answer is, you can't. But the point of a query letter isn't to get an editor to buy your novel; the point is to get them to ask to see more — a partial or complete manuscript — and invest some time in seeing if it's right for the publishing house. This is why it's important to craft a hook that will leave the agent or editor wanting to see more. Make your hook into something they must read. Practice makes perfect here, so don't craft your query letter and send the first hook you write. Keep trying, and use your critique group to hone that description until it shines.

Another common question is "If a house accepts queries, should I complete the manuscript before I submit?" No hard-and-fast rule applies to this situation, but I recommend having the book written for three reasons:

>> An editor's job isn't to vet your ideas.

>> Until you've actually started writing, you aren't going to know whether your story will really work the way you think it will.

>> If the editor asks to see your book, you want to be able to get it to them quickly. If you get a request for a complete manuscript, you don't want to have to scramble to finish the book.

If you need inspiration for writing your query letter, check out queryletter.com/post/161-examples-of-successful-query-letters-from-famous-authors for lots of helpful examples.

Deciding Whether You Need an Agent

If you decide, whether because you need or want one, to take on an agent, you're hiring a professional to represent you. An agent serves as your middleman (or woman) when submitting your manuscript, negotiating your contract, and dealing with any problems that may arise.

REMEMBER

Authors have two basic reasons for taking on an agent; one reason is a matter of necessity, and the other is a matter of choice.

>> All the major mainstream houses only take submissions that have been specifically requested (usually based on an author-editor appointment at a conference) and manuscripts that come in via an agent. For that reason, if you want to sell to a major mainstream publishing house, having an agent is pretty much a necessity.

>> If you're interested in writing for a series, an agent isn't necessary, because unsolicited submissions can still be made via query letter. Even so, many authors prefer having an agent. Not only does having an agent streamline the submission process (skipping the query stage and going straight to a partial or complete manuscript), but it also allows the author and the editor to maintain a creative partnership, letting the agent handle the complicated and occasionally contentious business details.

You will need to pay an agent if you are able to get one. Most literary agents take a 15 percent cut from your earnings. While this is a consideration, keep in mind it's much more likely you'll get a publishing deal if you have an agent, so you'll want to weigh your options and decide if working with an agent is right for you.

Understanding an agent's job

Every agent makes different arrangements with their authors, but the basic job description remains the same:

>> **Manuscript analysis:** Some agents, especially those who are former editors, give a great deal of editorial input to their clients, while other agents handle a manuscript basically as is. In either case, a big part of the job is deciding on the strengths and marketability of their clients' work, so they feel confident in its salability when they submit it.

>> **Market analysis:** Agents are always in touch with the market, keeping on top of who's publishing what and what particular editors are looking for. Your agent targets your submission effectively and gets it straight to the chosen editor's desk.

>> **Submission:** Agents have full authority to submit their clients' work to any house, and they can choose whether to submit a partial or complete manuscript. Although there's no guarantee that a house will buy a partial manuscript from a brand-new author just because it came in via an agent, they *will* look at it. In most cases, even if a book is rejected, an agent is given some basic information as to why and doesn't receive a simple form.

>> **Contract negotiation:** Agents are versed in contracts in general, and most houses' contracts in particular. They know what terms are fixed and which are open for discussion. Often they have pre-negotiated changes that are inserted in all their clients' contracts. Agents take care of all the ins and outs of negotiating on your behalf: the amount and payment terms of the advance; royalties, when those are negotiable; subsidiary rights, when those are held by the house; option times and terms; and so on. As your representative (and, essentially, your employee), your agent gets back to you at various points in the negotiation to get your thoughts and, ultimately, your approval.

>> **Subsidiary rights:** When the house doesn't hold subsidiary rights, your agent is the one who markets and negotiates them. The most common are film/TV rights, serialization rights, and foreign rights. Some agents handle subsidiary rights themselves or, if they work for a large agency, they hand them over to the agency specialists; others hand them off to a specialized subagent for handling.

>> **Finances:** In most (though not all) cases, the publisher sends all payments to your agent, who keeps their commission and pays the rest to you. Your agent also receives your royalty statements and goes over them looking for problems and questions. Most agents also keep financial records on their clients' behalf for tax purposes.

>> **Troubleshooting:** If problems occur (contradictions in a royalty statement, author-editor issues, major problems with a cover, or anything else), your agent steps in and handles those issues for you.

Finding an agent

Essentially, you need to look for an agent in much the same way you'd look for a publisher. You need to figure out who the players are, and then decide who would be a good match for you and your work. The following resources can help you find an agent:

>> **The Literary Marketplace (LMP):** The LMP is a vast publishing reference that comes out annually and is available in most major libraries. Or you can visit the website at `literarymarketplace.com`, which requires free registration and/or subscription. The LMP has an entire section on literary agents. Many

agents specify the types of projects they handle and their submission requirements.

>> **Online sites and searches:** Writers' websites like AgentQuery (agentquery.com) and QueryTracker (querytracker.net), as well as general Internet searches, can turn up helpful information, including insider info on different agents from authors who've worked with them.

>> **Writers' organizations and conferences:** Membership in writers' organizations gets you access to insider information and puts you in contact with other writers, who can be great sources of information. Writing conferences not only provide an opportunity to hear agents speak, but many agents also offer one-on-one appointments with aspiring writers, so you may actually pick up an agent on-site.

>> **Personal contacts:** Don't be afraid to ask your writer friends — published and unpublished — for advice and tips. A friend who has an agent can provide a valuable perspective. Even your unpublished writer friends may have gone through the submission process and have helpful information to share.

When you find an agent who expresses interest in your work, set up an appointment (in person, online, or on the phone) to discuss your work and your career aspirations, as well as how they work with authors, and make sure you ask questions (see the "Interviewing a potential agent" sidebar).

REMEMBER

Just because an agent offers to take you on doesn't mean that you have to go with that person unless, after a searching conversation, you think they are the right agent for you. When you take on an agent, you give that person a key role in your career. The right agent can help make you a star; the wrong one can stall you at Go. Agenting is a career that has very low barriers for entry, so make sure you're hooking up with one of the vast majority of highly able and professional agents, not someone who's just entered the field and has no credentials.

INTERVIEWING A POTENTIAL AGENT

The best way for you to find out about an agent is to ask questions:

- **Are they on their own or part of a larger agency?** How will that affect you, especially in terms of negotiating things like foreign-language and film/TV rights?

- **What are their credentials?** How long have they been an agent? If they're new, what's their background? Many agents used to be editors or other publishing

(continued)

(continued)

professionals. Have they sold a lot of books? Do they have additional relevant credentials? Some agents are also lawyers, for example.

- **What's their romance-industry experience?** Do they handle a lot of romance authors? If you're a would-be series writer, how familiar are they with category romances? What romance houses and editors have they worked with on behalf of their clients?

- **How big is their client list?** Many agents handle a lot of authors, because only a small number need their skills at any given time, while the rest are busy writing. Still, you want to get a sense that they're able to be there for you when you need them. As a new writer, you can't — and shouldn't — expect to be their only client, much less constant handholding, but you do need to know you can reach them and will have their attention when it's important.

- **What do they think about your book?** You need to know what they see as its — and, by extension, your — strengths and weaknesses. The two of you need to be on the same wavelength with storytelling, because they're not going to effectively represent you if they're not genuinely enthusiastic about your work.

- **How hands-on are they editorially?** The only right or wrong answer to this question lies in whether their approach is what you want and need. If you're looking for a lot of editorial feedback, then you want them to be hands-on. If you're not, you don't.

- **Do they have a plan?** Are they already thinking of an editor they suspect will love your book? A publishing house that's the perfect place for you to begin your career? Tell them a bit about what you have in mind for future books and the route you'd like your career to follow. Then talk to them about how they can help get you there.

Most of these questions don't have a right or wrong answer. Go by whatever makes you feel comfortable. For example, a brand-new agent, if they know their stuff and have genuine energy and enthusiasm for your book, can be a better choice than a veteran who has little time for you and may end up asking an assistant to handle everything. An agent eager to enter the romance market may be a perfect choice, because they'll work extra hard to make you a success — and themselves along with you. An agent who likes to offer editorial input can be great — as long as they don't make you spend months revising and re-revising and never actually submit your book. On the other hand, a hands-off agent may be great for your ego, but may end up sending your book out in less-than-optimum shape.

Sizing Up the Contract

Once you've been offered a contract from an editor, it's time to celebrate! Go out to dinner, get that special something you've been wanting, or eat some chocolate. However you want to celebrate, do it, because you deserve it for all your hard work. Then, it's time to buckle down and take a good look at what you're being offered.

Coming up with questions

First of all, understand that asking questions about the offer is fine. In fact, before you end the initial conversation with the editor, or when you call back to finalize things, ask all the questions you can think of, whether they're about the terms of the contract, your book, or the publishing process. You can ask your editor questions at any time, but after the first conversation, take some time to think of all the questions you can and then ask them all at once, so you don't have to interrupt their work day too often.

The first question that comes to your mind is almost certainly going to be what I always call the money question, so let's go over some of the relevant information for you.

Your offer is almost certainly for an *advance against royalties,* a kind of loan against your future royalty payments from book sales. (I discuss this subject in more detail in the "Understanding advances against royalties" sidebar.) Because of this setup, the amount of money that you get upfront — especially as a brand-new author — probably won't be break-the-bank large. Large advances do happen, but they are rare and certainly not the majority. If you're new, you're an unproven sales commodity, so the publisher probably won't want to throw tons of advance-against-royalties cash at you. The upside to all this? If your advance is relatively small, it's probably not the final amount you'll see on the book.

TIP

It may be a while until you see more money, so asking if there's room to increase the advance is okay. Just be prepared for the answer to be *no.* Your editor probably has little to no room to increase the offer, so don't be offended if that's the case. But it's also possible that your editor *can* go up on their original offer, and you won't know if you don't ask. So if — and only if — you feel it's warranted, go ahead and ask. Just be polite and treat your editor with the same professionalism you want them to show you.

TIP

If you've been offered a multi-book deal, even if there's no flexibility in the amount of the advance, you may find some in the *splits* (how much you're paid at different stages specified in the contract): signing, delivery and acceptance of proposal(s) and the complete manuscripts, and publication.

If you have an agent, they will be there for you during the negotiations. Their job is to help you through this process, although the editor will want to speak directly with you. Feel free to ask your agent any questions you have about the contract and what exactly you're being offered.

UNDERSTANDING ADVANCES AGAINST ROYALTIES

Most of the time, the advance you're offered is an advance against royalties. So what does that mean? You're getting paid money in advance. It's like a loan, with your book's future earnings as the collateral. Your publisher is giving you money before they can publish the book and it actually begins to earn money.

After your book is published, the various royalty rates covered by the terms of your contract kick in. Every copy sold, every foreign sale or condensation in a magazine or newspaper, or any use of the book in any other way covered by your contract, earns money for you. The first money the book earns for you, as specified by the royalty rates in the contract and up to the amount of your advance, goes back to the publisher as repayment for the "loan" they made you. After that's paid back, the money the book earns for you according to the terms of your contract goes to you in the form of royalty payments.

The schedule for paying royalties, or how often and in what months you see an accounting statement or a check, is laid out in your contract. Different publishers handle royalties in different ways, but most hold back what's called a *reserve*.

Because publishing houses pay royalties based not on the number of books printed or shipped but on the number actually sold, and because it takes quite a while to know how many books they can actually sell, most publishers hold back a reserve against returns for a period of time. Your contract and royalty statement should outline how much the house can withhold and for how long, and this amount determines how quickly you pay back your advance and how soon you start seeing additional money.

Note: There's no guarantee your advance will earn out and you'll see more money over time. However, given that most first-time authors don't receive huge advances (because publishers try not to offer a loan that can't be repaid), chances are that you'll eventually see additional money.

Though the money question may be the one most on your mind, it's probably not the only one. Here are some of the fairly big questions you may want to ask during that first call or a follow-up conversation:

» **How do you split the advance payments?** How much do you receive on signing, acceptance of the complete manuscript, publication, or at any other point?

» **What royalty rate(s) cover what types of sales?** Different royalty rates probably govern different editions (mass market paperback, trade paperback, hardcover, book-club edition, and so on), and rates may also escalate based on the number of copies sold.

» **What territories does the contract cover?** The contract may cover the United States only, North America, the world, or only specific other countries.

» **What languages does the contract cover?** Does the publisher plan to print your book in all English-language editions, specific foreign languages, or all major languages?

» **What subsidiary rights does the contract cover?** Subsidiary rights include everything from film and TV rights (they're glamorous, so everyone always thinks of them first) to audio rights, computer games, ebooks, condensation and serialization rights, and more. How does your publisher plan to divide the income from these sources?

» **Does the publisher want you to take a pseudonym?** If you've published in a different genre, it's possible they will want you to use a pseudonym. Can you take one if you want to? What strictures, if any, govern its use?

» **When can you expect your book to be published?** Your editor may be able to give you a specific date or just a general sense of one, but any estimate can be helpful when everyone who hears your news asks — and I promise you, they will — when your book's coming out.

» **How much time does your editor plan to give you to do revisions?** This question may or may not be a contractual point, but it's certainly something you need to know. At what point can you expect to receive a letter or a call outlining any necessary changes?

» **What are the terms of your option?** The option clause lays out the publisher's right to see your next work/next appropriate work, the length of time for which they get to see it exclusively, how much material (usually a complete versus a partial manuscript) you need to submit, and related issues.

Some of the questions racing through your head are minor enough that you may want to wait and see what the contract says. Here are some of the smaller ones that you don't need answered right away:

» **How many free copies of your book can you get?** Not an entirely unimportant question, because people are likely to start asking for signed copies. If you sell foreign rights, book-club rights, and so on, you also want to know how many copies you'll get of those editions. You should also ask about your author discount if you want to buy additional copies.

» **What kind of input, if any, do you have on the cover art and copy?** In most cases, you have little to no input, and you almost certainly don't have approval power. But you may be able to discuss things with your editor, at least, and they can incorporate any of your ideas that they like. Interestingly, you often have more input with a series book than with a single title.

» **What are your responsibilities in the editing and production process?** Will your editor give you a copy-edited manuscript to review? A galley proof (advance copy of your book)? What input do they allow you?

» **What else will your editor or your publishing house require from you?** It never hurts to ask a general question, because every house has different requirements and processes.

One last thing you need to ask: What's the specific information you need so you can contact your editor? The editor who called you — *your* editor — may not be the same editor you originally submitted your book to, so you want to be sure you have the correct spelling of that person's name, title, exact address, direct line or extension number, and email address. Just as they need to be able to contact you, you need to be able to get hold of them easily.

Reading (and rereading) the fine print

Reading your contract is a must, even if you have an agent. Your signature appears on your contract, and you're the one who's responsible for living up to all its terms. So even if you have an agent to do the negotiating for you, not to mention translate all the legalese into English, you need to read your contract yourself and know exactly what you're agreeing to. Where you have to, reread until you understand what you're reading.

Most clauses in your contract aren't negotiable and don't need to be. Don't try to prove you've read everything by asking for changes everywhere. It's possible you won't need or want to ask for any changes at all, but if you do negotiate, focus on the points that really matter.

Getting help

When the time comes to read, negotiate, and sign your first contract, having an agent really comes in handy. With an agent in tow, you have someone at the other end of the phone whose job involves answering your questions about publishing in general and contracts in particular.

TIP

If you don't have an agent, you have other resources to turn to who can help you understand the contract:

>> **A lawyer:** Use a lawyer who is familiar with publishing. They can advise on contract details and help you understand the legalese. Most lawyers charge by the hour.

>> **Romance Writers of America:** The RWA website (rwa.org) has a library of taped speeches from previous conferences, which may contain useful information about contracts. The website also has a library of back issues of the organization's monthly magazine, *Romance Writers Report,* which has published articles, including some about specific publishers' contracts, you may find helpful.

>> **Look online.** Although there can be a lot of misinformation on the Internet, you can find a lot of good information out there, too. By checking out writers' sites, you can find helpful discussions about negotiating. You may even be able to ask questions, though I caution you against revealing specific terms (of your advance, especially), because every contract's slightly different, and the specifics of your personal and financial business really should remain *yours*.

>> **Pick up** *The Essential Guide to Getting Your Book Published: How to Write It, Sell It, and Market It. . .Successfully* **(Workman Publishing Company).** This comprehensive title takes an in-depth look at the world of publishing in general. It includes dozens of interviews with agents, editors, bestselling authors, and booksellers. Plus it has sample query letters, a resource guide, and more.

Strategies for a Win-Win Negotiation

Compared to mainstream contracts, which are far more open to discussion, series contracts in romance publishing generally leave relatively little room for negotiation; it's simply the way the business works. If you've been offered a mainstream contract, here are some tips for making sure your contract negotiations are both successful and pleasant, and a win–win for all parties:

» **Remember that you and your editor have the same goal.** Unlike many other sorts of negotiations, where the negotiating parties have very different interests and often need to make major compromises, you and your publisher (represented by your editor) have the identical aim — to publish your book successfully, sell as many copies as possible, and make as much money as possible for both of you.

» **Be reasonable in your requests.** You can negotiate plenty of points, but not all of them, and not forever. Do you want more free author's copies of your book? Your editor can probably do another 10 or 15, but a 100 is probably pushing it. The same theory holds true for the tougher clauses, too, like the amount of your advance and various royalty rates; if you ask for reasonable increments of change, not huge ones, you're more likely to be successful.

» **Decide what's most important to you.** For example, is it more important that you get as much money as possible up front, keep your film rights, or negotiate a higher royalty on foreign editions? All or none of those specific things may be on the table, but a variety of things are likely to be under discussion in any negotiation. If the time comes when you have to choose when to push and when to give in, going in knowing what matters most to you helps.

» **Act professionally.** Negotiating with someone who threatens to walk over every point, however minuscule, or who takes everything personally, is very frustrating for the editor. Don't pull your financial hardships into the negotiation, and don't act as if everything's an insult. Remember, this is business. Your publisher is obviously a business, and now you are, too.

» **Be prompt in your responses.** You and your editor may naturally play phone tag sometimes, just because you're both busy, but don't let time go by just as a power play.

» **Accept that some things are the way they are.** Every house has clauses that it refuses to alter or delete, whatever the reason. If your editor says something's non-negotiable, don't keep fighting it. Move on, and don't dwell on the points you can't change. That said, if you have an issue with a non-negotiable clause to the point where it's a deal-breaker for you (and I'm assuming that neither you nor your editor wants anything to break the deal, and that you wouldn't threaten to walk away frivolously), then say so.

Working with Your Editor

The relationship between you and your editor is the most important one of your career. If you have an agent, that relationship probably runs a close second. The way you and your editor work together affects the progress and success of your book — and all your future books with that house.

Making the relationship work

The key to making the author/editor relationship work lies in realizing that from the moment they offer you a contract, they're your ally, the person who has chosen to make your book as strong as it can be and shepherd it through the publishing process so that it can be as successful as possible.

If they ask for revisions, as they're quite likely to do, it's because they think those revisions will make the book stronger. When they write copy or work with the art department on your cover, they're trying to create a cohesive, persuasive package so that your book sells as many copies as it can.

REMEMBER

The fact that you and your editor have the same goal (the successful publication of your book) in mind doesn't mean the two of you will agree on everything all the time, so don't worry if you don't always see eye to eye. Mutual honesty and respect can make your relationship a successful one. If you don't agree with a particular revision, for example, tell your editor so. Just explain your point of view and be polite. I know that should go without saying, but unfortunately, some new writers (and even some established authors) see their editor as the enemy and the process of working on the book as some kind of power struggle. If you want your career to be a long one, do not engage in that kind of attitude. Operate as if your editor is fair and open-minded.

TIP

What if you and your editor turn out to be a bad match? You can't make an informed decision in this regard until you've worked together for a while. Don't rush to a conclusion while you're doing revisions on your first book or at some equally early stage in the process. Give the relationship time to work. If you eventually realize that the two of you, despite both of your best efforts, aren't working well together, requesting a change of editor is perfectly fine. You have a few options:

>> If you have an agent, they can handle this request for you.

>> If you don't have an agent, you have to handle it yourself. If you have a good rapport, even if you don't see things the same way creatively, talk to your editor directly. If you don't feel comfortable taking the direct approach, talk to your editor's boss, explain the situation, and ask them to handle it.

REMEMBER

If you have to initiate that conversation with your editor, be polite and matter-of-fact, and keep your emotions in check by staying calm and professional. You aren't trying to bad-mouth your editor or (inadvertently) make yourself look like someone who's impossible to work with. You just want to create a better working situation for you both.

Revising your book one last time

Your first extended chance to get to know and work with your editor probably comes when you're asked to do revisions. Revisions at this stage are likely to be relatively minor compared to any revisions the editor asked you to do before they offered you a contract, because you wouldn't have been offered that contract unless your book was already close to publishable. If your editor asked you to do revisions earlier, those revisions were probably big-picture changes. Now you're likely to be dealing with smaller, more specific points.

TIP

When you become an about-to-be-published author, revisions are a collaborative process in a way they weren't before. Before you're signed, if an editor asked you to revise and resubmit, your only choice is whether to do it or not. Now you get to have an actual conversation. If you have a question about, or a problem with, something your editor has asked you to revise, go ahead and ask about it, because you can reach an easy compromise most of the time. The two-way communication and honest approach that make the author-editor relationship work also make the revision process go smoothly.

Line editing set straight

After you've done any last revisions, the line edit is the first time your editor picks up their pencil and starts working on your book. A *line edit* is a content edit, and a good editor does only as much as necessary to bring all the book's strengths to the fore. Your editor may edit so lightly that the manuscript looks almost untouched, or they may have edits on every page. Your editor will look for big concerns as they edit — for example, whether every character's behavior is believably motivated or whether the timeline makes sense. They will also keep smaller concerns in mind — whether every line of dialogue leads believably into the next or whether each chapter begins and ends effectively. They may also correct spelling and grammar when they find mistakes, but some editors leave that for the copy editor to handle.

Ideally, most problems get solved during the revision stage. But some small things always get missed and show up during the line-editing process, which by its very nature is a detail-oriented one, as the editor goes through the manuscript with a tight focus on every line.

Often, a book may need a new title because the title you gave it doesn't work for any number of reasons. Your publisher may think that title can't sell, or maybe it's too close to another book they're putting out. Whatever the reason, your editor may ask you to suggest other titles and collaborate with you on choosing one during the line-editing stage, or they may come to you with a suggestion the house likes to see if you like it, too. You may or may not have title approval, but most editors work with their authors to be sure everyone's happy with the final choice.

After line editing, your book will go through copy editing for another look at spelling and grammar. Feel free to discuss any questions or concerns you have with the copy editing as well. This will likely be the last time any changes will be made. Be prepared for tight deadlines at this stage of your book.

Chapter **18**

Handling Rejection

All writers face rejection at one point or another, whether it's through rejection letters or from negative reviews. Knowing it will come may help prepare you for it, and help you deal with it along your writing journey. The most important thing is to learn from it, and grow as a writer.

In this chapter, I discuss some aspects of the revision and rejection stages you'll almost certainly go through if you're trying to traditionally publish, including what an editor might be telling you in their rejection letter, how to revise your work if the editor requests it, and how to deal with rejection from an emotional standpoint.

If you're planning to indie publish, you may not have to deal with rejection letters, but most authors have to deal with bad reviews at some point in their career. In this chapter you learn how to handle them professionally. Remember, all books get them, and a bad review doesn't mean your book is horrible.

What the Rejection Letter Is Really Saying

After you send in your query letter or your manuscript (prepared according to the submission guidelines; see Chapter 17), you'll need to wait for a response. Plan to wait four to six weeks, and sometimes more. Agents and editors get hundreds if not thousands of query letters each year and they can get backed up. If, after six weeks, you haven't heard back, it's okay to send a follow-up email to the editor.

If you're sending in a query letter, you will get one of three responses: The editor will want to see either the full manuscript or a partial manuscript, or they will send a rejection letter. If they want to see the full manuscript, send it in, following their guidelines. The same thing goes for a partial manuscript request. You're hoping for a full manuscript request after they read your partial manuscript.

If you've sent in your manuscript, you'll get an acceptance letter, a rejection letter, or a revision letter from the editor. There are different types of rejection letters, and I'll talk about those in a minute. If you get an acceptance letter, it's time to celebrate. They want to publish your book! A revision letter means they want you to revise something in your manuscript and they'd like to see it again. This is not an acceptance, but you're close, and you can celebrate that they liked something about your book and want to see it after you've revised it.

REMEMBER

I've broken down the whole range of rejection and revision letters into relatively few types, but these letters exist on a continuum — especially when you're talking about any letter that contains a book-specific critique or encouragement at any level. The range of letters you may get and phrases you may need to interpret is huge. Editors are individuals. You can't judge a revision letter's intent based purely on its length, because a particular editor may consider a one-page letter that gets into specifics about your book as incredibly detailed, while to another editor, that's brief. Another editor may mention specifics or suggest revisions of any sort only if they intend the letter to be the highest form of encouragement.

All you, or anyone you ask for interpretive help, can do is take every factor you know into account — especially if you have other letters from the same editor as a comparison — and make your best guess as to what that editor intended.

REMEMBER

The bottom line: If an editor wants to see the book again, they will say so. If they don't, accept that and move on. To be traditionally published, you have to play the odds, using your time as wisely as possible — and that means recognizing both good and bad news for what it is. That approach increases the odds that one day you can hear the best news of all — that you've sold your manuscript.

Regarding rejections

The hard truth is that most manuscripts won't be accepted. Harlequin, for example, gets around 9,000 submissions each year, and takes on just 45 to 50 of those. You're reading this book and working on your craft to improve your odds of being one of the lucky ones whose work editors consider publishable, or at least worth commenting on. Even so, you need to know how to interpret every kind of possible response, starting with the worst:

» **The form reject:** This kind of rejection simply tells you the publisher found your manuscript unsuitable for publication at their house. It's a simple "no, thank you." It may list some common issues that led to the rejection, giving you examples, but they are not personal to your story and leave you wondering if your story has any of these issues, and if so, which ones. While it's frustrating to get a form reject, it simply means this project isn't right for this publisher.

» **Rejection, but hope for next time:** You may receive a rejection letter, but with a line that reads something like *Though this project isn't suitable for our needs, I would be happy to see future submissions from you.* This means this editor legitimately wants to see future work from you. Don't revise and resubmit the same book, but keep them in mind for another project. If this letter comes with specific information about why your book didn't work, take a close look at that. Writers often repeat mistakes in their work, and this will help you, not only with this project, but with future books as well.

Revising and resubmitting

The next-best thing to selling your book happens when an editor asks you to revise and resubmit. Even if the book doesn't ultimately sell, congratulate yourself on taking a considerable step forward toward your goal, a step relatively few would-be authors get to take. If you receive a request to revise and resubmit, it's a compliment to both your talent and the work you've put into studying your craft. Accept it gracefully and with pride.

There are a couple of variations on the revise-and-resubmit letter:

» **The top-line revise and resubmit:** This kind of letter gives you fairly broad comments, things to work on in your book, but they are big-picture issues like strengthening the conflict or making the characters' motivations clearer. You'll get this kind of letter when the editor feels your manuscript has potential — enough that it's worth their time to see it again — but it still needs quite a lot of work. What happens when you resubmit depends on your ability to take a big-picture view of your book and the editor's comments, and then do a thorough rewrite to address their concerns.

» **The detailed revise and resubmit:** This kind of response is the next-best thing to a contract offer. A letter like this can literally go on for pages, which makes it look quite daunting, but it really is good news. It means that the editor thinks your book is close to being publishable, and they're willing to invest a considerable amount of their time in writing a detailed letter to show you where the problems lie.

Understanding the Revision Process

The revision process isn't really all that different whether you have a top-line letter or a detailed one. Either way, you have to look at your book from a different angle, go back over what you thought worked, rewrite — sometimes substantially — and then go through the submission process all over again.

REMEMBER

The most important thing to know about any request to see a revised version of your book is that it's 100 percent sincere. Editors are busy people. Every editor I know is also a really nice person. But editors aren't so nice that they ask you to do extra work unless they see potential for a payoff. If an editor takes the time to write a personal, encouraging letter analyzing your text and suggesting changes, then offers to invest more time in reading the revised version, you can believe that they see potential in you and your book.

Similarly, don't ever think that an editor who sends you an encouraging letter isn't serious, and that they're really sending you the message "Put that book away and don't waste any more time on it." Editors don't put in the time on a long letter to drum your unworthiness into you, but rather to emphasize how much potential you have.

If an editor asks to see your book again, it's not a guarantee that the publishing house will eventually buy it, but such a request *is* a guarantee that you've made it one step closer to your ultimate goal: publication.

Addressing editor queries

When your editor asks for revisions, they are pointing out places in the book where something wasn't clear, didn't make sense, or took the book in the wrong direction. They're asking the author to revise and provide a clarification, an explanation, or a turn back onto the right path.

TIP

If you go through the book taking the editor's notes and turning them into questions you ask as you go, you can see where you need to make changes.

>> **Top-line revisions:** Top-line revisions are the big-picture issues. Take what the editor said, rephrase it, and start going back through your book. Ask yourself:

- **"Your heroine's motivations aren't always clear" becomes "Are my heroine's motivations clear in this scene?"** As you go through your book, asking that question scene by scene, you can make changes wherever you realize that you haven't made her motivations clear. By the time you're done, you've made your book stronger and taken care of the editor's concern.

- **"Your pacing lags toward the middle of the book" becomes "Does this scene slow the book down? How can I speed it up?"** With those questions in mind, you can look at the central section of your book and use the techniques I discuss in Chapter 10 to get things moving again in scenes where the pacing slows.

You can use this approach with anything an editor says, putting it into a form that helps you with your revisions.

Page-specific revisions: Sometimes the sheer number of the revisions in a lengthier, detail-oriented revision letter can be surprising, but remember that they're actually an editor's expression of enthusiasm and confidence. As you go through them page by page, most of them are likely to be specific and easy to deal with, but whenever something's not clear, turning it into a question can help. For example, "The transition between this scene and the next is jarring" becomes "How can I make this transition smooth and carry the reader along?"

The editor has already done a lot of the work for you by pointing out the specific places you need to look at. Address page-specific revisions in order and, even when you have quite a lot of them to wade through, they can be handled relatively quickly.

Using an incremental approach

Thinking about rewriting an entire book can be daunting. This is true even if a lot of the changes are page-specific and relatively finite, and it's particularly true if the editor made multiple big-picture suggestions for you to keep in mind.

TIP

Make the revision task seem less intimidating by breaking down the job into manageable increments. Handle one chapter at a time and then take a break. Or, look at one type of revision at a time — first pacing, then characterization, and so on. You may find focusing on and correcting problems that way easier. Work through the page-specific revisions as you go or as their own separate stage.

This incremental approach may not be the most time-efficient method, but if it helps you visualize the task and gets you working on the book rather than putting it off, it's worth whatever extra time it may take. Also, given how busy your day can be, working chapter by chapter may actually be the best approach. Fit a chapter in whenever you have time, instead of hoping to find a bigger block of free time. Find an approach that keeps you rewriting in a way that works for you.

Being timely

Time *does* count when you're doing revisions, for a couple of reasons:

>> **Every editor has a lot of projects going on at the same time.** Because editors are busy people, the sooner you can get your revised manuscript back on their desk, the more likely they are to remember it clearly, with the same enthusiasm that led them to request revisions in the first place.

>> **Doing revisions on spec is kind of like an audition.** You're doing your revisions in hopes of making a sale, so no contractual deadline is involved. But you're demonstrating to the editor that you're not only willing to revise, but also that you can do it in a timely fashion. Those are important things for them to know. If they buy one book from you, they're hoping to buy more in the future, and they need to know they can work with you. Returning your revisions quickly tells them that they can.

>> **Being quick may clinch the sale.** You may not know it, but when the editor asks you to revise, they may be looking at an upcoming hole in their schedule that they can fill with your book — if you get that book ready in time. Or they may see an opportunity to publish your book to tie in with a holiday or other upcoming event.

WARNING

Though time is of the essence, it's equally essential that you take enough time to revise thoroughly and effectively. If you do a hasty job, the editor will know it, and the fact that you were quick won't be enough to offset the fact that you were sloppy. Balance out both sides of the equation, finding a way to be as fast as you can while still keeping the quality of your work high.

When great minds don't think alike

What if you totally disagree with an editor's suggestions? This question is tough, because you're giving up the possibility of a sale if you decide not to revise. Before you make that determination — and sometimes it *is* the right one — analyze the situation and why you object to the suggested revisions.

>> **Minor points:** If you disagree over a few relatively minor points, make the rest of the revisions and resubmit, mentioning in your email the points you left alone and why. Be brief and don't be argumentative. A good editor is always open to discussing the need for changes, and such discussion doesn't burn any bridges.

>> **Major points:** What if the editor's vision of your book — who your characters are, where the story should go — is radically different from yours? Their approach may be just as interesting or valid as yours, but it requires telling a different story than you set out to tell. Does that new story resonate for you? It may be worth at least trying to revise along those lines and seeing whether it works. But if the suggested new direction genuinely doesn't make sense for you, if it's just not a story you can see yourself writing, then you don't have much of a choice. Don't make the revisions. Consider approaching that editor again with a project you think may appeal to them, but direct *this* project elsewhere.

TIP

If you decide you cannot revise the manuscript as asked, go ahead and send the editor a brief note thanking them for their interest, but let them know you're not going to resubmit. You don't want to sound like a prima donna, but you also don't want to burn any bridges by acting as if you're not appreciative of the help. So write the note, making sure you let the editor know how much you appreciate their interest in your work. Thank them for their time, but let them know you're taking the book in a different direction.

WARNING

If you find yourself reacting negatively to every editor's suggestions on every book you write, you probably need to take another look at yourself and start figuring out how to be more open-minded and flexible if you want to succeed in this business.

Handling the resubmission process

After you finish revisions, you've done almost everything you can do to try to sell your book. Now you just have to handle the actual resubmission of your manuscript. On the one hand, an editor read your manuscript and asked to see it again, so you have an "in," something you didn't have the first time around, which can reassure you. On the other hand, this time around — for that very same reason — you have a real shot at selling, so the pressure is turned up. It may feel as if everything's hanging in the balance, and that's *not* reassuring.

Go ahead and resubmit your manuscript, following the directions that your editor gave you. You have three possible outcomes to this resubmission. Either they will accept your manuscript for publication, they will ask for more revisions, or they will reject it. Even if they reject it, though, you've gained the interest of an editor who may want to see more work from you. Ask if they would be willing to look at another manuscript if you have one ready.

Identifying Common Issues

No one but the editor who wrote the letter can ever tell you exactly what they meant by a specific comment, but a lot of top-line revision letters talk about the same kinds of things. In the sections that follow, I outline common manuscript criticisms, my interpretations of what can spark those comments, and what you can do to fix the problem.

Your heroine isn't as sympathetic as she needs to be

As I discuss in Chapter 4, your heroine is the reader's alter ego. She needs to be approachable, someone the reader can empathize with. Would-be writers often try so hard to make sure their heroines don't act like wimps that they come on too strong. You may have made your heroine too shrill, for example, having her see an insult in every little thing and getting angry about it. Or she's so capable at every-thing that the hero looks like a wimp by comparison. Or maybe you've just made the heroine so beautiful and privileged, without a single insecurity, that no reader can identify with her.

Chances are you know (and like) your heroine so well that you're aware of all her insecurities, for example, and you think they're right there on the page. But you need to go back and add or emphasize (to the point that you may feel as if you're exaggerating) the missing qualities that can help your reader empathize with your heroine. Or you may need to actively change plot elements to create a greater sense of equality between the hero and heroine. Most readers are looking for a relationship of equals, not a complete reversal of the traditional sex roles.

Your pacing is erratic

A book with erratic pacing moves in fits and starts, like a car that keeps stalling out. Usually the author has a series of dramatic, tension-filled scenes that move well — maybe even actual action scenes, like a car chase or a fight — but the author hasn't figured out how to create a similarly strong pace in the scenes that connect them. In between these scenes, she may offer the reader a series of low-key dates, scenes of the heroine with her family or friends, scenes of her on the job, and so on.

TIP

If erratic pacing is your problem, you have to get rid of the filler scenes, which you can do in two ways (you may want to do both):

>> **Cut the slow scenes entirely.** Replace them with scenes where something *does* happen. Not every scene has to feature high drama, but every scene does need to move the romance and the plot forward. Think of it as a workout — you warm up before the intense exercise and then cool down afterward. Those warm-up scenes (and the cool-downs) should build on the more dramatic scenes, not exist in isolation from them.

>> **Inject drama into the scenes that you already have.** Give those ho-hum scenes not just text (the relatively boring stuff that's happening) but subtext, hidden tensions and passions that the reader sees and expects to explode at any minute. These components add drama to what may otherwise be a totally uninteresting scene.

Your hero's too strong/arrogant/tough

The editor may even say your hero comes across as nasty or rude. Given the popularity of the alpha hero (discussed in Chapter 4), a writer often goes too far in trying to create this hero type and comes up with a guy who's just too tough and really does come off as nasty, not appealingly strong. I frequently see this kind of hero in tandem with a too-strong heroine, and the result is two people who spend the whole book fighting with, yelling at, and competing with each other — but never actually meshing. They're equals, but not in an attractive way.

TIP

If your hero is described in a negative way, you need to tone down the tough-guy stuff and create a whole different side to him. You need to humanize him, to show his softer, more sympathetic streak (even if he hides it from the heroine). You may also find that using more of his point of view helps, because if you show the reader why he acts so tough, they will tolerate more gruff behavior than if his motivations are a mystery.

Your plot lacks the necessary complexity

The fact that a plot lacks the complexity necessary for the length of your novel makes itself evident in a variety of ways. For example, the romantic conflict gets settled several chapters before the end of the book, so suddenly a new — and totally unconnected — problem comes in from left field to keep the hero and heroine apart for another 40 or 50 pages.

If you receive this comment, you first need to analyze your book to figure out exactly why the editor made it. After you've done that, you can look at various ways to solve the problem. You may want to consider whether you can get away with a shorter book. In the first example above, perhaps you can cut the last few chapters and let the book end where the story naturally does.

TIP

If you need to beef up your central plot to avoid relying so heavily on a subsidiary story line, you need to complicate things for your characters. If you've written a romantic suspense novel, this is relatively easy, because most mysteries can handle another (believable) twist. Often, though, you need to look to your characters for complexity. If you deepen and complicate their conflict, you give yourself additional building blocks for their scenes together, and you give them issues that take longer to work out. Both those additions allow you the freedom to add scenes that feel dramatic and relevant, and that lengthen your book without padding it.

Your characters' motivations aren't clear

This is a fairly common issue. Particularly (but by no means exclusively) in books with a lot of action, like a romantic suspense novel, much of the focus goes to what's going on but not as much goes to why. An author may explain plot developments, but they frequently overlook emotional ones. Characters get mad or frustrated, and the reader never gets any — or enough — sense of why they feel that way. Or the heroine thinks that she loves the hero, but the reader just sees the two of them at odds, even if they are irresistibly physically attracted to each other, so all that emotion seems to come out of nowhere.

You may think you've been clear about what's going on in your characters' heads. Because you know them so well, you don't spell out what they're thinking because you're thinking it right along with them. The reader, though, is meeting these characters for the first time when they start on page one, so they need more to go on. You may feel as if you're hitting your reader over the head with a sledgehammer by spelling things out, but you aren't; you're just giving them what they need to know.

TIP

I talk in more detail about using your characters' points of view in Chapter 9, but this tip can help you open your characters' minds to your reader: Let your heroine wonder why she suddenly sees the hero in a different light (or vice versa). Point out the small shifts in perception and emotion that ultimately lead to love. Emotions — especially love — are often illogical, so sometimes you just need to have the character ask the same question that's running through the reader's mind: Why do I like him so much? Why did I just get mad at her when I really want to kiss her?

Your characters seem more like types than real people

Editors most often direct this comment toward secondary characters, but heroes and heroines aren't immune. They too can feel as if the author hasn't fully formed them as individuals; instead, simply assigning them suitable traits. As I discuss in Chapter 4, any character who has more than a walk-on part should feel like a real person, but often they seem to come straight from central casting: the kindly grandmother who's always baking cookies; the gay hairdresser; the surly, trash-talking teenager; the outwardly sweet but secretly mean — and always glamorous — other woman.

TIP

With the secondary characters, you need to go back and mix up their traits a bit. You don't want them to be so interesting that the reader pays too much attention to them and wonders too much about their lives and fates, but you do want them to seem like individuals.

REMEMBER

If you have the stereotype problem with your hero or heroine, fixing it may be tougher than the same problem with your secondary characters. Go back to the beginning and start thinking about your couple as emotional individuals, not just in terms of their physical descriptions and outward characteristics. Delve deeper into their backgrounds, their hopes, and their insecurities to create a more complete picture, and let their emotions drive their actions as much as possible.

Maximizing Your Chance of Success

No matter how hard you work, chances are you're going to rack up some rejections and bad reviews along the course of your writing career. That's generally the rule for most authors seeking traditional publishing, not the exception. Enjoying the writing process and the fulfillment that creating compelling characters and story lines brings can go a long way toward helping you cope with rejection.

Keeping a positive attitude

Rejection is never fun, but keeping a healthy and positive mindset is imperative to succeeding in this industry. If your manuscript isn't right for a particular publisher, keep going. Submit another one. The only way you fail is if you quit. Thinking of your rejection letters as another process you need to go through in your publishing journey turns a negative into a positive.

Keeping a positive attitude, even in the face of rejection, can help you in the end. No one wants to work with an author with a poor attitude, and this can come through in your interactions with editors and agents. Remember to smile and keep thinking of the good things that will come to you because of your hard work. Always be professional in your dealings. This will carry you far.

Dealing with rejection, emotionally and professionally

It's understandable — even expected — that rejection hurts. No editor doubts that every submission they see represents someone's hard work, but despite that, most of the time their job is to tell someone that their book didn't make the grade. Given how personally invested you feel in your work, you're totally justified in being upset by rejection. No one says you have to put rejection out of your mind as if it never happened, and get back to work on your newest project five minutes after you read your rejection letter. But consider this: Dealing with rejection can make the difference between having a successful writing career and giving up when you shouldn't.

REMEMBER

Part of being a writing professional is dealing with rejection. Even published authors get rejected. Authors who have an editor and a career still sometimes come up with a project that isn't right for the market. If you ask them, I'm sure they can tell you that it's never easy. But it's a fact of the writing life, they've figured out how to deal with it, and you need to figure it out, too.

After the rejection letter comes and you've gotten over your first moments of pain, give yourself some time to come to terms with the fact that this book wasn't *the* book, then deal with rejection like the professional you plan to be. Here are some tips:

>> **Expect it.** I'm not saying that the minute you send a manuscript, you should start mourning the fact that the publishing house will reject it, but in terms of your overall career and all the submissions you'll make over the years, you can expect to face rejection. If you factor in that possibility, it loses the power to surprise you when it comes, and that preparedness takes away a big part of its power to hurt you.

>> **Analyze objectively.** You may find such analysis hard, especially the first few times, but by the time you get a rejection letter, you've probably been away from the manuscript for a few months, at least. Try to think about it as if you're looking at someone else's book, and think about possible reasons why an editor may have turned it down. If the editor gave you feedback, use that as your basis for analysis. You'll probably start to see flaws you didn't see when you first sent it off.

>> **Seek support.** Do you have friends who are writers, or have you become part of a writers group? Call them or get together for coffee, and talk about what happened. They've all probably gotten rejection letters before, and no one can offer support like someone who's been through the same thing. As a benefit, if your letter contained book-specific criticism, they may be able to help you analyze the manuscript in light of that.

>> **Get some distance from your book.** Sometimes it helps to put a manuscript away for several months and work on something else. You'll often come back to it with fresh eyes and a new perspective.

REMEMBER

>> **Keep writing!** If you're a writer, not just a dabbler, you need to write the same way that you need to breathe. You may be a little distracted when you first sit down at the keyboard again, second-guessing yourself for a little while, but don't let that stop you. Keep writing, and soon you'll find yourself caught up in your latest characters and their story.

It's also important to deal well with rejection emotionally. You still have family and friends, and quite possibly co-workers, counting on you, so you don't have the luxury of falling apart. You're the best judge of how you deal with adversity, so call on your usual coping techniques to help you now. Here are a few suggestions:

>> **Remember that your book was rejected, *you* weren't.** It's easy to take rejection as a personal indictment, but that's a huge mistake. Ninety-nine percent of the time, the editor is not passing judgment on you at all; they've judged your manuscript and nothing more. It's all too easy to extrapolate from a rejection letter and decide that you're worthless on every level of your life, but you're not — and you need to remind yourself of that.

>> **Indulge yourself.** Get your mind off what happened by doing something you enjoy. Get a manicure, go to a movie (a comedy, a tearjerker, something to shift your mood), or cook the kind of gourmet dinner you haven't had time to make while you've been busy writing.

>> **Give yourself a reward.** I'm not saying to break the bank and buy yourself something extravagant, but it takes courage to submit a manuscript. Whatever the outcome, you've passed a milestone; do something to commemorate it. Reward your bravery and determination. Just don't stop being courageous. As soon as the next book's ready, go ahead and submit it, too.

Analyzing your book in light of the rejection itself, in tandem with editorial feedback, gives you insights as you move forward in your career. You get important insights — of mistakes you've made and don't intend to make again, and also of strengths you bring to the writing process — as your reward for submitting your book. It's not the reward you wanted, but it *is* something you can take forward and use.

WHEN IS ENOUGH ENOUGH?

For most would-be writers, a point comes with a book — sometimes, with book after book — when you've done all you can. You've submitted to every publisher you can find, you've revised as much as you can based on general lists of potential problems, and you're still getting form rejects. The hard truth is that you probably need to table that project. Not every book sells, and even a lot of bestselling writers have manuscripts that never sold and never will. When that time comes for your book, accept it, move on, and apply what you learned to your next manuscript.

If traditional publishing isn't in the cards, you can indie publish your book, Many authors have gone on to successfully indie publish manuscripts that were rejected by traditional publishers. Just because your book isn't right for a publishing house doesn't mean it won't sell for you. Check out Chapter 16 for more on indie publishing.

REMEMBER

Coping with the news gives you the composure to accept that reward, see it objectively, and make use of it. A constructive outlook leads directly to the final step: moving on. You need to put rejection behind you. You'll probably have to deal with rejection again, but you can't let the fear of it control you. Move on, whether to the next book or the next potential publisher. Moving on may not be easy, but if you want to be a published writer, it's the only way.

Dealing with bad reviews

Similar to manuscript rejection letters, bad reviews come with the territory. Every author gets them, even the most famous authors. If you don't believe me, go search online for any author you know and love and take a look at their reviews. It doesn't matter how many books they've sold or how many five-star reviews they have, there will be some bad reviews.

The easiest way to deal with bad reviews is not to read them. You never have to worry about them getting you down if you just ignore them. But, practically speaking, that's not very helpful advice, and I'm not a big believer in sweeping things under the rug. Just realize that bad reviews will come, and it's not necessarily an indicator that your writing is bad or that your book is terrible.

REMEMBER

No matter what, don't respond to a bad review. You want to treat this business with professionalism, and bad reviews are simply a part of it all. Responding negatively online to a bad review can hurt you in the end. Ignore the bad reviews, even if they say misleading things, or get details of your book wrong. You'll be better off.

Different people like different things. It's okay if someone reads your book and doesn't like it. Don't dwell on the bad review, and don't take it personally. Instead, focus on the good reviews you have. Many people will love and be entertained by your work. You will touch lives. Let that be your focus, and carry you forward.

A FEW WORDS FROM A PRO

USA Today bestselling romance author Michelle Pennington was kind enough to share \with me her thoughts on bad reviews:

"No matter how good an author is at their craft, there's no escaping the torment of bad reviews. In my experience, the percentage of bad reviews I have received has remained roughly the same even as my skills as a writer have improved. Why is this? I believe it's because reviews aren't always a reflection of a story's quality, but of the kind of experience the reader had with it.

"When reading a bad review, it's important to know how to process it. Begin with accepting your emotions. Thick skin is a fallacy. The only true way to survive criticism is to view it through a business perspective — one that firmly excludes your inner creative. Take what is constructive and use it for your benefit. Anything that is simply an opinion based on that person's experience with the story should be immediately let go so that it doesn't creep into your psyche and cause damage.

"No reader will ever experience your story the way you did because they read it through the filter of their own perceptions, traumas, biases, and opinions. This is one reason why readers can have different experiences with the same book. They also have different desires that they are looking for your book to fulfill. So when you get reviews that sting, remind yourself that the story simply wasn't for them and that's okay.

"But when logic doesn't help, just know that venting to a trusted person in privacy is incredibly helpful. Learning to have a sense of humor about bad reviews is also absolutely vital. One of my favorite reviews on any of my books is a one-star review that said my heroine needed a binkie and a time out. Laughter takes away the sting."

6

The Part of Tens

Discover the most popular tropes in romance writing.

Come up with a winning title.

Understand the most common writing mistakes beginners make.

Learn the questions every romance writer needs to ask herself.

Beat writer's block.

Chapter **19**

Ten Tropes Every Editor Knows — and Why They Still Work

One of the most common criticisms of romance novels is that they're all the same. As a romance reader and aspiring writer, you know that this criticism isn't true. What *is* true is that certain plot types (called *tropes*) are so effective that they have names that every editor and most writers know. However, these plot types aren't actual plots, because they don't lay out the middle and end; all they lay out is the beginning. These common tropes really consist of *setups,* and they're different every time because each writer brings their own spin to them.

The reason these tropes are so effective is that they all contain the seeds of emotional conflict — a must for a well-written romance — which gets your reader invested in your characters' lives and relationship. It's that investment on the reader's part that keeps them turning the pages. If you begin with a plot that has that emotional component built in from the start, you're already ahead of the game. In this chapter, I lay out some of the best-known tropes, and any one of them may give you an idea for your next book.

REMEMBER

You bring your own voice, imagination, and characters to any trope — one only *you* can create. Whether you use a setup that's earned a name through frequent use or one that's never been seen before, your job as a writer is to make that plot your own.

Marriage of Convenience

Decades ago, a marriage-of-convenience plot was usually financially motivated. For example, the heroine's wealthy grandfather stipulated in his will that she had to marry — sometimes the man of his choice, sometimes the man of her choice — in order to inherit the family wealth. These days, women are more than capable of earning their own living, and it takes more than a will to make a marriage-of-convenience plot believable.

Today, a marriage of convenience is more likely to be motivated by nonmercenary means. For example, the hero's chance of maintaining custody of a beloved foster child would be improved if he were married, or the heroine's dying grandmother's final wish is to see her married. The marriage may even be a sham, but with genuine emotional consequences; for example, the hero and heroine are under-cover cops who have to pose as a married couple in order to bring down a baby-stealing ring.

REMEMBER

What makes this trope work is that it involves marriage — the most intimate of human relationships — to someone who's essentially a stranger, which sets up a sense of emotional and sexual tension right from the start.

Stranded with a Stranger

This trope most commonly strands the hero and heroine together via some kind of disaster, like a snowstorm, avalanche, plane crash, or shipwreck. Similar to a marriage of convenience, the plot puts two strangers in a state of forced intimacy, with all the tension that implies. To really up the ante, don't stop at making them strangers; make them strangers who have a good reason — maybe even more than one reason — not to get along. Whether they're just very different types — maybe a corporate CEO who's decided he needs a mountain cabin as a retreat versus a wolf researcher who's totally at home in the wild and has no use for weekend nature boys. Or maybe they are two people with a specific gripe — rival ranchers feuding over the piece of property where they're now stranded. Whatever the circumstances, you add a specific source of tension to the obvious discomfort of being locked up with an attractive stranger of the opposite sex, a romantic equation that adds up to more the sum of its parts.

Runaway Bride

The heroine in this story line literally runs away on her wedding day and ends up in the arms of the hero, whether because she hitches a ride in his car, hides in the back of his truck, or runs out of gas in front of his house. A variation of this plot is the kidnapped bride, which involves the hero kidnapping the heroine on her wedding day — for what will turn out to be good and acceptable reasons. Again, the characters are in a forced-intimacy situation, with the two of them getting caught up in each others' lives in emotionally fraught circumstances. The fact that all this happens on her wedding day — often with her still in her wedding dress — adds extra drama, with one dream ending and another, even better one beginning as she meets the hero.

Secret Baby

The secret baby isn't necessarily an infant, although babies or very little kids tend to work better in romances than surly teenagers. The basic setup is that the hero got the heroine pregnant (they may even have been married at the time) but never knew it, and then they were separated. Now he shows up to find she had his child or maybe that she's pregnant with his baby. Whether they want to reunite or not, their lives are now connected, and they have to find a way to deal with the issues that caused their original separation. In real life, babies usually bring a couple together. In a secret-baby romance, at first the baby seems to drive a wedge between them, because the hero's furious that she never told him about the baby or the pregnancy. He may even threaten to sue for custody. But ultimately, the baby becomes the key to their reconciliation.

Second-Chance Romance

In this trope, ex-spouses, or ex-lovers, are brought back together and fall in love again or discover that they never stopped loving each other. As with the secret-baby story line, the hero and heroine need to find a way to overcome the issues that drove them apart before. A twist on this plot has them discovering that their divorce was never final. You can even apply the stranded-together setup with great effectiveness. The very fact that they were once intimate but have become emotional strangers creates tension any time they meet, and that tension is ratcheted up even higher the longer they're forced to be together.

Back from the Dead

This plot is another type of second-chance romance. One of the characters — usually the hero — was declared dead. The heroine has rebuilt her life and is usually on the verge of remarrying when he appears. Suddenly she's torn between two loves and two lives. As an added twist, he may find a child he never knew about, who was born after his "death." In some cases, the new guy turns out to be a creep, so the hero's timely return saves the heroine from genuine unhappiness. In other cases, the new guy is a genuinely good man, adding to the emotional impact of the story (readers often enjoy shedding a tear or two along the way to a happy ending) and possibly providing you with a character worth spinning off into his own story.

Mistaken Identity

This trope has several variations. A hero and heroine who have the same last name but are otherwise strangers can be mistakenly assigned to the same cabin on a cruise (which is also a version of being stranded with a stranger). Or a heroine with a unisex name can be hired under the assumption that she's a man, finding herself the lone woman on an oil rig, a ranch, or some other bastion of masculinity. Once again, forced intimacy is the name of the game.

Woman in Jeopardy

This trope is an especially good way to showcase an alpha hero (as described in Chapter 4). Many romantic suspense novels feature this plotline, starring a heroine in danger and the hero whose job it is — or who makes it his job — to protect her. She doesn't need to be a wimp, either. She can be strong and capable, but just caught up in a situation where she needs some help — and ends up finding love.

The Dad Next Door

He may not be literally next door, and he may even be the heroine's boss. The basic setup is that he's suddenly a single dad, maybe with a baby he never knew about left on his doorstep, or maybe he's inherited a baby (or a bunch of kids), and he needs the heroine's help. This plot works equally well with an alpha or a beta hero (see Chapter 4).

Even Sketchier Setups

Other tropes are recognizable by name but are even less specific in terms of plot elements. The names of the following setups are pretty self-explanatory, and any one of them can provide an opening for your story:

>> Boss/secretary or boss/employee

>> Amnesia

>> Virgin heroine

>> On the run

>> Rancher/cowboy and the city girl

Chapter **20**

Ten Tips for Coming Up with a Successful Title

Along with cover art, a good title is a crucial part of getting a reader to pick up your book, so it pays to know everything you can about creating a title that works for you. In this chapter, I share tips for making sure your title stands out to a reader in an appealing way, finding a title that suits your book, and titling connected projects. I also lay out the pros and cons of using titling tricks like alliteration, single-word titles, and common expressions.

Speak the Reader's Language

Accept the fact that no title can appeal to every reader. In fact, you may find that impossibility to be a good thing, because it takes a lot of pressure off you. You want to — and you *can* — create a title that appeals to the bulk of the readers most likely to be interested in your book. The first key to creating the perfect title lies in knowing who your readers are and what they like. If you've written an historical romance, you don't have to worry that readers looking for paranormal romantic suspense may pass your novel by. Focus on getting historical readers to notice you.

Use K-lytics reports (k-lytics.com/romance) and the bestseller lists as your resources. Take a look at the names of other books in your segment of the market and think about what those titles have in common, which ones work for you, and which ones are selling best. Many books on bestseller lists are there because of the authors' name, not their titles, but newer authors do sometimes make the lists, too. And, either way, checking out the most successful players never hurts. If you want to indie publish, it's important to also look at all the bestselling indie titles. K-lytics reports will tell you who the bestselling indie authors are in your genre.

Know the Long and the Short of It

Winning titles can be long or short. (*Long* is a relative term, given the physical limitations created by fitting your title, your name, and the art into the confined space of a book cover.) There are pros and cons to both:

>> **Longer titles come with design challenges but often grab the reader, because she hasn't seen anything else like them.** If you are poetic and let the words flow, you may find that coming up with something unique is easier when you have more words at your disposal. A longer title also gives you more space to state your case and "explain" what your book's about. But remember that a long title can sound flat and rhythmless.

>> **Shorter titles are punchy because they pack a lot into a small space.** They can be easier to remember — a plus if a reader wants to ask for your book in the store or tell a friend about it — simply because they have fewer words to remember (and get right). But they can also be so short that they don't say enough to the reader to interest them.

TIP

Longer titles often work best on historical romances or books that focus solely on the relationship. Shorter titles often fit contemporary romances, especially romantic suspense novels, whose fast pacing makes a good match for a shorter, snappier title. Most books fall somewhere in the middle ground, with titles of three or four words.

Try Single-Word Titles

One-word titles go in and out of favor, and they represent the extremes of the short-title pros and cons (as seen in the preceding section). Finding a word that actually says enough to sum up an entire book is the biggest problem with one-word titles. Plus, the one word you choose has to be memorable and stand out from all the other single-word titles. When a one-word title works, it *works*. It has a real bang to it, and it hits the reader like a wake-up call. But when it fails, it really fails, because it says nothing and doesn't stand out from all the books around it.

Match Title and Tone Perfectly

Your title needs to reflect your book's plot and tone. If you've written a romantic suspense novel, give it a title that reflects the suspenseful, tense, danger-filled tone of the book, not a flowery and generically pretty title. If you've written a historical romance, choose a title that reflects that fact (royal and noble titles always give the reader a good clue), and avoid contemporary phrases that don't fit the period. A paranormal title should sound eerie or a little bit weird, while a romantic comedy should have a light title.

TIP

When you're titling your book, don't pick something so generic that it can fit on any romance. (You know the kind of title I mean — *Love's Perfect Passionate Embrace* and the like.) Instead, think about the specifics of your plot and the tone of your book, and create a title to match.

Use Keywords

A lot of titles, particularly series titles, rely heavily on keywords or tropes to indicate the type of story: marriage of convenience, amnesia, pregnant heroine, and so on. (See Chapter 19 for more about the most common tropes in romance novels.) A trope-based title does clearly define the story, so any reader looking for that kind of book knows she has found it. It's hard to misunderstand *An Inconvenient Marriage, Missing Memories,* or *Baby on Board.* When you work the trope in cleverly, your title becomes both accurate and memorable. If you don't phrase it cleverly, though, one hook-based title can sound an awful lot like a bunch of others, so a reader may wonder whether she's read this book already. And some titles try to fit in so many keywords that they end up sounding like shopping lists (*The Cowboy's Pregnant Teenage Secret Bride,* for example).

TIP

Using keywords in your title can also make your book come up higher in searches on Amazon. Your title is indexed and is heavily rated for search results. If you choose a catchy title that also is something many people search for when looking for a particular trope, your book could be what comes up first. The key is to find a clever title that also uses keywords.

Consider Alliteration

An alliterative title fits together well, and it usually has something catchy about it. Alliterative titles also often flow — especially if the initial repeated letter is soft: an *s* or soft *c*, an *f* or an *m*. But alliteration can sound too affected and self-conscious, or more like a tongue twister (*Peter Piper Picked a Passionate Pair*).

Coin a Cliché

Clichés and other recognizable expressions, as well as common phrases, frequently make for good titles. Readers may like them because the recognition factor makes them feel comfortable, or it may also be because everyone knows what they mean. You can use one exactly as everyone knows it — *Wolf in Sheep's Clothing* (which, depending on the cover art, can come off as suspenseful or humorous) or *Killer Smile* (suspense all the way). Or you can play with the familiar phrase for effect, like *High Crimes and Miss Demeanor* (probably humorous, maybe even historical, depending on when the phrase entered the language).

Name Names

You can really make your title unique by using one of your characters' names in it, especially if you can work in a full name, since first names alone are less likely to be unique, but a full name will stand out to the reader (think *Jane Eyre*). That puts a lot of pressure on you to give your characters names worthy of being included in a title, but this strategy can win you readers if you choose the right name.

Make Connections

If you're writing a *miniseries* — a series of books connected by plot, characters (often family members), or setting — you may want to give each book a title that implies the connection. Whether they all contain the same word (*fire* or *heart*), related words (four connected books that use the four basic elements — earth, air, fire, and water), a family name (the books all feature related characters), or some other connecting theme, this gimmick can help readers find the books on the shelf and solidify the connection between them — but only if you make each individual title strong. If you have to make a choice, choose unrelated but salable titles instead of related weaker ones.

Follow in Others' Footsteps

You can't copyright titles, so don't worry if your title turns out to duplicate someone else's or someone else's title duplicates yours. This situation happens less often than you'd expect, given how many romances are published every year, but it does happen. Be careful not to choose a well-known title for your book (sorry, but *Gone with the Wind* is unavailable) or knowingly duplicate another title, especially a current or recent bestseller. You want to avoid confusion when you can. Make your book stand out to readers — don't leave them wondering whether they've read your book or not just because the title sounds familiar to them.

Chapter **21**

Ten Tips for Avoiding Common Writing Mistakes

Every writer was a first-timer once, and many still admit to first-timer-style jitters with each new book. Those jitters don't need to hurt you, even when you *are* a first-time writer. When an editor or customer is reading your romance novel, all they care about is the book. In this chapter, I give you some tips you can use — and some tips for what you should avoid doing — so your book doesn't announce on every page that you're new to the game and still learning your craft.

Remember the Reader's Expectations

If you remember only one thing, remember this: Give the reader what they want or find another career. All successful genre publishing is based on knowing what the reader wants and then providing it. This expectation is never truer than it is for romance. Be thinking about your reader the minute you decide whether to write a contemporary or historical romance, a series or mainstream novel, and then make it your goal to satisfy your reader's expectations from page one until the end.

Don't Overwrite

A pro knows exactly what they want to say and says it. An amateur loads adjectives and adverbs into every sentence. The simplest idea ends up being as complex (and about as interesting) as a physics textbook. Pare down your prose; make every word count. Too many adjectives say nothing; one carefully chosen adjective says everything. Only describe what's important to describe. If you lavish equal time on everything, nothing stands out and nothing matters. Be careful of getting too cutesy in your writing, constantly slipping in puns, inside jokes, and clever turns of phrase. You'll only turn your reader off.

Love It or Lose It

If you don't love romance and — especially — love your characters, you're in the wrong business or, at the very least, you're writing the wrong book. In a genre that's focused on emotion, don't even think about faking it. If you're not enjoying yourself as you write, if you don't empathize with your characters and care deeply that they get together for that key happily-ever-after moment, you can bet your reader is not going to care, either. You have to believe love is wonderful, possible, and worth working for, or every word you write will be a lie, and any reader (and editor) will see right through it.

Let Your Characters Drive the Plot

Make sure that your hero and heroine, in particular, are complex and interesting, and that your reader can identify with your heroine and fall in love with your hero. Introduce your characters — not just to the reader but to each other — early in the book. Get their conflict out on the table, and let them drive the plot, not be driven by it. (For all the ins and outs of creating sympathetic heroines and irresistible heroes, check out Chapter 4.)

Know That Effective Conflict Comes from Within

If a reader wants talking heads debating the issues of the day, she'll turn on a cable news channel. Your reader chooses a romance novel because she wants emotional drama that comes from — and touches — the heart, not the head. Let conflict come from within your characters because of who they are, not what they think. (In Chapter 5, I provide additional insight on including conflict — especially emotional conflict — in your manuscript.)

Make Sure You Have Enough Plot

Whether you're writing a 55,000-word Harlequin Romance novel or a 150,000-word mainstream romantic suspense novel, make sure that you have enough plain old story to support the length of your book. If you're showing every scene from multiple points of view, writing scenes that don't move the plot and romance forward, or digressing into subplots and the details of your secondary characters' lives, you need to go back and complicate your plot so you can focus on the central love story.

Keep Your Story on Track

The reader doesn't want to hear your every thought or even your characters' every thought. Your reader also doesn't care how much research you did or how fascinating you found it. Your job is to focus on the romance, not digress into nonessential information, however interesting it may be. Every scene needs to move the story forward, to take the romance one step beyond where it's been, so don't let your mind or your writing wander. An outline may be just what you need to help keep your story on track, and I talk about creating one (and using it effectively) in Chapter 7.

Keep Your Reader Interested

Your reader may be scared, and you may even make her cry, but never let her get bored. Everything you do should be geared toward entertaining your reader. If you keep your reader happy and entertained, when she reaches the end of your book, she'll be sorry that the story is over and will go looking for your next novel.

Don't Forget the Details

Don't move from A to C or D without making it clear what B is. Everything has to add up. Motivations need to be clear, and your plot has to be logical. Your book is fiction, but it has to make just as much sense as if it were real. Make your characters' motivations believable (I talk about creating motivation in Chapter 5), keep your timeline consistent, check your facts (I talk about research in Chapter 13), watch out for contradictions, and don't ever think you can get away with something because "no one will notice." Your readers *will* notice, and they won't like it.

Keep the Story Moving

Pacing is key. Know where to start, when to stop, how to intercut scenes, and how to create and resolve cliffhangers. Know how to use language to get your reader's heart racing and her hands flipping pages, and then know how to give her a breather before ramping up the tension again. Give your reader everything she thinks she wants, then make her want more and keep her reading until she gets it. Grab her attention and hold it until she reaches the final page. (I show you how to set the pace in Chapter 10, and how to start, stop, and create cliffhangers in Chapter 12.)

Chapter **22**

Ten Questions Every Romance Writer Needs to Ask Herself

Because writing is such a solitary process, you're going to face a lot of times when you have to ask yourself hard questions — and provide your own answers. Even knowing what to ask can be tough, and having some guidance for figuring out the answers can certainly help. So, in this chapter, I provide some questions and considerations that may help you in the writing process.

Should I Write Romance Novels?

You may have a tough time with this question, because everything you're hoping for depends on your answer. But look at the bottom line: If you don't like reading romances, if you don't buy into the fantasy and feel happy every time a hero and heroine get together, or if you're only thinking about writing a romance because you want to make some money, then romance isn't the genre for you. Better to recognize this fact right away and figure out what you *should* be writing.

Why Can't I Get Started?

If you're having problems getting the writing process underway, a number of things could be going on. First, you may not have found the right kind of romance for you yet. Check out Chapter 2 and go through the process of narrowing things down. A change of scene or subgenre may get you on track.

You may also be facing simple fear. Thinking about making your dream come true is scary, and it becomes even scarier when you start working on it, because doubts can creep in: What if I can't pull it off? A lot of times, just recognizing your fear helps you deal with it.

If recognizing why you're afraid isn't enough, you need to just make yourself write without expecting too much. Set a reasonable number of pages as a target and don't judge those pages too harshly after you've written them. Just keep going, and you can probably find your rhythm as your natural bent for storytelling takes over. You can go back later and revise what you've written, but for now, just get the momentum going.

What Can I Do When the Ideas Don't Come?

Sometimes you feel like you've hit a wall. Nothing's coming together, and no idea feels right or interesting enough to get you going. In this situation, you just have to stop pressuring yourself. Get out into the world and do something fun — read a book that you've been looking forward to but haven't had time for, watch TV, rent a movie, go to the beach and daydream . . . anything to relax and open your mind so that you can recognize a good idea when it comes. And a good idea *will* come. You just need to be receptive to it.

How Can I Focus and Stay Positive When Things Go Wrong?

Problems with your writing can often leave you in a slump. But insecurity and depression can strike at any time, often causing your writing train to go off the rails even when your story's not having any obvious problems. When things go wrong and you feel negative (or you feel negative and then things go wrong), remind yourself that every writer goes through phases like this one, so you shouldn't beat yourself up about it. You can give yourself a breather, a day or two to just have fun with life and rejuvenate your mind.

Or you can follow the same advice I suggest in the earlier section about having trouble getting started: Just keep writing, as much as possible without judging, and force yourself through the bad patch. You can go back later and revise — assuming you even need revision. Often, the writing's fine — it's your perceptions that are off.

Finally, reward yourself for your accomplishments, whether that means taking time to cook your favorite meal (or going out to eat), watching your favorite movie from the comfort of your couch, or shopping for a new pair of shoes. Hitting yourself with a stick doesn't help your writing, but holding out a carrot may be just what you need.

When Is It Research and When Is It a Waste of Time?

Get tough on yourself. If you're discovering all kinds of really interesting stuff that you can't honestly say belongs in your book, you're wasting time. Stop it right now and start writing! Procrastination is a cardinal sin. Check out Chapter 13 for more information on drawing the line.

When Should I Publish or Submit My Manuscript?

Is your manuscript done? Have you polished and rewritten and polished again? Has your critique group told you it's great? Are you just making work for yourself by going over the book again? As terrifying as it is to pronounce your book done and ready to submit to a publisher or publish it yourself (and believe me, I know it's scary), you need to do it. Whether you send a query letter, a full or partial manuscript, or send to a freelance editor for indie publishing, the time has come. Be proud of yourself for getting to this point, and then take that crucial next step. You can never sell if you don't.

Do I Need an Agent?

If you want to sell a mainstream romance novel, you almost always need an agent. Check out each particular publisher's requirements, but in general, expect to find out that you will need an agent. Series romance is still wide open to authors who want to submit on their own, but a lot of writers choose to work with an agent so that they have an advocate, as well as someone who knows the business side of publishing and can handle all the negotiating. With series submissions, the decision is a personal one, and no answer is wrong. I cover the agent question in more detail in Chapter 17.

How Do I Handle a Friend's Success?

As the Golden Rule says, "Do unto others . . ." You may be hurting inside, even feeling jealous (a totally human reaction), but practice your acting skills and hide those feelings because, deep down, you know that you *are* happy for your friend. And remember: The odds of your book finding success haven't changed and depend entirely on the strength of your book — which you control.

When and How Do I Follow Up on My Book's Status?

As frustrating as it is, be patient. Wait at least three months after you submit a manuscript, and when you do follow up, make a response as easy for the editor as possible. Provide all the relevant information about your book (its title, your pseudonym if you used one, and whether it was a complete or a partial manuscript) and when you submitted it. Most prefer getting an email inquiry, but check with the submission guidelines for the publishing house to make sure you're contacting the right person and going through the proper channels.

When Do I Let Go of a Book?

If you've submitted to, and been rejected by, every publisher you can think of, if you've revised the book in every way that makes sense to you, if you can't think of anything else to do that doesn't smack of vain hopefulness, it might be time to stop. If you've decided a book can't be published traditionally, and if you believe it has a market, you do have the option to indie publish it. (Chapter 16 covers indie publishing in detail.) But keep writing. You can always submit your next manuscript to traditional publishers and try again.

IN THIS CHAPTER

» **Writing your way through a block**

» **Skipping ahead**

» **Changing views**

» **Rereading your outline**

» **Working on a different project**

Chapter **23**

Ten Ways to Beat Writer's Block

First, a word on what writer's block *isn't*. Writer's block isn't the stage that many writers go through when the book is still forming in their minds — when they may start and stop, rethink, replot, take a break, and then sit down and start writing in earnest, sometimes repeating that sequence several times until they finish the book. If that's your writing process and it works for you, you don't have writer's block, because you don't have a problem. Writer's block isn't the culprit every time you take a break in the writing process — only when that break becomes paralyzing. The longer you give in to writer's block, the harder it can be to get yourself writing again.

Most writers experience writer's block at some point. It helps to know that it's normal, and many authors go through this. There are different ways authors deal with writer's block. If you're finding yourself at a crossroads in your writing, the practical tips in this chapter may help you get moving again.

Work Your Way Through It

This may seem obvious, but the best way to keep writing is to . . . keep writing! Just sit down at the computer and start typing. At the end of the day, you may decide that 99 percent — or even 100 percent — of what you've written is lousy, and you'll throw it out. But as you keep writing, sooner or later you'll hit on something — even if it's just one thing — that works for you, and then you have something to run with.

Select a Different Scene

In general, writing a book from Chapter 1 straight through to the end makes sense, because the elements you planned in your outline may change as you write, affecting what happens next. But if you're having trouble with a particular scene, try moving on to the next scene or writing a scene that happens later in the book. A love scene is a particularly good choice, because it's less likely to change radically.

Look at the Last Scene You Wrote

Sometimes the problem isn't the scene you're trying to write, but the previous scene that sets that one up. The setup scene may be further back — maybe even a few scenes ago, if you took a radical turn. You may need to get a little distance from that earlier scene, and then look at it again, and you'll see what you did wrong. Fix that, and suddenly your characters and story are back on track. Often this relates to tension. If you have destroyed the tension between your two characters, go back to the place where that tension dispersed and rework it.

Write a Scene That You Won't Use

If you feel like you're losing touch with your characters, write an easy scene with them — one that you'll never use but one that will help you get in touch with their voices again. Write about their honeymoon or the birth of their first child. Write about a normal date for them — the kind romance-novel couples never get to have — where they talk all about who they are and discover how much they have in common. Get to know them all over again, and then go back to your story armed with that new knowledge.

View the Scene from a Different Angle

Sometimes just getting another perspective gets your creative juices flowing again. For example, you can do the scene entirely via description from a third character's point of view. What does the observer see, and what does she think is going on in the characters' minds? You can do the scene entirely in dialogue, so the conversation carries the burden of explanation. Or write the entire scene from your hero or heroine's point of view, as if he or she is remembering what happened and is analyzing what it all meant. Using any one of those treatments as a basis, you can go back and look at the scene with fresh insights as you start writing.

Don't Focus on Perfection

Sometimes "good enough" really *is* good enough — for now. You'll have an opportunity later to do a second draft or even a third, so don't expect things to be perfect right away. Get the basics of the scene down, and then move on. Later, you can go back and polish, totally rewrite, or even cut the scene, if you want to. In the meantime, don't let one scene hold you up — keep writing.

Stop in the Middle

If you find yourself constantly stuck when you sit down to write, try stopping before you've ended your chapter. This way, when you sit down to write, you automatically know where you're going and how to finish the chapter, which gets your juices flowing. It's much easier to keep going once you've already started writing. I'll sometimes even stop mid-sentence to remind myself where I was going with my scene so I can easily pick it back up.

Analyze Your Outline

If you're an outliner, take another look at what you planned to do and ask yourself whether everything makes sense in terms of plot and character. When you look at your outline again from start to finish, you may see gaps and problems you missed, and those issues may be what's hanging you up now. Fix those issues, and suddenly your writing starts moving again. In Chapter 7, I talk about how to create your outline, and I give you some tips on keeping it a part of the writing process.

Re-energize Your Creative Instincts

Try thinking about what drew you to this story in the first place. The characters? The chance to try your hand at romantic comedy? The fun of creating a complicated suspense plot? Whatever kind of story you're telling, try taking a break from writing and go watch a movie or read a book that tells a similar story, whether plot- or tone-wise. Lose yourself in that story and just enjoy it. Let yourself remember why you started your own book in the first place, and then go back to writing with that enthusiasm fresh in your mind.

TIP

Brainstorming with another person can help get the juices flowing again. Even if you don't have someone else to brainstorm with, take a few minutes and write down every possible way your story could go, even if it's silly, or a direction you'd never go. Writing them all down can sometimes unlock new ideas that will work for your story. After you come up with twenty or so new ideas for your story, put a star by the ones with the most tension. Those are the ideas that you should pay the most attention to.

Start Another Project (If All Else Fails)

Sometimes you just need a break from a certain story or character. Maybe you hit a plot snag and need to think about how to solve it before you can move on. Or maybe you've tried everything, nothing has worked, and you just can't get back into the rhythm of the book. In that case, you may have no option but to stop working on it, but don't stop writing altogether. Start working on your next book, whether planning it or actually writing it, but don't let yourself be controlled by writer's block.

Index

contractions, use of, 146

contracts

on allowing you to self-publish, 271

as difficult to get with large publishing house, 267

indemnification in, 240

making negotiations successful and pleasant, 308

marketing budgets in, 264

option clause in, 305

reading/rereading fine print in, 306

resources to help you understand them, 307

role of agent in, 299, 300

RWA for information about, 307

series contracts, 307–308

sizing up of, 303–307

subsidiary rights in, 300, 305

understanding advances against royalties, 304

unfavorable clauses in, 265

with vanity presses, 269

warranties and indemnification in, 240

control issues, as faced by romance characters, 97

conversation, use of, 158

copyright, registering yours, 289–290

copyright information, 275

cover art, from traditional publishers, 306

cover copy

importance of back-cover copy, 74

from traditional publishers, 306

creativity, listening to yours, 127

Critique Circle, 53

critique groups

examples of, 53

pros and cons of, 53–54

cute meet

defined, 207

pros and cons of, 207–209

D

Dabble (software), 48

dad next door (trope), 335

dangling prepositions, use of, 245

dark moments, most romance novels as having, 105

Dawson, Mark (founder of SPF Community), 263

Day, Sylvia (author), 36

The Deluxe Transitive Vampire: The Ultimate Handbook of Grammar for the Innocent, the Eager, and the Doomed (Gordon), 245

description

avoiding talking too much in, 143–144

as showcasing author's voice, 137

dialect, effective use of, 155–156

dialogue

avoiding pitfalls in over-use of, 182–183

being careful with unattributed dialogue, 158–160

good dialogue as one of the make-or-break elements every editor looks for, 154

harnessing power of, 181–182

putting it on paper, 158–160

as technique for conveying characters' voices, 149

use of to convey information naturally, 157–158

using dialect and accents effectively, 155–156

writing great dialogue, 154–160

dialogue tags, use of, 159

discovery writing

defined, 122

described, 127–128

letting characters guide you, 128–129

methods of, 123–124

versus outlining, 121–132

plotting as you go, 129–131

rewriting trap, 132

dreams, of love, as romance writer's device, 101–102

E

Eats, Shoots & Leaves (Truss), 245

ebook

Advanced Reader Copy (ARC) as, 280

defined, 260

editing, line, 310–311

editorial reviews, 284

editors

addressing queries from, 316–317

common manuscript criticisms from, 320–323

disagreeing with suggestions from, 318–319

working with, 14, 309–311

The Elements of Style (Strunk and White), 50, 245

ellipses, use of, 247–248

em dashes, use of, 247, 248–249

EmailOctopus, 286

emotional conflict

as always internal, 95

creation of, 91–96

highlighting of, 92–94

versus intellectual conflict, 91–92

as single most important factor driving plot and creating reader's interest, 89

emotional intimacy, 19, 72, 87–88, 98, 100, 101, 171, 219

emotional moments, reaching key ones, 174

emotional tension

creation of, 91–96

as driving force of romance, 11–12

as one of five basic expectations of romance readers, 19

emotionally involving love scenes, 11

as needing to be heroic, 11

playboy hero, 73

showing of as heroine's equal, 68

softer side of, 68–69

strengths of, 68

strong, irresistible hero as one of the five basic expectations of romance readers, 19

types of, 69–74

western heroes, 34

heroine

imperfection of, 63–64

as key to every romance, 61–66

and love scenes, 193

making her complex, 63

making her feel real, 61–62

naming of, 64–66

physical appearance of, 63

as reader's alter ego, 11, 60, 61

sympathetic heroine as one of five basic expectations of romance readers, 19

heterosexual romance, 11, 36, 66

Heyer, Georgette (author), 32

historical romance

alpha heroes in, 71

arranged marriage in, 130

contemporary versus, 9, 22–23, 28

describing typical meal in, 229

doing research for, 227, 228, 237

as having cutoff date, 24

immersing yourself in rhythms and events of day-to-day life, 235

inspirational romances as, 30

keeping track of new theories and discoveries about historical periods, 234

making names specific to time period, 65, 75, 78

Native American heroes as particularly popular in, 75

need for accuracy in, 34

pace of life in era you've chosen as influencing, 185

as reflecting vocabulary and speech patterns of time period, 154

Regency romances as subgenre of, 31

as represented in category romance series, 27

social mores as dictating behavior of sexes in, 101

speaking reader's language in, 337

time period in, 114

titles of, 338, 339

word count in, 32

holiday, as milestone, 173

homosexual romance, 66

hook, 87, 203, 204–205, 217, 277–278, 297, 298

humor

having sense of humor about bad reviews, 327

power of, 69

hybrid author

as best of both worlds, 271–272

defined, 271

hybrid publishing companies, 269

I

"I love you," saying it at the right moment, 102–103

icons, explained, 3

images, using professional ones, 277

in medias res ("in the middle of things"), 209

inciting incident, in first quarter of book, 130

indemnification, in publisher contracts, 240

indentation, formatting of, 254

indie publishing

anthologies in, 31

best practices of, 14–15

as changing landscape in Regency romances, 32

choosing of, 13–14

creating a professional product in, 275–279

defined, 259–260

finding success in, 273–294

finding top indie author groups, 40

formatting for, 255

options for book covers in, 276

point of view in, 164

pros and cons of, 269–270

writing in series, 28

IngramSpark, 288, 289

inspirational romance

deciding if this is your subgenre, 39

described, 30

expectations for, 20

importance of explicit commitment to marriage in, 103

Liz Isaacson as author of, 35

as not focusing on physical relationship, 40, 101, 102, 172, 196

slower-paced, thoughtful scenes in, 185

as sweet romance, 10

Instagram, showcasing book on, 293

intellectual conflict

versus emotional conflict, 91–92

taking care with, 94–95

internal conflict, versus external conflict, 95

internal monologue

defined, 165

as technique for conveying characters' voices, 149

tips for writing effective ones, 166–167

use of, 165–166

international locations, 111

Internet, as great for information and misinformation, 233–235

intimacy

emotional intimacy, 19, 72, 87–88, 98, 100, 101, 171, 219

physical intimacy, 19, 87–88, 98, 100, 101, 126

About the Authors

Victorine Lieske was a young mother, who, after injuring her back, was not willing to sit idle during recovery. She decided to write a book . . . and she did it in a week. Then came four years of honing her skills and all the rewrites it would take to get the novel ready. Victorine studied the market and self-published her story. Her willingness to follow trends paid off; that first novel hit *The New York Times* bestseller list. Since then Victorine has published more than 30 titles (detailed at victorinelieske.com). Her commercial success in sweet romance led to another novel on the *USA Today* bestseller list. Victorine stays on the forefront of trends in the business of writing. She is a sought-after speaker and instructor and is part of *The Writing Gals* collaborative. When she's not writing, Victorine enjoys travel, crochet, Korean dramas, and designing book covers through Blue Valley Author Services.

Leslie Wainger wrote the first edition of *Writing a Romance Novel For Dummies*. After a long, successful, and fulfilling career as an editor, Leslie retired from publishing and moved west — well, to western New York. She followed up on her years of volunteer work at the Bronx Zoo and Connecticut Humane Society by becoming a pet adoption counselor. She retired for real in early 2022, though she still volunteers. Most of her time is spent enjoying her own pet population, trying to read all the ebooks she's amassed, and enjoying time with family and friends.

Dedication

Victorine Lieske: I would like to dedicate this book to my husband, who is kind enough to travel with me, who always supports me in everything, and who watches Korean dramas with me even when they are sappy and romantic.

Authors' Acknowledgments

Victorine Lieske: I'm so thankful for everyone who has helped me over the years. I couldn't have done any of this without all of you. I have had countless beta readers and critique partners who have taught me all about romance writing, way too many to name, but believe me, if you've been a reader for me, know that you're included in this. I'm very thankful for my family who lets me spend hours on my laptop, getting my work done. You all are the best.

I especially want to thank my readers. You inspire me to keep going, even when it's difficult. A huge thank you to Michelle Pennington, who so eloquently wrote her feelings on handling bad reviews and allowed me to use it in this book. I also want to thank Laura Burton, Anne-Marie Meyer, and Judy Corry for always being there for me. You gals are the best. A massive thank you to my editors, Laura Walker, Rachel Camp, and Cara Seger, who always make me look good. And a special thank you to Elizabeth Stilwell, Lynn Northrup, and Cynthia Helms for helping me through this process.

Publisher's Acknowledgments

Executive Editor: Steven Hayes

Project Editor: Lynn Northrup

Copy Editor: Lynn Northrup

Technical Editor: Cynthia Helms

Production Editor: Saikarthick Kumarasamy

Cover Image: © LightField Studios/Shutterstock